BREASTFEEDING

Biocultural Perspectives

EVOLUTIONARY FOUNDATIONS OF HUMAN BEHAVIOR

An Aldine de Gruyter Series of Texts and Monographs

EDITED BY

Monique Borgerhoff Mulder, *University of California, Davis*
Marc Hauser, *Harvard University*

Richard D. Alexander, **The Biology of Moral Systems**

Laura L. Betzig, **Despotism and Differential Reproduction: A Darwinian View of History**

James S. Chisholm, **Navajo Infancy: An Ethological Study of Child Development**

Russell l. Ciochon and John G. Fleagle (eds.), **Primate Evolution and Human Origins**

G.A. Clark and C.M. Willermet (eds.), **Conceptual Issues in Modern Human Origins Research**

Lee Cronk, Napoleon Chagnon, and William Irons (eds.), **Adaptation and Human Behavior: An Anthropological Perspective**

Martin Daly and Margo Wilson, **Homicide**

Irenäus Eibl-Eibesfeldt, **Human Ethology**

Richard J. Gelles and Jane B. Lancaster (eds.), **Child Abuse and Neglect: Biosocial Dimensions**

Kathleen R. Gibson and Anne C. Petersen (eds.), **Brain Maturation and Cognitive Development: Comparative and Cross-Cultural Perspectives**

Frederick E. Grine (ed.), **Evolutionary History of the "Robust" Australopithecines**

Barry S. Hewlett (ed.), **Father-Child Relations: Cultural and Biosocial Contexts**

Kim Hill and A. Magdalena Hurtado, **Ache life History: The Ecology and Demography of a Foraging People**

Warren G. Kinzey (ed.), **New World Primates: Ecology, Evolution, and Behavior**

Jane B. Lancaster, Jeanne Altmann, Alice S. Rossi, and Lonnie R. Sherrod (eds.), **Parenting across the Life Span: Biosocial Dimensions**

Jonathan Marks, **Human Biodiversity: Genes, Race, and History**

Lewis Petrinovich, **The Cannibal Within**

Richard B. Potts, **Early Hominid Activities at Olduval**

Eric Alden Smith, **Inujjuamiut Foraging Strategies: Evolutionary Ecology of an Artic Hunting Economy**

Eric Alden Smith and Bruce Winterhalder (eds.), **Evolutionary Ecology and Human Behavior**

Barbara Boardman Smuts, **Sex and Friendship in Baboons**

Patricia Stuart-Macadam and Susan Kent (eds.), **Diet, Demography, and Disease: Changing Perspectives on Anemia**

Wenda R. Trevathan, **Human Birth: An Evolutionary Perspective**

James W. Wood, **Dynamics of Human Reproduction: Biology, Biometry, Demography**

BREASTFEEDING

Biocultural Perspectives

Patricia Stuart-Macadam and Katherine A. Dettwyler
EDITORS

Routledge
Taylor & Francis Group
LONDON AND NEW YORK

About the Editors

Patricia Stuart-Macadam is Associate Professor of Anthropology at the University of Toronto. Her research focuses on an evolutionary and biocultural perspective of health, disease and nutrition in prehistoric and contemporary human populations. She is the editor (with Susan Kent) of *Diet, Demography, and Disease: Changing Perspectives on Anemia* published by Aldine de Gruyter in 1992.

Katherine A. Dettwyler is Associate Professor of Anthropology at Texas A&M University. Her research focuses on the biocultural interactions between infant feeding beliefs and practices and the growth and health of children. She is the author of *Dancing Skeletons: Life and Death in West Africa* (1994).

First published 1995 by Transaction Publishers

Published 2017 by Routledge
2 Park Square, Milton Park, Abingdon, Oxon OX14 4RN
711 Third Avenue, New York, NY 10017, USA

Routledge is an imprint of the Taylor & Francis Group, an informa business

Library of Congress Cataloging-in-Publication Data

Breastfeeding : biocultural perspectives / Patricia Stuart-Macadam and
Katherine A. Dettwyler, editors.
; cm. — (Foundations of human behavior)
Includes bibliographical references and index.
ISBN 0-202-01191-7 (cloth). — ISBN 0-202-01192-5 (paper)
1. Breast feeding—Cross-cultural studies. I. Stuart-Macadam, Patricia, 1951- II. Dettwyler, Katherine A. III. Series.
RJ216.B776 1995
649'.33—dc20 95-18089
CIP

ISBN 13: 978-0-202-01192-9 (pbk)

This volume is respectfully dedicated to
Derrick B. Jelliffe and *Niles R. Newton*
for their lifelong commitment to
promoting maternal and child health
through breastfeeding

Contents

Foreword

In the 1880s, more than 95% of infants in the United States were breastfed, and were weaned only after they had reached 2–4 years of age. In the 1990s, only about one-half of infants in the United States are breastfed, and three-quarters are weaned by 6 months. As there is no biological or psychological evidence that artificial infant feeding is a better or even an equal substitute, the decline in the initiation and duration of breastfeeding reflects a profound biocultural crisis. *Breastfeeding: Biocultural Perspectives* fills critical gaps in our understanding of the biological and cultural realities of this crisis.

As a practicing obstetrician who actively promotes breastfeeding, I have experienced the frustration of challenging cultural norms. Contrary to the prevailing, egocentric belief of the medical profession, physician advice has little direct effect on whether a woman will breastfeed or not; most women have already decided their mode of infant feeding before pregnancy or in the first few weeks after the pregnancy has become apparent. A woman's decision to breastfeed is determined by her personality, education, experience, family, friends, and the larger political/advertising community. Cultural forces that conflict with breastfeeding include loss of family support, lack of easily identifiable role models, an increasing emphasis on self-actualization, with concomitant rejection of the unique mutually dependent relationship of the breastfeeding dyad; real and/or perceived needs for women to work outside the home, psychological/psychiatric theory that can easily misinterpret prolonged breastfeeding as being psychologically detrimental to the child, and overemphasis on the role of the breasts in sexuality.

That the medical profession can indeed counteract adverse cultural forces by acting as an opinion leader is testified to by their success in this role on issues such as public sanitation, pediatric vaccination, and the antismoking campaign. These successes have been due to a clear, distinct message of biologic advantage. Although the biologic advantages of breastfeeding are clear and distinct to students of lactation, the differences between breastfeeding and artificial feeding are sufficiently narrow and/or underrealized that the public receives a message that can be obscured by adverse cultural forces.

The medical profession needs to strengthen its advocacy of breastfeeding in the community by enhancing the narrow, provincial, and meager knowledge of the biocultural aspects of breastfeeding transmitted in the usual education and training provided to health care professionals. I believe that *Breastfeeding: Biocultural Perspectives* is a seminal work in this regard and should be the first textbook read by students and advocates of breastfeeding. This book brings together an enormous body of anthropological, archaeological, behavioral, historical, cultural, and animal studies, to offer a multifaceted perspective on the subject of human breastfeeding. Breastfeeding is viewed as a defining behavior of the order Mammalia; it is considered in archaeological, historical, and cross-cultural contexts, and variations in breastfeeding are explored in terms of their impact on population health and function.

Breastfeeding: Biocultural Perspectives presents a well-organized, cogent argument that breastfeeding should last 3–4 years rather than the 0.5–1 year duration found in modern U.S. culture. The responsibility for this artificially shortened period of breastfeeding lies both with the culture and with the *medicalization* of breastfeeding. The medical profession plays a greater role in determining the duration of lactation than in the initiation of breastfeeding. Its influences may be direct (e.g., lactation management) or indirect (e.g., obstetric or neonatal care). As with other normal physiological events (e.g., labor, delivery, and the newborn transition), breastfeeding has undergone tremendous *medicalization* in the last 50 years. Women who, in earlier times, would have based their decisions concerning breastfeeding on the norms of their family, friends, and community, now turn to health professionals for answers and advice. This shift has resulted from at least five major cultural phenomena: (1) a loss of community/family knowledge, role models, and support of breastfeeding; (2) a greater tendency to hand over responsibility for personal health to the medical profession; (3) an increasingly more patronizing attitude toward patients by the medical professions; (4) a greater reliance on institutions such as hospitals, which demand conformity, regulation, and scheduling for efficient function; and (5) an indication that, because most women deliver in the controlling environment of the hospital, premature clinical application of poorly conceived and poorly tested medical theory has great adverse impact. Continuous electronic fetal monitoring and routine feeding supplementation of the newborn are two prominent examples.

The alarming frequency of ill-advised clinical protocols stems from a variety of causes. First, although American medical and nursing schools fail to educate their students adequately concerning the physiology of lactation and nursing behavior, it is to these very health care providers—nurses and physicians—that our culture directs women for expert, authoritative answers to their breastfeeding questions. Having had little or no clinical observation of healthy, well-established breastfeeding dyads during their clinical training, the health professionals' ignorance and lack of experience may exaggerate adverse biocultural influences on breastfeeding. Second, physicians and nurses are notoriously eager to provide advice, even if their knowledge of, or experience with, the subject is limited. Many questions may seem purely cultural in nature, but answers to these questions can result in subtle biological outcomes, e.g., when to wean or when to feed solid food. Finally, health care providers practice in a consistently high-stress environment and often exhibit a demanding personal work ethic. The results of these combined stresses can be seen in their own interpersonal relationships, and in the statistics concerning the higher divorce rates, increased incidence of drug abuse, and shorter duration of breastfeeding among health professionals. Small wonder, then, that these stressed, pressured professionals shy away from advising women either to breastfeed in the first place, or to extend breastfeeding for a prolonged period of time.

There are several textbooks, such as those by Lawrence and by Riordan and Auerbach, that provide solid biological knowledge and information on the principles of breastfeeding management for the self-education of health care providers. *Breastfeeding: Biocultural Perspectives* is an essential complement to these clinically oriented textbooks. The broad scope of its presentation allows the student of breastfeeding to understand the biology more fully and provides the reader with the basis for a multifactorial conviction to support the clinical and management issues described in the other textbooks.

Breastfeeding: Biocultural Perspectives is appropriately dedicated to two giants in the field of breastfeeding: Derrick Jelliffe, M.D. and Niles Newton, Ph.D.—my mother. Students and friends of my mother will easily concur with the appropriateness of the dedication. As a research psychologist, my mother had a multifaceted view of medical issues, whether they concerned breastfeeding (her first and central focus), female surgery, labor management, or the role of oxytocin. She scoured the animal, anthropological, and historical, as well as the clinical literature to raise questions and support her theories. Her publications reflect her far-reaching approach: primary work with Margaret Mead, Ph.D., experimental research with mice, controlled, observational studies of women, and controlled, experimental trials with lactating women. As I read *Breastfeeding: Biocultural Perspectives,* I could almost hear my mother talking. The book embodies her style and perspective. She would have deeply enjoyed and admired the scholarly and broad-minded handling of an issue so dear to her life's work. Thank you.

Edward Newton, M.D.

Acknowledgments

We would like to thank all those individuals who contributed their assistance and encouragement during the preparation and production of this volume. The authors of the chapters, in particular, deserve an extra thanks for their hard work and patience. Patricia Stuart-Macadam would like to especially thank Dr. Roy Stuart for his prompt and thorough editing of all the manuscripts. Annette Chan of the Department of Anthropology at the University of Toronto and Paul Vlasschaert provided welcome technical assistance. Thanks also go to Margaret Beasley, Judy Cobb, Linda Stewart, and Loanne Tremain, my special friends in Duncan, Oklahoma, who supported me during all the ups and downs of editing this book. Katherine Dettwyler, thank you so much. You were always there when I needed you and you went beyond the call of duty in all the work you put into this book! An enormous thank you goes to James Macadam for his unfailing love and support and to Leila, Anne, and Jamie Macadam, whose existence provided the inspiration for this book. For their many and varied contributions to the tasks involved in the editing of this volume Katherine A. Dettwyler would like to thank Helen Danzeiser Dockall, Constance K. Judkins, and Joyce Bell, of the Anthropology Department, as well as the staff of interlibrary services at Evans Library and at the Medical Sciences Library of Texas A&M University. We also appreciate the suggestions made by Sarah Hrdy and the anonymous reviewers and the help provided by Richard Koffler, executive editor at Aldine de Gruyter, and his friendly staff, particularly Arlene Perazzini and Diana McDermott.

Patricia Stuart-Macadam
Katherine A. Dettwyler

1

Biocultural Perspectives on Breastfeeding

Patricia Stuart-Macadam

INTRODUCTION

The biological anthropologist has a unique way of viewing the world: a cross-cultural and evolutionary perspective that acknowledges that there are both biological and cultural components to human behavior. A survey of the existing breastfeeding literature reveals that, in general, this perspective has not been widely adopted. For example, much of the literature has focused either on cultural aspects, such as the style of breastfeeding, and the cultural milieu in which it occurs, or biological aspects, such as breast milk properties and composition. As biological anthropologists, the editors of this volume feel that it is essential to approach the topic of breastfeeding with a perspective that views breastfeeding within a biocultural, cross-cultural, and evolutionary framework. The main goal of *Breastfeeding: Biocultural Perspectives* is to use this type of approach, both to explore a number of issues relating to human lactation and breastfeeding and to illustrate the perils of ignoring the "bio"factor of the biocultural equation. Another goal of the book is to integrate data from diverse fields to present a more holistic view of breastfeeding. These goals are accomplished through the inclusion of the work of researchers involved in a number of different disciplines, including biological anthropology, cultural anthropology, history, nutrition, and medicine. The contributors to this volume have different attitudes and opinions, depending on their philosophy, training, and research interests, but all are aware of the biocultural nature of breastfeeding and strive to put this message across in their writing.

In Chapter 2, "A Time to Wean: The Hominid Blueprint for the Natural Age of Weaning in Modern Human Populations," Dettwyler examines comparative mammalian data on weaning age and comes to some conclusions that refute the commonly held beliefs on the "natural" weaning age of humans. According to Dettwyler, the range of weaning age for humans, variously estimated by gestation length, as a function of birth weight, adult weight, or adult body dimension, or by timing of eruption of first permanent molar, should be between 2.5 and 6 years, depending on the method used. This is substantially different from the weaning age of between 9 months and 1 year that has, until now, been cited as the "natural" weaning age of humans. Dettwyler says that human cultural traits, such as the modification of food with heat, or the processing of cereal products, would have resulted in a weakening of the strong association between biological variables such as the eruption of the first permanent molar and weaning age. However, as she states "It is reasonable to assume that 5–7 million years of evolution as hunting and gathering hominids on the East African savannah has resulted in genetic coding that leads the human infant to expect nursing to continue for several years after birth, and for the urge to suckle to remain strong for this entire period."

Acknowledgment and understanding of this fact are important, particularly in light of the peculiar bias against, and even disparagement of, "extended" nursing prevalent in contemporary North American society. This discrimination has also occurred in other times and cultures; Wickes (1953) describes the case of a woman living in nineteenth-century Britain who suckled a child for three and a quarter years and then developed epilepsy. The attendant physician wrote: "The worst symptoms of debility at last attended this monstrous proceeding."

In my chapter (Chapter 3), "Breastfeeding in Prehistory," I synthesize data from a number of sources including bone chemistry, history, ethnology, and demography to develop a picture of breastfeeding patterns and practices in prehistory. Some data, such as that obtained from chemical studies on archaeological bone, are highly technical and probably new to the reader; some, such as that obtained from historical and ethnographic sources, are more general in nature and widely known. I show that culture, in the form of differing infant feeding practices, can have an enormous impact on the health, morbidity, and mortality of contemporary infants, and that undoubtedly there was a similar effect for infants in prehistoric times. A synthesis of the various types of data brings me to the conclusion that, as in modern and historical times, breastfeeding practices in prehistory must have varied according to temporal, geographic, cultural, and even idiosyncratic factors. However, it does appear that in many prehistoric cultures substantial supplementation with foods other than breast milk, if not actual weaning, took place between 2 and 3 years of age.

In Chapter 4, "The Culture and Biology of Breastfeeding: An Historical Review of Western Europe," Fildes presents a fascinating survey of breastfeeding practices in preindustrial and industrial western European societies. She argues that although there are a number of factors that affect the health of mothers and infants, the method of infant feeding was not only one of the most important determinants of early childhood morbidity and mortality, but it also affected maternal health. She focuses on several infant feeding variables that have had an impact on health and disease patterns of mothers and infants throughout history: whether or not an infant was breastfed, and if breastfed, for how long; and the timing and type of supplemental and weaning foods. She concludes that there are very complex interactions between the biology and culture of breastfeeding that can have a profound effect on both maternal and infant health.

Quandt's chapter (Chapter 5), "Sociocultural Aspects of the Lactation Process," puts breastfeeding into the context of a feeding behavior that is regulated by the social and structural milieu in which the participants interact. She considers three important dimensions of breastfeeding: (1) whether or not, and when, breastfeeding is initiated, (2) the duration of exclusive breastfeeding, and (3) the frequency, duration, and timing of breastfeeding episodes. Quandt reviews the biobehavioral interactions of breastfeeding, and illustrates how these have been shaped by social and cultural factors into a diverse array of contemporary infant feeding practices. She touches on breastfeeding behaviors and birth-spacing, "breastfeeding style," and the "insufficient milk" controversy. Finally, she proposes a model that links the biology of lactation to social and cultural factors through specific breastfeeding behaviors.

Van Esterik takes a political stance to breastfeeding and tackles the advocacy issue head-on in Chapter 6, "The Politics of Breastfeeding: An Advocacy Perspective." She traces the development of infant feeding as a public policy issue and follows the path of the struggle against obstacles to breastfeeding that began at a grass roots level and resulted in global initiatives leading to the Innocenti Declaration. She describes a number of issues and organizations that arose along the way, including La Leche League, INFACT (the Infant Formula Action Coalition), and IBFAN (the International Baby Food Action Network). Van Esterik concludes with a discussion of advocacy and anthropology and says that "Breastfeeding is simultaneously biologically and socially constructed, deeply embedded in social relations, and yet cannot be understood without reference to varying levels of analysis including individual, household, community, institutional, and world industrial capitalism."

In Chapter 7, "Beauty and the Breast: The Cultural Context of Breastfeeding in the United States," Dettwyler reminds us that we, are, indeed, mammals. The class Mammalia actually derives its name from the mammae, or mammary glands, which distinguish mammals from other classes of animals. The function of mammae is to nourish young with the secretions of the gland. Dettwyler poses the question "Why do women have breasts?" and illustrates how far women in Western, particularly North American, culture have drifted from their mammalian heritage in terms of the function of breasts. In that culture, breasts are not considered to be organs for the feeding of young, but, instead, sexual objects for the titillation of men. This underscores how cultural beliefs can mask biological function. Dettwyler explores a number of assumptions underlying beliefs about breasts and emphasizes that North American attitudes toward breasts (and, as a consequence, breastfeeding) are the result of learned, not innate, behavior. As she says, "breastfeeding is both a 'simple and natural' process that flows from our human biological status as mammals, and a heavily culturalized behavior that can be so modified by cultural perceptions away from a 'natural process' as to be almost unrecognizable." Dettwyler ends with a discussion of ways in which North American women can "take back their breasts" so that both mothers and infants can enjoy the benefits of breastfeeding.

In Chapter 8, "Baby-Controlled Breastfeeding: Biocultural Implications," Woolridge presents data on the physiological repercussions of imposing arbitrary schedules on the process of breastfeeding. He supports the concept of "baby-controlled" feeding on the premise that infants are individuals who have differing nutritional requirements and are capable of regulating their own food intake. Data from his studies show that not only the volume but also the quality of milk is amenable to manipulation. By taking an individual rather than a populational approach, he is able to identify a number of predictors (behavioral) of the fat concentration of milk (physiological). He shows that feed frequency and duration have a direct effect on milk fat concentration.

In Chapter 9, "Breastfeeding: Adaptive Behavior for Child Health and Longevity," Cunningham presents a summary of the health advantages of breastfeeding and the potential health problems associated with formula feeding. Data from a number of studies show that formula-fed babies are at increased risk in terms of morbidity and mortality. For example, in Latin America, the risk of mortality for bottle-fed infants is at least 10 times higher than for breastfed infants. Even in the western world, where living conditions are generally good, the risk of fatal and nonfatal respiratory infections is 2- to 5-fold higher among bottle-fed infants. Cunningham shows that otitis media, bacteremia, and meningitis occur more frequently among infants who are not breastfed. The relative risk for bottle-fed infants in sudden infant death syndrome (SIDS) is more than fivefold, which translates into 4000 crib deaths every year in the United States. He observes that autoimmune diseases, subtle immune deficiencies, systemic vasculitis, and allergic diseases are immunoregulatory diseases that are influenced by the method of infant feeding, and can be triggered by exposure to cow's milk (in the form of infant formula) early in life. Cunningham also presents evidence that psychomotor and neural development are advanced in breastfed babies relative to formula-fed babies. Although there are some contraindications for breastfeeding, primarily related to the mother's diet or use of drugs, there is a long list (Table 9.3) of threats to the health of formula-fed babies that can result from errors in the manufacture or preparation of formulas. In conclusion, Cunningham still feels that "breast is best."

McKenna and Bernshaw's chapter (Chapter 10), "Breastfeeding and Infant–Parent Co-sleeping as Adaptive Strategies: Are They Protective against SIDS?," presents a detailed discussion of the relationship between SIDS and infant feeding practices, one of the issues raised by Cunningham in Chapter 9. They point out that the physiological effects on infants of breastfeeding and adult proximity during sleep have not been appreciated by researchers. They show that populational differences in SIDS incidence, knowledge of the disorder itself, and an understanding of infant physiology can provide clues to why some infants die from SIDS and others do not. McKenna and a co-investigator have been actively involved in laboratory research monitoring physiological processes of mother–infant co-sleeping and breastfeeding. They have discovered that co-sleeping and breastfeeding infants spend less time in deep stages of sleep, and that co-sleeping creates more variable physiological experiences for the infant. These observations have important implications for understanding the complex etiology of SIDS.

Ellison, in Chapter 11, "Breastfeeding, Fertility, and Maternal Condition," writes about the relationship between breastfeeding and lactational infertility. It is astounding to realize that modern science has only recently elevated this phenomenon from "old wives tale" to acceptable dogma. This, even though the relationship between breastfeeding and temporary infertility appears to have been known for centuries; it was acknowledged by Aristotle (Anderson, 1983), and was well known in later historical times (Fildes, 1986). However, as Ellison states, it was not until the 1970s (Tyson, 1977), that the endocrinological basis for this relationship began to be understood. Every time a baby stimulates the nipple by sucking, prolactin is released by the hypothalamus. It was recognized that prolactin was linked to the suppression of ovarian function in lactating women. Ellison states "As Henry (a French demographer) had originally suspected, natural fertility variation appeared to be a reflection of variation in biological functions, albeit an aspect of reproductive biology intimately connected with behavior." Using data from a number of studies, Ellison identifies some of the cultural factors that can affect the duration of lactational amenorrhea, including the frequency with which the infant is fed, the duration of breastfeeding, whether night feeding occurs, and when supplementary food is introduced. Depending on these cultural factors, menses can resume almost immediately, within a few months, or be delayed for between 1 and 2 years. Once again, culture is shown to have a profound effect on biology.

In Chapter 12, "Breast Cancer, Reproductive Biology, and Breastfeeding," Micozzi illustrates that overall breast cancer risk is associated with a very complex array of cultural and biological factors. Breastfeeding appears to confer protection against breast cancer in two major ways: first, through being breastfed as an infant, and second, through breastfeeding as an adult. The first follows from Micozzi's observation that dietary events relevant to breast cancer risk probably occur early in life. If a woman was not breastfed, there is a risk of overnutrition associated with bottle feeding and early supplementation. Overnutrition is associated with larger body size and early menarche, both of which are known risk factors for breast cancer. Animal studies have shown that increased dietary protein can lead to tumor production, and, in human studies, breast cancer has been related to high protein diets, particularly those containing animal protein. Many infant formulas are based on cow's milk, which has several times more protein than human milk. Total caloric intake can also be a risk factor, and there is a greater possibility for formula-fed babies to consume excess calories. As well, Micozzi postulates that breast cancer rates are related to consumption of milk and dairy products, based on the observation that lactase-deficient populations have lower levels of breast cancer, and most infant formulas are based on cow's milk. Another factor may be that as they have missed out on the immunities conferred by breast milk, formula-fed infants have inferior immune systems compared to those of breastfed infants, leading to a greater susceptibility to carcinoma. This is supported by the study by Davis, Savitz and Graubard (1988) on lymphoma.

If a woman breastfeeds her own children, she may experience protection against breast cancer on two levels, hormonal and microenvironmental. Nonpregnant, nonlactating women have higher levels of estrogens, which appear to be associated with breast cancer risk. Prolonged lactation produces a microenvironment that is less carcinogenic for breast tissue, and avoids conditions of stasis in the breast. The longer a woman breastfeeds, the more she will benefit in terms of reduced cancer risk. This is confirmed by studies on Asian women, who traditionally nurse their infants for long periods (Tao, Yu, Ross and Xiu, 1988; Yoo, Tajima, Kuroishi, Hirose et al., 1992), and a study on North American women by Newcomb, Storer, Longnecker, Mittendorf et al. (1994).

As Micozzi says, probably one of the reasons that breastfeeding has not been identified as a stronger protective factor in North American studies is that few women breastfeed in the "ancient pattern," that is, on demand, at night, and for periods longer than 1 year.

SYNTHESIS

Humans have two basic modes of responding to change: cultural and biological. One of the great strengths of our species is our capacity to respond to environmental challenge through cultural means rather than having to rely on the much slower biological–genetic pathway. Even so, we cannot deny our mammalian heritage. Biology and culture are inextricably related, and an alteration in a behavior can have a reciprocal effect on biology. Nowhere is this more apparent than in the story of breastfeeding. Breastfeeding is the ultimate biocultural phenomenon; in humans breastfeeding is not only a biological process but also a culturally determined behavior. We have lived as hunters and gatherers for almost our entire time on earth; we have known plant and animal domestication, providing the potential for alternatives to breast milk, for less than 1% of our evolutionary history (Eaton, Shostak and Konner, 1988). This means that for more than 99% of our existence all human infants have obtained their main nutrition through breastfeeding and as mammals we have an evolutionary history of lactation that is even more ancient. So it is that humans have evolved as both biological entities and social creatures. Breast milk and breastfeeding have become intricately linked to physiological processes and health and disease patterns of both mothers and infants. Alterations of this age-old pattern can have profound implications for the physiology, growth and development, and health of human infants and children as well as for the physiology and health of women. This has not been appreciated by members of the medical profession, social scientists, and the general public (an exception is the excellent book by Jelliffe and Jelliffe, 1978). As the authors of this volume make clear, understanding the implications of breastfeeding for both mothers and infants provides a key for understanding health and disease patterns of both ancient and modern populations.

Throughout our evolutionary history, the mother–infant relationship has been forged and sustained by the breastfeeding link. The millions of years of intimate contact between mothers and infants consequent on breastfeeding have resulted in what is basically a physiologic interdependence—each relying on the other for optimum functioning of various physiological processes. Interference with this link by adopting cultural practices that hinder or prevent it from occurring can have detrimental consequences on the health of both the mother and infant. It is extremely important to realize that behavior can affect biology and that nature has crafted a unique two-way process for enhancing the health and survival of mothers and infants.

MOTHER–INFANT PHYSIOLOGIC INTERDEPENDENCY

Introduction

What did nature craft? From the moment a newborn infant is put to its mother's breast a chain of events is triggered that affects the physiology, and ultimately the health, of both mother and child. As the infant suckles, the nerve endings in the nipple and areola are stimulated, signaling the pituitary gland to release two important hormones, prolactin and oxytocin. Although the mechanisms are not well understood, prolactin promotes the production of milk, and oxytocin contracts the cells lining the alveoli in the breast, squeezing the milk into the ducts and making it available to the infant. Prolactin has been called the "mothering hormone." It is said to have a relaxing effect on the mother and enhance the desire for mother infant proximity (Lawrence, 1989; Sobrinho, 1993). Prolactin is also linked to the suppression of ovarian function in lactating women, which results in lactational amenorrhea. Oxytocin has been called the "hormone of love" because of its relationship to orgasm, birth, breastfeeding, and bonding (Newton, 1978). Oxytocin has another important function—to contract the uterus (experienced as "afterpains" when the contractions occur as the baby nurses within the first few days after birth). These contractions begin the process of returning the uterus to its prepregnancy size, and help to expel the placenta along with excess tissue and blood. Oxytocin and prolactin are also involved in numerous other metabolic processes, many of which are only beginning to be understood. Metabolic efficiency appears to be enhanced in lactating women, so that the energy cost of milk production may be compensated for by a reduction in overall maternal energy expenditure (Illingworth, Jung, Howie, Leslie and Isles, 1986; Prentice and Whitehead, 1987).

For a period of time before and after childbirth the breasts secrete a substance called colostrum. Among other functions, colostrum acts as a purge, aiding in the elimination of meconium (the dark-green tar-like substance in the gastrointestinal tract of babies) by stimulating peristalsis. Human colostrum and breast milk are rich in substances, ranging from immunoglobin A to lactoferrin, which confer immunities on the recipient child (Hooton, Pabst, Spady and Paetkau, 1991; Lawrence, 1989). The contact between mother and child through breastfeeding provides an elegant system whereby the mother's body manufactures antibodies to microorganisms that the infant is exposed to and transmits these antibodies to the infant via the breast milk (Lawrence, 1989). Human milk also contains species-specific concentrations of hormones and other bioactive compounds including peptides, amino acids, glycoproteins, prostaglandins, and prolactin, which may be responsible for the optimum development of the gastrointestinal tract, pituitary gland, pancreas, and brain of the human infant (Sheard and Walker, 1988; Ellis and Picciano, 1992). It is likely that our hunter and gatherer ancestors would have put their infants to the breast whenever they cried in what has been termed "unrestricted" or "on demand" style of breastfeeding and that breastfeeding would have continued for a number of years.

This is our evolutionary inheritance; this is what our bodies have become accustomed to after millions of years of evolutionary history as mammals. We can use this inheritance to our advantage, or we can squander it through behaviors that delay, inhibit, or even prevent the physiological processes mentioned above from occurring. These behaviors are primarily culturally mediated and evolved because of individual, familial, or societal pressures, customs, or beliefs. These factors have a profound effect on infant feeding practices, from the very basic decision of whether or not to breastfeed to the "style" of breastfeeding and the timing and type of supplemental foods. For example, as Dettwyler points out in Chapter 7, some North American women may decide not to breastfeed partly because of inhibitions related to the common perception of breasts as sexual objects. Or as Fildes (Chapter 4) has shown, an upper class woman of fifteenth-century England would have hired a wet nurse rather than breastfeed her own infant. In this case the infant would derive the benefits of breastfeeding, but the mother would not. In historical times, and even today, babies in some societies are denied colostrum, with all its beneficial properties, in the belief that it is a poisonous substance dangerous for the newborn. There are many other culturally determined behaviors that can affect these physiological processes; the following discussion illustrates some of the biological consequences of these behaviors for both mothers and infants.

Some Effects on the Mother

There is a distinct physiological difference between a lactating and nonlactating woman. As Peaker says: "The secretion of milk . . . markedly affects the whole maternal organism" (1976:87). For example, heart function is affected by lactation; cardiovascular changes occur including high blood flow to the mammary glands, alimentary tract, and liver, and high cardiac output, particularly to the mammary glands, gastrointestinal tract, and skin (Peaker, 1976). There is also a generalized response to lactation that includes an increase in body temperature and rhythmic contractions of the uterus (Newton, 1971). Lactating women have been shown to have higher levels of serum parathyroid hormone, 1,25-dehydroxyvitamin D_3, and phosphorous, and these differences may persist even after weaning; urinary calcium excretion decreases rapidly in early lactation, and declines further as lactation continues (Feldblum, Zhang, Rich, Fortney and Talmage, 1992). There is an increase in the gastrointestinal endocrine system during lactation and hormones such as gastrin, cholecystokinin (CCK), insulin, glucagon, and somatostatin are affected (Silber, Larsson and Uvnäs-Moberg, 1991). These hormones enhance digestion and stimulate anabolic metabolism by promoting insulin release. In animal studies, it has been shown that the size of the gastrointestinal tract, liver, and pancreas actually increases during lactation (Widström, Winberg, Werner, Svensson et al., 1988; Widdowson, 1976) although it is not known whether this occurs in women.

Lactating women have higher levels of prolactin and oxytocin than nonlactating women (Leake, Waters, Rubin, Buster and Fisher, 1983; Widström, Winberg, Werner, Hamberger et al., 1984; Silber, Larsson and Uvnäs-Moberg, 1991). If an infant is put to the mother's breast within minutes of birth, the oxytocin that is released stimulates contraction of the uterus and the constriction of uterine blood vessels, thus accelerating delivery of the placenta and reducing postpartum bleeding and the possibility of uterine hemorrhage (LaCerva, 1981). Precisely what these higher levels of hormones mean in terms of differences in human behavior, if any, is uncertain, but animal studies have shown that these hormones enhance nurturing behavior in females such as retrieval, nest-building, licking, and proximity to pups in rats and are associated with reduced levels of aggression toward other animals (Carter and Getz, 1993; Insel and Shapiro, 1992; Newton, 1971, 1978; Pederson, Caldwell and Jurkowski, 1988). As Silber et al. say: "Although oxytocin has been suggested to promote maternal behavior in different animals, it is unlikely that any maternal behavior in humans is entirely hormonally regulated. There are indications, however, that vestiges of such behavior exist and that also in humans, hormones such as oxytocin do play a part in the preparation of the female for maternity" (1991:287). Although many factors may be operative, one study has shown that anxiety levels are lower in breastfeeding women (Uvnäs-Moberg, Widström, Nissen and Björvell,

1990); the researchers found correlations between prolactin and oxytoxin levels and scores on the Karolinska Scales of Personality. Lawrence (1989) has suggested that high levels of prolactin may be physiologically soothing to the mother. She says: "The long-term psychophysiologic reaction of unrestricted nursing is a more even mood cycle compared with the mood swings associated with ovulation and menstruation" (1989:155). It is possible that the high levels of oxytocin and prolactin produced during breastfeeding have an enhanced positive effect on the mother–infant relationship.

There is evidence that breastfeeding is associated with a reduced risk of women's cancers (Eaton et al., 1994) including ovarian cancer (Schneider, 1987; Gwinn, Lee, Rhodes, Layde and Rubin, 1990), breast cancer (Micozzi, Chapter 12), and possibly endometrial cancer (Pettersson, Adami, Bergstrom and Johansson, 1986). Until recently, it was widely believed that lactation had no effect on the incidence of breast cancer (Kelsey and John, 1994). However, since the 1980s several case-control studies have suggested that lactation, particularly for long periods, is associated with a reduction in the risk of breast cancer in premenopausal women (Byers, Graham, Rzepka and Marshall, 1985; McTiernan and Thomas, 1986; United Kingdom National Case-Control Study Group, 1993; Yuan, Yu, Ross, Gao and Henderson, 1988; Micozzi, Chapter 12). Before this time there had been some hints that breast cancer and breastfeeding are related. Ing, Ho and Petrakis (1977) published a study on breast cancer in Hong Kong women who customarily breastfeed only with the right breast. The data indicated that in postmenopausal women who have breastfed unilaterally, the risk of cancer is significantly higher in the unsuckled breast, and that breastfeeding may help to protect the suckled breast against cancer. A 1969 publication by Schaefer noted that breast cancer was extremely rare among Inuit women and that up to 1969 there had been only one definite case of mammary carcinoma in a Canadian Inuit. This occurred in a woman who, although she had nursed seven of her children for up to 2 years each, had never nursed on the carcinomatous breast since the "nipple on that side did not work" (Schaefer, 1969). This suggests that there is a predilection for dysfunctional breasts to develop breast cancer. Population surveys indicate that breast cancer rates are low in women in populations where it is common to breastfeed, including Asia, the far North, and Africa (Post, 1982).

The most recent study on the association between breast cancer and breastfeeding is a multicenter, population-based, case-control study of 6888 women (Newcomb et al., 1994). After adjustment for a number of factors, lactation was found to be associated with a slight reduction in the risk of breast cancer among premenopausal women. For premenopausal women with a cumulative total of more than 24 months of lactation, the risk of breast cancer was 0.72 relative to that for women who had never lactated (Newcomb et al., 1994). The researchers concluded that if all women with children lactated for 24 months or longer, the incidence of breast cancer among parous premenopausal women might be reduced by nearly 25%. Another study (Layde, Webster, Baughman, Wingo, Rubin, Ory and The Cancer and Steroid Hormone Study Group, 1989) concluded that women who had breastfed for more than 2 years had a 43% lower risk of breast cancer than women who had never breastfed. In Chapter 12, Micozzi suggests that breastfeeding reduces breast cancer risk either because of hormonal reasons and/or differences in the microenvironment of the breast.

Studies assessing the relationship between bone mineral density and reproductive factors, such as breastfeeding, have been contradictory; some show a protective effect, some show a detrimental effect, and some show no effect. However, there have been weaknesses in most of these studies, with small sample sizes, and deficiencies in addressing specific issues relating to lactation, such as duration, timing, and intensity. In many of the studies any differences between ever breastfed and never breastfed groups may have been minimized because the women who breastfed did so for very short periods. Or as Hreshchyshyn, Hopkins, Zylstra and Anbar (1988) found, if all women who had breastfed are compared with those who had not, there are no significant differences in development of osteoporosis, whereas if only parous women are considered, those who breastfed had a higher lumbar spine bone mineral density than those who did not. Their data showed that there was a 1.5% increase in bone mineral density per breastfed child. Cumming and Klineberg (1993) found a similar trend; parous women who had not breastfed had twice the risk of hip fracture as nulliparous women. An increased average duration of breastfeeding per child was associated with a greater reduction in risk of hip fracture. Feldblum et al. (1992) found that women who had breastfed had an estimated 41 mg/cm^2 higher lumbar bone mineral density after controlling for parity, body mass index, physical activity, and menopausal status. Kreiger, Kelsey, Holford and O'Connor (1982) found a 40% reduction in the risk of hip fracture for each 12 months of breastfeeding during a woman's lifetime. Alderman, Weiss, Daling, Ure and Ballard (1986) found a similar magnitude among women who had breastfed for longer than 12 months overall. Studies by Aloia, Cohn, Vaswani, Yeh, Yuen and Ellis (1985) and Kelsey, Browner, Seeley, Nevitt and Cummings (1992) have shown that breastfeeding protects against fractures of the vertebrae. Although not all studies in the past 10 years have found evidence for a protective effect of lactation on bone mineral density, the fact that some animal studies (Feldblum et al. 1992; Lamke, Brundin and Moberg, 1977) and several well-designed human studies have suggests that this relationship may exist.

It is well documented that formula-fed children in developing countries have higher rates of lethal illnesses than breastfed children (Cunningham, Chapter 9). However, data show that children in both developing and developed countries also suffer more frequent and severe bouts of acute illness, ranging from intestinal disorders to SIDS to respiratory conditions (Cunningham, Chapter 9) and chronic illness, such as juvenile diabetes and Crohn's disease (Cunningham, Chapter 9; Stuart-Macadam, 1993). What is seldom mentioned is the enormous financial, emotional, and energetic costs to parents involved in caring for a sick child. An extreme example would be the emotional strain on the Pakistani mother in Figure 1.1, whose daughter was dying, in part because she was not breastfed (and because in this culture traditionally males are favored over females). A less extreme example would be one of the possibly millions of North American mothers whose child suffers from frequent episodes of otitis media (middle ear infection) as the result of not being breastfed (among other factors). There is unequivocal evidence that breastfed children develop fewer and less severe ear infections than formula-fed babies (Cunningham, Chapter 9). For example, Schaefer (1971) found that bottle feeding increased the risk of chronic otitis media in Inuit children by more than fivefold and that there was an inverse relationship between incidence of chronic ear disease and duration of lactation. Individuals breastfed for more than 12 months had the lowest incidence of otitis media. In a sample of 348 infants from the state of New York, Cunningham (1979) found that those who were formula fed were 2 1/2 times as likely to develop acute otitis media than those who were breastfed. Saarinen (1982) studied the incidence of otitis media in a group of 237 children. Recurrent otitis media was strongly associated with early formula feeding; the longer exclusive breastfeeding continued, the fewer episodes of otitis media occurred. Breastfeeding was shown to have a long-term protective effect up to 3 years of age. In a study on Swedish children, Aniansson, Andersson, Hakansson and Larsson et al. (1994) showed that the first episode of acute otitis media occurred earlier in children who were weaned before 6 months of age, and that the frequency of acute otitis media was significantly lower in the breastfed children than in the nonbreastfed children in every age group.

In the United States alone there are an estimated 30 million annual office visits to pediatricians for treatment of earaches, with an annual cost for diagnosis and treatment of over $2.2 billion (Jacobs, 1992). This takes a enormous toll on parents in terms of emotional stress, time spent in doctors' offices and hospitals, and money, and otitis media is

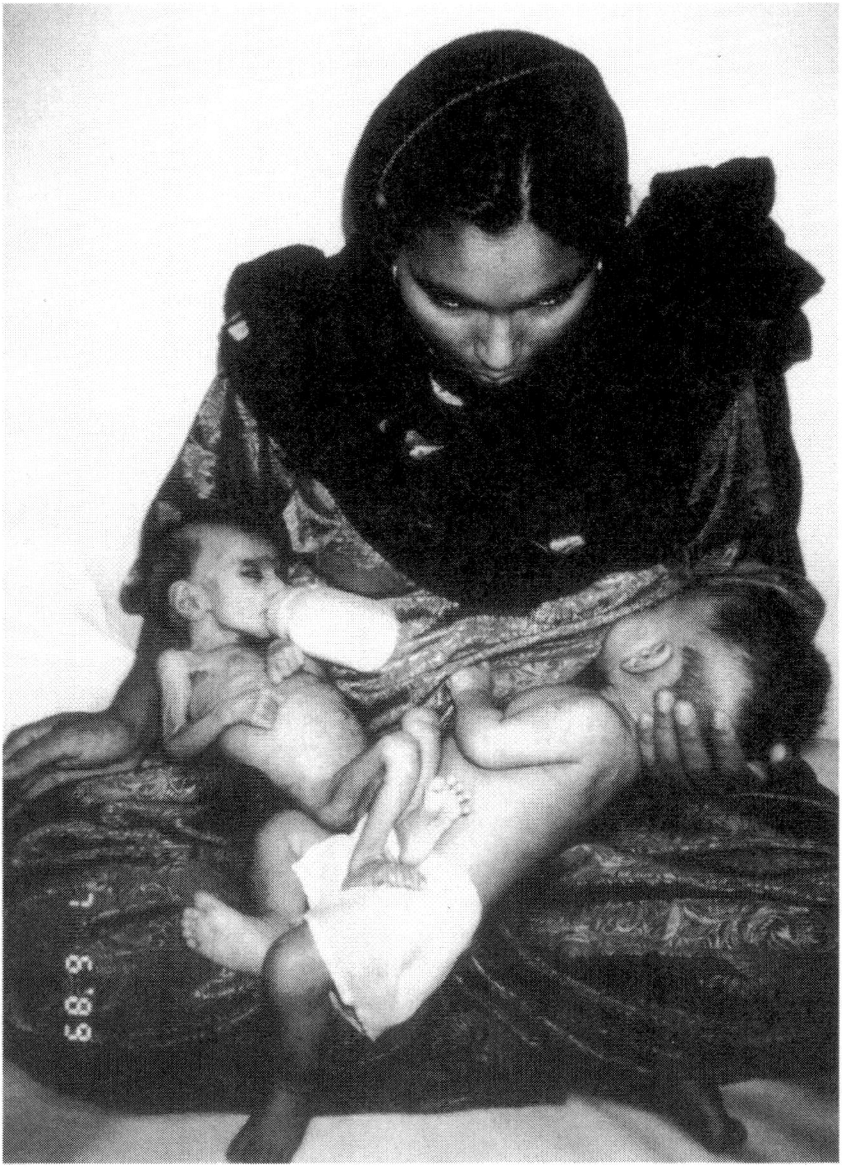

Figure 1.1. Five-month-old twins from Islamabad, Pakistan. The bottlefed twin, a girl, was malnourished and suffered from frequent bouts of diarrhea. (Courtesy of Dr. Mushtaq A. Khan, Pakistan Institute of Medical Sciences, Islamabad.)

only one of a number of acute and chronic diseases to which formula-fed infants are more susceptible. The mother who breastfeeds has an advantage over the mother who formula feeds because she has a healthier child, thereby decreasing her level of emotional stress and saving time, money, and energy.

In conclusion, there are distinct physiological and metabolic differences between lactating and nonlactating women. The long-term effects of these differences on human females are unknown; however, studies are beginning to show that not breastfeeding may have detrimental consequences later in a woman's life. Women who have never breastfed have an increased probability of developing premenopausal breast cancer, ovarian cancer, and possibly endometrial cancer and senile osteoporosis. It appears that experiencing lactation during her reproductive cycle may confer short- and long-term health benefits to a woman.

Some Effects on the Infant

> breast milk not only prevents many ailments, softens and cools the gums when inflamed, forwards dentition, and prevents its fatal consequences, but even lays a lasting foundation for a robust and healthy constitution. (Jean Astruc, 1746)

As the previous quotation illustrates, the beneficial effects of breast milk for infants have been known for generations. For example, seventeenth- and eighteenth-century European physicians noted that a breastfed child was less likely to develop rickets, have less trouble with teething, and was less likely to die (Fildes, 1986). However, it has only been in the past 50 years, with greater understanding of the properties of breast milk and increased knowledge of the acute and chronic health problems associated with the use of infant formulas, that the full extent of the benefits of breastfeeding on infant health is becoming known. The beneficial qualities of breast milk become apparent within moments after the first breastfeed and continue over the lifetime of an individual.

For example, in the days immediately after birth the elimination of meconium is accelerated in babies who receive colostrum. Babies breastfed within a short time after birth pass their first stool earlier and have lower levels of bilirubin [a waste product formed by the destruction of red blood cells (Rosta, Makoi and Kertesz, 1968)]. Since high levels of bilirubin in the blood cause jaundice, breastfed babies fed on demand are less likely to suffer from jaundice than formula-fed babies. A study by Carvalho, Klaus and Merkatz (1982) showed that hospital policies that reduce or limit the number of breastfeeds may interfere with the normal processes that eliminate bilirubin from the newborn infant. More frequent breastfeeds resulted in lower serum bilirubin levels, suggesting that babies who are breastfed frequently in the first few days after birth would be least likely to suffer from jaundice.

Human milk contains hormones, peptides, amino acids, and glycoproteins that may play a role in the maturation of the small intestine. These include epidermal growth factor (EGF), nerve growth factor (NGF), somatomedin-C, insulin growth factor, insulin, thyroxine, cortisol, taurine, glutamine, and amine sugar (Sheard and Walker, 1988). Studies have shown that animals fed breast milk have greater mucosal mass, DNA, and protein content of the small intestine than artificially fed animals (Bines and Walker, 1991). This, and other data, suggests that breast milk provides an important stimulus to the development of the human intestine. On the basis of their research, Bines and Walker (1991) suggest that the duration of lactation appears to influence the degree of breast milk stimulated intestinal growth and maturation. Since the epithelial surface of the gastrointestinal tract has an important role in digestion and absorption and acts as a protective barrier against microorganisms, antigens, and enterotoxins, this could have important implications for the development of the human immune response (Bines and Walker, 1991). This may explain why formula-fed babies are at increased risk for allergies and chronic gastrointestinal disorders such as Crohn's disease and ulcerative colitis (Cunningham, Chapter 9; Stuart-Macadam, 1993).

Although a controversial issue, an association between bottle feeding and malocclusion (malposition of the teeth that interferes with the maximum efficiency of the masticatory process) has been postulated ever since bottle feeding started to become a popular infant feeding alternative in North America (Labbok and Hendershot, 1987). A number of factors are involved in the ultimate size and shape of the oral facial region including facial symmetry, jaw size and position, palate height, overbite and overjet, tooth size and shape, and muscle function (Sanger and Bystrom, 1982). With the exception of tooth size and shape, all of these are influenced by both genetic and environmental factors [which include oral practices such as the use of artificial nipples, soothers (dummies), and digit sucking] (Sanger and Bystrom, 1982). Studies investigating the relationship between method of infant feeding and malocclusion have produced contradictory results but there have been a number of methodological problems including small sample sizes. One major problem is that few babies in these studies have been exclusively breastfed for long enough (without the use of bottle or soother) to provide a good control sample. For example, a study by Ogaard, Larsson and Lindsten (1994) found no difference in the frequency of posterior crossbite between bottle-fed and breastfed Norwegian children, but breastfeeding was not defined, nor was duration mentioned. The authors did say that "the frequency and duration of breastfeeding in these populations is extremely low compared with the situation among so-called primitive people" (1994:164).

Two large population-based studies do support a relationship between bottle feeding and malocclusion. A retrospective study by Adamiak (1981) surveyed a group of 748 4- to 6-year-old children. There was a clear negative association between the duration of breastfeeding and the incidence of occlusal anomalies, with 24.2% of children breastfed longer than 6 months having occlusal anomalies compared to 36.4% of children who were breastfed less than 3 months or not at all. Labbok and Hendershot's 1987 survey of a sample of 9698 U.S. children showed that the longer a child had been breastfed, the lower was the incidence of malocclusion. This trend was constant for all variables tested and remained even when adjusted for age and maternal education. The relative risk of malocclusion for children breastfed from 0 to 3 months was 1.84. The authors concluded that 44% of the malocclusion experienced by children in this study was attributable to less than prolonged breastfeeding. Whether an increase in malocclusion is the result of the different sucking technique of bottlefed and breastfed babies [the tongue action of a breastfed baby is a "rolling" or peristaltic motion as opposed to the "piston-like" action in the bottle-feeder (Lawrence, 1989)], the forces produced by the pressure of an artificial nipple on the roof of the mouth, or other factors, are unknown.

Data from several studies have indicated that breastfed newborns exhibit more body activity, are more alert, and have stronger arousal reaction than bottle-fed babies (Newton, 1971; Davis et al., 1948; Bell, 1966). This may have implications for future physiological and behavioral development. In fact, some studies have suggested that motor and cognitive development is superior in breastfed babies (Cunningham, Chapter 9). For example, several studies have shown that, on average, breastfed babies walk earlier than bottle-fed babies (Hoefer and Hardy, 1929; Biering-Sorensen, Hilden and Biering-Sorensen, 1983; Martorell and O'Gara, 1985).

Although studies have shown conflicting results, there is increasing evidence for a relationship between nutrition in early infancy and later neurodevelopment. One of the first studies to suggest this relationship was published 65 years ago by Hoefer and Hardy (1929). More recent studies have shown that even when a number of factors are controlled for, there is a tendency for breastfed children to have higher test scores in intelligence and language tests (Fergusson, Beautrais and Silva, 1982; Young, Buckley, Hamza and Mandarano, 1982; Bauer, Ewald, Hoffman and Dubanoski, 1991; Lucas, 1990; Lucas, Morley, Cole, Gore et al., 1989a,b; Lucas, Morley, Cole, Lister and Leeson-Payne, 1992; Rogan and Gladen, 1993; Temboury, Otero, Polanco and Arribas, 1994). The studies by Lucas et al. (1989a,b, 1992) are of particular interest because all the children were premature and had originally been tube-fed their mother's milk. The researchers concluded that the advantage in cognitive test scores was provided by the breast milk itself rather than the process of breastfeeding. There was also a dose–response relationship between the proportion of mother's milk in the diet and subsequent test score; the more the milk, the higher the test score. These researchers were able to follow these children up to 7–8 years of age and found that even at this age the children who had consumed breast milk had a significantly higher IQ (8 point advantage) than those who had received no maternal breast milk. Major growth activity in the human brain is not complete until 2 years of age and it is possible that optimum development of the human brain is dependent upon the many hormones and bioactive substances found in human milk (Ellis and Picciano, 1992).

There are myriad factors involved in the expression of any disease, some of which are genetic, some environmental. It appears, however, that disease can occur in susceptible nonbreastfed individuals either because of the lack of the benefits of breast milk, and/or the detrimental aspects of infant formulas based on cow's milk. It is undeniable that the breastfed infant has an immunological advantage over a formula-fed infant. As Cunningham points out in Chapter 9, there is overwhelming evidence supporting the advantages of breastfeeding in generally unhealthy environments. Lawrence (1989) states that in the third world deaths among newborns not suckled at the breast are at least five times higher than among those who receive colostrum and mother's milk. Fildes points out in Chapter 4 that the mortality of nonbreastfed infants was well known in antiquity, and weaker or more "prized" children were breastfed for prolonged periods. Chapters 9 and 10 also include evidence that the health benefits of breast milk are apparent even in babies living in modern industrialized countries. The immunological advantage enjoyed by breastfed infants lasts not only for the first year of breastfeeding (Cunningham, 1979, 1981) but on into subsequent years (Wray, 1990), and even continues after weaning (Gulick, 1986).

In some cases, not being breastfed is only one of a number of risk factors that can lead to disease. This is certainly the case with conditions such as idiopathic juvenile diabetes mellitus (where there is a relationship between genetic predisposition, infectious diseases, and consumption of cow's milk (Karjalainen, Martin, Knip, Ilonen, Robinson,

Savilahti, Akerblom and Dosch, 1992; Kostraba, Cruickshanks, Lawler-Heavner, Jobim et al., 1993), SIDS (McKenna and Bernshaw, Chapter 10), chronic gastrointestinal disease such as ulcerative colitis (where there is a relationship between genetic predisposition, environment, diarrheal illness in infancy, and consumption of cow's milk (Koletzko, Sherman, Corey, Griffiths and Smith, 1989), or atopic disease [where there is a relationship between genetic predisposition, environmental factors and consumption of cow's milk (McConnochie and Roghmann, 1986)]. Not being breastfed, and/or being fed cow's milk, could for some individuals be "the straw that broke the camel's back." Since, unlike genetic factors, breastfeeding is a protective measure that can be controlled, it is worth considering for infants who have a family history of diabetes, gastrointestinal conditions, or atopic disease. In other cases being breastfed or not can possibly be a matter of life or death. This is poignantly illustrated by the picture of the Pakistani twins (Figure 1.1), and documented in a study of liver disease by Udall, Dixon, Newman, Wright, James and Bloch (1985). In that study, data were collected on 32 children who were born with a gene that leads to a deficiency of α_1-antitrypsin, a serum protease inhibitor. Children with α_1-antitrypsin deficiency are at increased risk for the development of liver disease; approximately 10 to 20% develop liver dysfunction (Udall et al., 1985). The liver disease may progress to cirrhosis and death. Severe liver disease occurred in eight (40%) of the bottlefed and one (8%) of the breastfed infants, and all eight infants who died as the result of their disease were bottle fed. In such cases breastfeeding could possibly have saved lives.

There is a growing awareness that early childhood nutrition can have long-term effects on the health of individuals (Hahn, 1987; Lucas, 1990). For example, Osborn (1967) examined the coronary arteries of 109 young people under the age of 20 who died from a variety of causes. He divided his sample into three groups based on whether they had ever been breastfed, or had been breastfed for less than 1 month or for more than 1 month. He then determined whether there had been any reduction in the size of the lumen of the arteries (an indication of atherosclerosis and potential heart problems later in life). Although the children who had been breastfed were not immune from lumen reduction, 69% of those who had never been breastfed were considered to have bad coronary arteries (as opposed to 26% of those who had been breastfed for over 1 month). Forty-five percent of those children who had been breastfed for over 1 month had coronary arteries classed as normal compared with only 17% of those who had never been breastfed. Preliminary data from a study by Lucas (1990) suggest that the way a preterm infant is fed, in just the early weeks postpartum, may have a major impact on later growth and development.

There is also tentative evidence for an association between childhood cancer and early nutrition. A case-control study of 201 cases and 181 controls from Denver by Davis et al. (1988) assessed whether inadequate exposure to the immunological benefits of human milk leaves infants more susceptible to childhood malignancies. The results showed that children who were artificially fed or breastfed less than 6 months were at increased risk for developing cancer, particularly lymphoma, before the age of 15. The risk for artificially fed and short-term breastfed infants was approximately twice that of infants breastfed longer than 6 months. Cunningham (1986) found a negative correlation between breastfeeding and Hodgkin's disease in the United States, using regional data from a 1966 survey of hospital nurseries and 1970–1974 mortality rates supplied by the National Center for Health Statistics. Micozzi (Chapter 12) is probably the first researcher to suggest that early childhood nutrition, in particular formula feeding as opposed to breastfeeding, may have an effect on a woman's breast cancer risk later in life. A recent case-control study by Freudenheim, Marshall, Graham, Laughlin, Vena, Bandera, Muti, Swanson and Nemoto (1994) provides the data to support Micozzi's views. These researchers found a 25% lower risk of breast cancer among women who had been breastfed as infants compared with those who had been formula fed.

It is sometimes forgotten that breast milk is actually a food (Quandt, Chapter 5). There is a difference in the nutritive qualities of breast milk and infant formula that can actually be recognized in infants. A breastfed infant is said to have firmer flesh and feel more solid than a formula baby (Eiger and Olds, 1987). This is not surprising, since endocrine and metabolic responses in infants apparently differ depending on the type of feeding. For example Lucas, Boyes, Bloom and Aynsley-Green (1981) found that in comparison to breastfed infants, formula-fed infants have a greater insulin and GIP (basal plasma gastric inhibitory polypeptide) response to feeding, lower levels of basal and postprandial blood ketones, and a greater postfeed rise in both lactate and pyruvate concentrations. Human milk contains a vast array of bioactive compounds including immunological factors, enzymes, growth factors, and hormones that are either *not* found in infant formula or occur at very low levels (Ellis and Picciano, 1992). Some of these compounds, which may be particularly important for the optimum development of the human infant, are epidermal growth factor (EGF), prostaglandins, and prolactin. As Ellis and Picciano say, "The presence of hormones and other bioactive components in milk (human) may aid in formation of proper development or maturation of structures and/or set the proper level of functioning of physiological systems" (1992:13). It is obvious then that in terms of nutrition, there are qualitative and quantitative differences between breast milk and infant formula. This may be comparable to the difference between freshly squeezed juice from oranges straight off the tree and powdered artificial orange drink. Vitamins and minerals are present in both, but what a difference! Like fresh orange juice, breast milk is a vibrant, dynamic fluid that varies in flavor and proportions of nutrients. Like powdered orange drink, infant formula can be affected by errors or omissions in its manufacture and preparation. However, the consequences for the infant who receives nutrient-deficient or improperly prepared formula are much more serious than for an adult who consumes inferior or improperly prepared orange drink (Chapter 9).

Common bacteria that cause pneumonia, ear infections, and many other diseases are evolving into forms untreatable by all known medicines, threatening a chilling postantibiotic era that would be "nothing short of a medical disaster" according to Alexander Tomasz of Rockefeller University (*Duncan Banner*, 1994). For example, as previously mentioned, there are an estimated 30 million office visits annually to American pediatricians for treatment of earaches alone (Jacobs, 1992). The pneumococcus bacteria, which is responsible for perhaps half of these 30 million visits, is currently treatable by only one antibiotic, vancomycin. Without alternative antibiotics, a vancomycin-resistant pneumococcus would mean that effective treatment for many cases of ear infection would not be available. In this situation breastfed babies have an advantage on two fronts; not only will they develop fewer and/or less severe ear infections than formula-fed babies (Cunningham, Chapter 9), but their general immune system is superior to that of formula-fed infants (Gulick, 1986). If the scenario of antibiotic-resistant bacteria becomes as widespread a reality as has been suggested then the breastfed child will have an enormous advantage over the formula-fed child.

Iron status also differs between breastfed and formula-fed infants. As early as 1928 McKay noticed that exclusively breastfed infants had higher hemoglobin values than artificially fed babies (Oski and Landaw, 1980). The advantage began to disappear when the breastfed babies were given other foods. Since that time a number of other researchers have commented that iron dificiency is rarely observed in breastfed infants, but is common in infants fed cow's milk or unfortified cow's milk-based infant formula (Woodruff, 1958; Fransson and Lonnerdal, 1980; Calvo and Gnazzo, 1990; Lehmann, Gray-Donald, Mongeon and Di Tommaso, 1992; Shrestha, Chandra and Singh, 1994). Researchers now know that there are several factors that contribute to higher levels of iron-deficiency anemia in formula fed babies. First, there is little iron in cows' milk and it is less bioavailable to the infant. Infants absorb 50–70% of the iron in breast milk compared to 10% of the iron in cow's milk and 3–5% of the iron in iron-fortified proprietary formulas (Oski and Landaw, 1980). The introduction of supplemental foods in early infancy also has a detrimental effect on iron status because it impairs the bioavailability of iron from human milk. Infants who are breastfed exclusively for periods of 6–9 months maintain normal hemoglobin values and normal iron stores (Oski and Landaw, 1980). Second, intolerance of cow's milk or cow's milk-based infant formula can cause gastrointestinal bleeding in infants (Calvo and Gnazzo, 1990; Dallman, 1992; Shrestha et al., 1994). Third, the high levels of calcium in cow's milk can depress the absorption of both heme and nonheme iron in other foods by about 50% (MacPhail and Bothwell, 1992).

Iron-fortified infant formulas have been introduced to prevent iron-deficiency anemia in artificially fed infants, but there are risks associated with this. Too much iron can also cause problems. The much larger quantities of available iron in the diet of iron-fortified formula-fed infants has been associated with a higher susceptibility to salmonellosis, botulism, and SIDS (Weinberg, 1994). A number of infant formulas produced in the United States contain extremely high concentrations of iron, some three times higher than the maximum quantity recommended by nutritional scientists (Weinberg, 1994). Human milk is rich in an iron-binding protein, lactoferrin, which is an important aspect of the body's defense system for preventing the growth of iron-requiring toxigenic bacteria such as *Salmonella, Clostridium, Bacteroides, Escherichia,* and *Staphylococcus* (Weinberg, 1994). As Weinberg says (1994:49): "Is it prudent to augment formulas for infants less than six months of age with as much as 155 times the quantity of the metal that is present naturally in breast milk?"

Since the devastating occurrence of widespread AIDS many members of the medical establishment have come to the realization that the key to health and longevity lies with a strong and vital immune system bolstered by excellent nutrition and preventative medicine, rather than with increasingly sophisticated technology and an ever expanding arsenal of drugs. Both from a nutritional and an immunological standpoint, breast milk has been shown to be superior to infant formula. In view of the increasing evidence of acute and chronic conditions associated with *not* being breastfed, breastfeeding should be considered as an inexpensive, widely available, and highly effective form of preventative health care.

To conclude, there are physiological and metabolic differences between a breastfed and a formula-fed infant; these differences can affect the growth, development, and the short- and long-term health of infants and children.

Reciprocal Effects on Both Mother and Infant

Different ideas or customs about how often, how long, and when an infant is put to the breast, and whether and when supplemental fluids, foods, and/or pacifiers will be given can have an effect both on the nutritive quality of the milk that the infant receives and the amount of milk that the mother produces (Woolridge, Chapter 8). For example, there may be a twofold effect when an infant is given less access to its mother's breast either because access is regulated according to some arbitrary schedule, or the infant is given early supplemental feedings. First, a reduction in suckling means reduced stimulation of the mother's nipple and lower levels of oxytocin and prolactin. This leads to a corresponding reduction in the amount of milk produced. Second, as Woolridge has pointed out in his chapter, frequency of feeding influences milk fat concentration, and an infant who suckles more frequently will receive milk with a higher fat content. It may be then that cultural practices can be directly linked to what is perceived as "lactation failure" (Quandt, Chapter 5; Woolridge, Chapter 8).

As Ellison discusses in Chapter 11, a number of factors can affect the duration of lactational amenorrhea, including individual variation, nutritional status, work patterning, and the frequency and duration of breastfeeding. There appear to be advantages for both mother and infant from an extended period of lactational amenorrhea. For example, it is evident that for humans, as for nonhuman primates and other mammals (Anderson, 1983; Short, 1983), lactational amenorrhea acts as a natural birth spacer. Closely spaced births have been shown to have a negative impact on the survival probabilities not only of the first-born child in a sequence, but also of the second. In his chapter Ellison cites a study by Hobcraft, McDonald and Rutstein (1983) that shows that a birth in the 2 years prior to the birth of the index child increased that child's risk of dying by over 50% in 13 of 23 countries included in the study. In developing countries a child whose own birth is followed quickly by another is at increased risk of death, as much as 77%, when the second birth follows within 12 months of the first (Berg and Brems, 1990). Ellison speculates that closely spaced births in some way deplete maternal reserves, producing a negative effect on the health of current and future offspring, as well as on the woman herself. That this was also known in historical times is demonstrated by Fildes in Chapter 4. Breastfeeding was said to benefit the mother in several ways, including reducing the likelihood of her dying from pregnancy-related problems or childbirth. In 1719, Pierre Dionis (cf. Fildes, 1986) noted that pregnant women often died, whereas death was rare among nursing mothers.

Style of breastfeeding not only affects survival probabilities of mother and child, but also has demographic consequences. Any cultural practices that have the effect of reducing the intensity, duration, and/or frequency of infant suckling can result in a decrease in the duration of lactational amenorrhea, thus increasing fertility. Short (1983) writes that fertility rates seem to have increased as our hunting and gathering ancestors adopted agriculture and became more settled, probably because animal milk and cereal products were used as supplements for infants. If the !Kung can be used as an example of our hunting and gathering ancestors (an extrapolation that must be made with caution), it is possible to use data on their cultural practices and demography in a case study. According to Lee (1980), the nomadic !Kung diet is deficient in suitable weaning foods such as milk and porridge, which are easily digested by infants and toddlers. Solid foods are introduced by 6 months of age, but mother's milk is an important food source into the third year of life. In more settled !Kung villages cow's milk and cultivated grains are available, reducing the child's need for breast milk. The decrease in nipple stimulation that ensues results in lower levels of prolactin and an earlier resumption of ovulation. Lee calculated that the mean length of birth interval for a 10-year period (1963–1973) was 44.11 months for nomadic !Kung women compared to 36.17 months for sedentary !Kung women. As he states, "This 8-month difference would significantly increase both the birth rate and completed family size for the sedentary women" (Lee, 1980:336).

This relationship between breastfeeding and fertility was also known in historical times, if not earlier. Fildes (1986) collected comments of three types from historical sources dated between 1500 and 1800 that indicate a knowledge of the relationship: (1) that the wish to have more children quickly was a valid reason for a woman not to breastfeed, (2) that women who breastfed had fewer pregnancies, and (3) that women should breastfeed to avoid pregnancy (Fildes, 1986:108). She also quotes a remark made by Newcome in 1695 that suggests that breastfeeding was actually discouraged among the aristocracy to ensure that more children would be born. Pierre Dionis (1719) noted that in France, married women usually had a child every year for years, but those who suckled had only two or three at most. He advised women who wished to avoid pregnancy to breastfeed.

For societies whose members regularly use various types of contraception, the contraceptive effects of breastfeeding are not so critical, however, many people around the world do not use such measures. According to Berg and Brems (1990), breastfeeding is perhaps the principal factor influencing the length of the birth interval for the 83% of couples in developing countries who do not use modern forms of contraception. Family Health International has estimated that breastfeeding reduces total possible fertility by an average of 34% for 5 countries in Africa, 30% for 12 countries in Asia, and 16% for another 12 countries in the Americas (Thapa, Short and Potts, 1988). Data from the mid-1970s suggest that lactational amenorrhea provides about one-third more protection against pregnancy in developing countries than all family planning program contraceptive methods combined (Berg and Brems, 1990). Short (1983) has also stated that breastfeeding may prevent more pregnancies than all artificial forms of contraception. He even goes so far as to say "The changing history of breast-feeding is the history of the human population explosion" (Short, 1983:38).

CONCLUSION

The biocultural, cross-cultural, and evolutionary perspective to breastfeeding adopted in this book illustrates how behavior can and does affect biology and highlights the physiological interdependence between mother and infant. Studies are beginning to show that there are physiological, metabolic, and possibly even psychological differences between a breastfeeding mother–infant pair and a nonbreastfeeding mother–infant pair. Ellis and Picciano go so far as to say: "Since many bioactive compounds found in human milk are absent from formula preparations, the possibility exists that formula-fed infants may indeed follow a different path of postuterine development" (1992:13). It is possible that the hormonal and physiological processes triggered by breastfeeding can also result in a different biological path for women. There is increasing evidence that these differences can have a significant impact on the short- and long-term health of both mothers and infants.

The close physiological interdependency between mothers and infants is illustrated by two recent studies on breast cancer. One study (Freudenheim et al., 1994) found that a woman who was *breastfed* as an infant has a 25% reduction in risk of breast cancer as an adult. The other study (Newcomb et al., 1994) found that women who *breastfeed* their infants have a 25% reduced risk of premenopausal breast cancer. Thus, in breastfeeding a daughter, both mother and infant benefit from a significant reduction in breast cancer risk. When an infant breastfeeds frequently, the stimulation of the mother's nipple releases oxytocin and prolactin in high enough levels to result in lactational amenorrhea. Lactational amenorrhea benefits both the mother and infant; it acts as a natural birth spacing mechanism that allows the mother to recover from the energy depletion of pregnancy, prevents conception, and improves the survival probabilities of the child. Studies that include duration of breastfeeding as a variable are beginning to show that there is an increasing dose–response in health benefits, that is, the longer the duration of breastfeeding the more health benefits are accrued by both mother and infant (Fredrickson, Chapter 15; Newcomb et al., 1994; Hreshchyshyn et al., 1988; Kreiger et al., 1982).

Awareness of these dynamics around behavior and biology permits women to make better informed decisions regarding themselves and their infants. In an ideal world all mothers would be encouraged to breastfeed their infants, and conditions would be such that both would reap the health benefits breastfeeding evolved to provide. However, it is not an ideal world and we cannot turn back the clock. Sometimes, for example, in conditions of desperate poverty, political and economic factors mean that staying home to breastfeed a baby may ultimately lower the health status of mother and baby because of lost wages (Vitzthum, 1994). Even given a change in cultural perceptions toward breasts, as Dettwyler advocates in Chapter 7, unless there is also change in United States legislation making women eligible for paid maternity leave for a sufficient length of time, it will be difficult for women working outside the home to breastfeed as they wish. From the beginning of recorded history, and no doubt earlier, some women have chosen to or have been forced to provide alternatives to their own breast milk for their infants. However, in prehistoric and early historic times virtually all infants received breast milk for some period of time. If not, they would have died. Modern women have many more choices than did women in antiquity: they may choose to have their labor induced by drugs, have a caesarean section instead of vaginal birth, or bottlefeed their infant with formula instead of breastfeeding it themselves or hiring a wet-nurse. These are all choices that may be valid and necessary. However, it is vitally important that both men and women realize that there can be a price to pay for their choices.

For example, they need to know that the drugs used for analgesic or anesthetic purposes during labor can enter the bloodstream of the infant and produce drowsiness, which may make it difficult for the infant to "latch on" to the nipple and initiate lactation. It has been shown that when mothers received a single 200 mg dose of a sedative, secobarbital, during labor their infants sucked at significantly lower rates and pressures and consumed less nutrients for up to 4 days compared to infants whose mothers received no medication (Lawrence, 1989). This could prolong the time taken for involution of the uterus in the mother and be associated with an increased risk of jaundice in the newborn. They need to know that an infant's early introduction to cow's milk-based formula in the hospital, whether because the choice has been made not to breastfeed at all or not to breastfeed at night, or because a nurse wants to placate a crying baby in the nursery, could trigger the development of juvenile diabetes, atopic disease, or gastrointestinal disease later in the life of a genetically susceptible child. A formula-fed baby is also at greater risk of developing acute conditions such as otitis media, respiratory infections, or SIDS. They also need to know that there is increasing evidence that not breastfeeding her child could increase a woman's risk of developing ovarian cancer or breast cancer in the premenopausal period.

Women who make choices that optimize their own health and the health of their infants need to be acknowledged and supported by their families, the public, and the medical profession. If they choose to breastfeed in public, or for a longer period than the perceived norm, they should not be discriminated against. If they wish to breastfeed their newborn infant "on demand" in hospital, then medical personnel should not sabotage their efforts by giving these infants pacifiers, bottles of water, or formula without the mother's consent. This practice can lead to "nipple confusion" or jaundice, and can even trigger disease in genetically susceptible individuals.

Breast milk is not a magic potion, not a panacea for all human ills. It is a vital, dynamic substance that can transmit both beneficial (such as immunoglobins and nutrients) and detrimental (such as nicotine and alcohol) substances to the infant. The benefits of breastfeeding or the disadvantages of formula feeding for mothers and infants no doubt vary depending upon the individual, family, ethnic group, living situation, environment, and time period. For example, the ancient practice of dry-nursing infants in some northern European countries was associated with a much lower mortality rate than dry-nursing in other countries during the same time period presumably because the environment was less hospitable to pathogens than in warmer countries. Not being breastfed will probably not have as much impact on healthy infants without genetic predisposition to serious disease born into a good environment. These infants should suffer few, if any, deleterious consequences if not breastfed, although there is the possibility of some effects, such as greater frequency of acute infections or inferior motor and cognitive abilities. However, for infants born with some genetic defect or genetic predisposition to serious or chronic disease, or into a disadvantaged or unhygienic environment, breastfeeding can confer critical advantages. Similarly, not breastfeeding will probably not have much of an effect on a healthy women who has no predisposition to breast cancer or senile osteoporosis and is living in a good environment. However, for a woman who is genetically susceptible to breast cancer, or a nutritionally deprived woman not on contraceptives and living in a third world country, the decision not to breastfeed may have a significant impact on her health.

The development of the artificial infant food industry, beginning in the mid-nineteenth century, has made it possible for large numbers of infants to survive without breast milk for the first time in human history. However, it was not until around the mid-twentieth century (in North

American and western Europe) that these products began to be used on a widespread basis. It is only now, almost 50 years later, that researchers are beginning to understand the short- and long-term health implications of *not* breastfeeding for both mothers and infants. We now know that mothers who do *not* breastfeed are at increased risk for conditions such as postpartum hemorrhage, premenopausal breast cancer, ovarian cancer, and possibly endometrial cancer and senile osteoporosis. Babies who are *not* breastfed are at increased risk for acute and chronic disorders including SIDS, gastroenteritis, ulcerative colitis, allergies, juvenile diabetes, otitis media, lymphomas, and, in females, premenopausal breast cancer. They may have impaired intestinal maturation, slower motor development, inferior cognitive development, and more dental malocclusion. Feeding babies infant formulas is equivalent to a nutritional experiment on a mass scale, unlike anything in human history since the agricultural revolution; it is not surprising that alteration of such an ancient pattern of behavior should have some adverse biological consequences.

It is important for all of us to realize that because of our evolutionary history mothers and infants are physiologically linked in ways that many of us never imagined; that nature has crafted a unique two-way system for the health and survival of mothers and infants; that, because behavior can affect biology, alterations of the age-old mother–infant breastfeeding duality can have biological consequences for both mothers and babies; that breastfeeding can confer health advantages or prevent health problems even for infants living in the best of conditions. Only then will it be possible to make informed decisions about the choices involved in the processes of labor, childbirth, postnatal care, and infant feeding.

For any number of reasons, personal, medical, sociological, political, or societal, women may not want to or be unable to breastfeed their infants. Nevertheless, whatever the reason, this does not negate the potential biological consequences for both mother and infant. It does not negate the fact that for the foreseeable future breast milk is going to be immunologically and nutritionally superior to infant formula. Nor does it negate the importance of breastfeeding on the fertility, morbidity, and mortality of modern and ancient human populations. Women need to breastfeed to ensure their optimum health potential; babies need to be breastfed to achieve their optimum health potential. Because of our evolutionary history mothers and infants *need* each other for optimum physiologic and metabolic functioning and breastfeeding provides the key to achieve this.

Ellison (Chapter 11) refers to the mother–infant breastfeeding relationship as "the choreography of mother and child." Yes, it is an intimate dance, choreographed by nature and culture, that has been performed through the ages and is vital for the optimum health and well-being of both mother and child.

REFERENCES

Adamiak, E.
1981 Occlusion anomalies in preschool children in rural areas in relation to certain individual features. *Czasopismo Stomatologiczne* 34:551–555.

Alderman, B. W., N. S. Weiss, J. R. Daling, C. L. Ure, and J. H. Ballard
1986 Reproductive history and postmenopausal risk of hip and forearm fracture. *American Journal of Epidemiology* 124(2):262–267.

Aloia, J. F., A. N. Vaswani, J. K. Yeh, P. Ross, K. Ellis, and S. H. Cohn
1983 Determinants of bone mass in postmenopausal women. *Archives of Internal Medicine* 143:1700–1704.

Anderson, P.
1983 The reproductive role of the human breast. *Current Anthropology* 24(1):25–45.

Aniansson, G., B. Alm, B. Andersson, A. Hakansson, P. Larsson, O. Nylen, H. Peterson, P. Rigner, M. Svanborg, H. Sabharwal, and C. Svanborg
1994 A prospective cohort study on breast-feeding and otitis media in Swedish infants. *Pediatric Infectious Disease Journal* 13:183–188.

Astruc, J.
1746 cited in Fildes, V. (1986) *Breasts, Bottles, and Babies*. Edinburgh: Edinburgh University Press.

Bauer, G., L. S. Ewald, J. Hoffman, and R. Dubanoski
1991 Breastfeeding and cognitive development of three-year old children. *Psychological Reports* 68:1218.

Bell, R. Q.
1966 Level of arousal of breastfed and bottlefed human newborn infants. *Psychosomatic Medicine* 18:177–180.

Berg, A., and S. Brems
1990 *A Case for Promoting Breastfeeding in Projects to Limit Fertility*. World Bank Technical Paper Number 102, The World Bank, Washington, D. C.

Biering-Sorensen, F., J. Hilden, and K. Biering-Sorensen
1983 Breastfeeding and infant health in Copenhagen 1941–72. *Danish Medical Bulletin* 30:36–41.

Bines, J., and W. A. Walker
1991 Growth factors and the development of neonatal host defense. In *Immunology of Milk and the Neonate*, edited by J. Mestecky, C. Blair, and P. Ogra, pp. 31–39. New York: Plenum Press.

Byers, T., S. Graham, T. Rzepka, and J. Marshall
1985 Lactation and breast cancer: Evidence for a negative association in premenopausal women. *American Journal of Epidemiology* 12:664–674.

Calvo, E. B., and N. Gnazzo
1990 Prevalence of iron deficiency in children aged 9–24 mo from a large urban area of Argentina. *American Journal of Clinical Nutrition* 52:534–540.
Carter, C. S., and L. L. Getz
1993 Monogamy and the prairie vole. *Scientific American* 268(6):100–106.
Carvalho, M., M. Klaus, and R. Merkatz
1982 Frequency of breast-feeding and serum bilirubin concentration. *American Journal of Diseases of Children* 136:737–738.
Cumming, R. G., and R. J. Klineberg
1993 Breastfeeding and other reproductive factors and the risk of hip fractures in elderly women. *International Journal of Epidemiology* 22(4):684–691.
Cunningham, A. S.
1979 Morbidity in breastfed and artificially fed infants. *Journal of Pediatrics* 95:685–689.
1981 Breastfeeding and morbidity in industrialized countries: An update. In *Advances in Maternal and Child Health*, Vol. 1, edited by D. B. Jelliffe and E. F. P. Jelliffe, pp. 128–168. Oxford: Oxford University Press. 1986 Letter to the editor. *Lancet* 2:520.
Dallman, R.
1992 Changing iron needs from birth through adolescence. In *Nutritional Anemias*, edited by S. J. Fomon and S. Zlotkin, pp. 29–37. Nestle Nutrition Workshop Series, Vol. 30. Nestec Ltd. New York: Vevey/Raven Press.
Davis, H. V., R. R. Sears, H. C. Miller and A. J. Brodbeck
1948 Effects of cup, bottle and bottlefeeding on oral activities of newborn infants. *Pediatrics* 2:549–558.
Davis, M. K., D. A. Savitz, and B. I. Graubard
1988 Infant feeding and childhood cancer. *Lancet* 2:365–368.
Dionis, P.
1719 Cited in Fildes (1986).
Duncan Banner
June 5, 1994.
Eaton, S. B., M. Shostak, and M. Konner
1988 *The Paleolithic Prescription*. New York: Harper & Row.
Eaton, S. B., M. C. Pike, R. V. Short, N. Lee, J. Trussell, R. Hatcher, J. Wood, C. Worthman, N. G. Blurton Jones, M. J. Konner, K. Hill, R. Bailey, and A. M. Hurtado
1994 Women reproductive cancers in evolutionary context. *Quarterly Review of Biology* 69(3):354–367.
Eiger, M. S., and S. W. Olds
1987 *The Complete Book of Breastfeeding*. New York: Workman.
Ellis, L. A., and M. F. Picciano
1992 Milk-borne hormones: Regulators of development in neonates. *Nutrition Today* 27(5):6–14.
Feldblum, P. J., J. Zhang, L. E. Rich, J. A. Fortney, and R. V. Talmage
1992 Lactation history and bone mineral density among premenopausal women. *Epidemiology* 3(6):527–531.

Fergusson, D. M., A. L. Beautrais, and P. A. Silva
1982 Breastfeeding and cognitive development in the first seven years of life. *Social Science and Medicine* 16:1705–1708.

Fildes, V.
1986 *Breasts, Bottles, and Babies*. Edinburgh: Edinburgh University Press.

Freudenheim, J. L., J. R. Marshall, S. Graham, R. Laughlin, J. E. Vena, E. Bandera, P. Muti, M. Swanson, and T. Nemoto
1994 Exposure to breast milk in infancy and the risk of breast cancer. *Epidemiology* 5(3):324–331.

Graber, T. M.
1963 The "three M's": Muscles, malformation, and malocclusion. *American Journal of Orthodontics* 49:418–450.

Gulick, E.
1986 The effects of breast-feeding on toddler health. *Pediatric Nursing* 12(1):51–64.

Gwinn, M., N. C. Lee, P. H. Rhodes, P. M. Layde, and G. L. Rubin
1990 Pregnancy, breastfeeding, and oral contraceptives and the risk of epithelial ovarian cancer. *Journal of Clinical Epidemiology* 43(6):559–568.

Hahn, P.
1987 Obesity and atherosclerosis as consequences of early weaning. In *Weaning: Why, What, and When?*, edited by A. Ballabriga and J. Rey, pp. 95–113. New York: Vevey/Raven Press.

Hallberg, L., L. Rossander-Hulten, and M. Burne
1992 Prevention of iron deficiency by diet. In *Nutritional Anemias*, edited by S. J. Fomon and S. Zlotkin, pp. 169–181. Nestle Nutrition Workshop Series, Vol. 30. Nestec Ltd. New York: Vevey/Raven Press.

Hobcraft, J., J. W. McDonald, and S. Rutstein
1983 Child-spacing effects of infant and child mortality. *Population Index* 49:585–618.

Hoefer, C., and M. C. Hardy
1929 Later development of breastfeeding and artificially fed infants. Comparisons of physical and mental growth. *Journal of the American Medical Association* 92:615–619.

Hooton, J. W. L., H. P. Pabst, D. W. Spady, and V. Paetkau
1991 Human colostrum contains an activity that inhibits the production of IL-2. *Clinical Experimental Immunology* 86:520–524.

Hreshchyshyn, M. M., A. Hopkins, S. Zylstra, and M. Anbar
1988 Associations of parity, breast-feeding, and birth control pills with lumbar spine and femoral neck bone densities. *American Journal of Obstetrics and Gynecology* 159(2):318–322.

Illingworth, J., R. T. Jung, P. W. Howie, P. Leslie, and T. E. Isles
1986 Diminution in energy expenditure during lactation. *British Medical Journal* 292:437–441.

Ing, R., J. H. C. Ho, and N. L. Petrakis
1977 Unilateral breast-feeding and breast cancer. *Lancet* 2:124–127.

Insel, T., and S. Shapiro
1992 Oxytocin receptors and maternal behavior. *Annals of the New York Academy of Sciences* 652:122–141.

Jacobs, J.
1992 The homeopathic approach to acute otitis media. *The Health Care Letter* 3(2):3–4.
Jelliffe, D. B., and E. F. P. Jelliffe
1978 *Human Milk in the Modern World*. Oxford: Oxford University Press.
Karjalainen, J., J. Martin, M. Knip, J. Ilonen, B. H. Robinson, E. Savilahti, H. K. Akerblom, and H. M. Dosch
1992 A bovine albumin peptide as a possible trigger of insulin-dependent diabetes mellitus. *The New England Journal of Medicine* 327(5):302–307.
Kelsey, J., and E. John
1994 Lactation and the risk of breast cancer. *The New England Journal of Medicine* 330(2):136–137.
Kelsey, J., W. Browner, D. Seeley, M. Nevitt, and S. Cummings
1992 Risk factors for fractures of the distal forearm and proximal humorus. *American Journal of Epidemiology* 135:477–489.
Koletzko, S., P. Sherman, M. Corey, A. Griffiths, and C. Smith
1989 Role of infant feeding practices in development of Crohn's disease in childhood. *British Medical Journal* 298:1617–1618.
Kostraba, J. N., K. J. Cruickshanks, J. Lawler-Heavner, L. F. Jobim, M. J. Rewers, E. C. Gay, H. P. Chase, G. Klingensmith, and R. F. Hamman
1993 Early exposure to cow's milk and solid foods in infancy: Genetic predisposition and risk of IDDM. *Diabetes* 42:288–295.
Kreiger, N. J. L. Kelsey, T. R. Holford, and T. O'Connor
1982 An epidemiologic study of hip fracture in postmenopausal women. *American Journal of Epidemiology* 116:141–148.
Labbok, M., and G. Hendershot
1987 Does breast-feeding protect against malocclusion?
An analysis of the 1981 child health supplement to the National Health interview survey. *American Journal of Preventive Medicine* 3(4):227–232.
LaCerva, V.
1981 *Breastfeeding: A Manual for Health Professionals*. New York: Medical Examination Publishing Co., Inc.
Lamke, B., J. Brundin, and P. Moberg
1977 Changes of bone mineral content during pregnancy and lactation. *Acta Obstetricia et Gynecologica Scandinavica* 56:217–219.
Lawrence, R. A.
1989 *Breastfeeding: A Guide for the Medical Profession*. St. Louis: C. V. Mosby.
Layde, P. M., L. Webster, A. Baughman, P. Wingo, G. Rubin, H. Ory, and The Cancer and Steroid Hormone Study Group
1989 The independent associations of parity, age at first full term pregnancy, and duration of breastfeeding with the risk of breast cancer. *Journal of Clinical Epidemiology* 42:963–973.
Leake, R. D., C. B. Waters, R. T. Rubin, J. E. Buster, and D. A. Fisher
1983 Oxytocin and prolactin responses in long-term breastfeeding. *Obstetrics and Gynecology* 62(5):565–568.
Lee, R.
1980 Lactation, ovulation, infanticide, and women's work: A study of hunter-

gatherer regulation. In *Biosocial Mechanisms of Population Regulation*, edited by M. Cohen, R. S. Malpass, and H. G. Klein, pp. 321–348. New Haven, CT: Yale University Press.

Lehmann, F., K. Gray-Donald, M. Mongeon, and S. Di Tommaso
1990 Iron deficiency anemia in 1-year-old children of disadvantaged families in Montreal. *Canadian Medical Association Journal* 146(9):1571–1577.

Lucas, A.
1990 Does early diet program future outcome? *Acta Paediatrica Scandinavica* 365:58–69.

Lucas, A., S. Boyes, S. R. Bloom, and A. Aynsley-Green
1981 Metabolic and endocrine responses to a milk feed in six day old term infants: Differences between breast and cow's milk formula feeding. *Acta Paediatrica Scandinavica* 70:195–200.

Lucas, A., R. Morley, T. J. Cole, S. M. Gore, J. A. Davis, M. F. M. Bamford, and J. F. B. Dossetor
1989a Early diet in preterm babies and developmental status at 18 months. *Lancet* (335):1477–1481.

Lucas, A., R. Morley, T. J. Cole, S. M. Gore, J. A. Davis, M. F. M. Bamford, and J. F. B. Dossetor
1989b Early diet in preterm babies and developmental status in infancy. *Archives of Diseases in Children* 64:1570–1578.

Lucas, A., R. Morley, T. J. Cole, G. Lister, and C. Leeson-Payne
1992 Breast milk and subsequent intelligence quotient in children born preterm. *Lancet* 339:261–264.

Mackay, H. M. M.
1928 Anemia in infancy: Its prevalency and prevention. *Archives of Diseases in Children* 3:1175–1191.

MacPhail, P., and T. H. Bothwell
1992 The prevalence and causes of nutritional iron deficiency anemia. In *Nutritional Anemias*, edited by S. J. Fomon and S. Zlotkin, pp. 1–12. Nestle Nutrition Workshop Series, Vol. 30. Nestec Ltd. New York: Vevey/Raven Press.

Martorell, R., and C. O'Gara
1985 Breastfeeding, infant health, and socioeconomic status. *Medicial Anthropology* 9(2):173–181.

McConnochie, K. M., and K. J. Roghmann
1986 Breastfeeding and maternal smoking as predictors of wheezing in children age 6 to 10 years. *Pediatric Pulmonology* 2:260–268.

McTiernan, A., and D. B. Thomas
1986 Evidence for a protective effect of lactation on risk of breast cancer in young women: Results from a case-control study. *American Journal of Epidemiology* 124:353–358.

Menard D., and P. Arsenault
1988 Epidermal and neural growth factors in milk: Effects of epidermal growth factor on the development of the gastrointestinal tract. In *Biology of Human Milk*, edited by L. A. Hanson, pp. 105–120. New York: Vevey/Raven Press.

Newcomb, P. A., B. E. Storer, M. P. Longnecker, R. Mittendorf, E. G. Greenberg, R. W. Clapp, K. P. Burke, W. C. Willett, and B. MacMahon
1994 Lactation and a reduced risk of premenopausal breast cancer. *The New England Journal of Medicine* 330(2):81–87.
Newcome, H.
1695 cited in Fildes, V. *Breasts, Bottles, and Babies*. Edinburgh: Edinburgh University Press.
Newton, N.
1971 Psychologic differences between breast and bottle feeding. *American Journal of Clinical Nutrition* 24:993–1003.
1978 The role of the oxytocin reflexes in three interpersonal reproductive acts: Coitus, birth and breastfeeding. *Clinical Psychoneuroendocrinology in Reproduction*. Proceedings of the Serono Symposia, Vol. 22, pp. 411–418. New York: Academic Press.
Ogaard, B., E. Larsson, and R. Lindsten
1994 The effect of sucking habits, cohort, sex, intercanine arch widths, and breast or bottle feeding on posterior cross-bite in Norwegian and Swedish 3-year-old children. *American Journal of Orthodontics and Dentofacial Orthopedics* 106(2):161–166.
Osborn, G. R.
1967 Stages in development of coronary disease observed from 1500 young subjects. Relationship of hypotension and infant feeding to aetiology. *Colloques internationaux sur le rôle de la paroi artérielle dans l'atherogenese*, pp. 93–129. Paris: Editions de Centre National de la Reserche Scientifique.
Oski, F. A., and S. A. Landaw
1980 Inhibition of iron absorption from human milk by baby food. *Journal of Diseases of Children* 134:459–460.
Peaker, M.
1976 Lactation: Some cardiovascular and metabolic consequences, and the mechanisms of lactose and iron secretion into milk. In *Breastfeeding and the Mother*, edited by Ciba Foundation. Ciba Foundation Symposium 45 (new series), pp. 87–101. Amsterdam: Elsevier Science Publishers.
Pedersen, C., J. D. Caldwell, and G. F. Jirikowski
1988 Oxytocin and reproductive behaviors. In *Recent Progress in Posterior Pituitary Hormones 1988*, edited by S. Yoshida and L. Share, pp. 141–149. Amsterdam: Elsevier Science Publishers.
Pettersson, B., H-O. Adami, R. Bergstrom, and E. Johansson
1986 Menstruation span: A time-limited risk factor for endometrial carcinoma. *Acta Obstetricia et Gynecologica Scandinavica* 65:247–255.
Post, R. H.
1982 Breast cancer, lactation, and genetics. *Social Biology* 29:357–386.
Prentice, A. M., and Whitehead, R. G.
1987 The energetics of human reproduction. *Symposium of the Zoological Society of London* 57:275–304.
Rogan, W., and B. Gladen
1993 Breastfeeding and cognitive development. *Early Human Development* 31:181–193.

Rosta, J., Z. Makoi, and A. Kertesz
1968 Delayed meconium passage and hyperbilirubinaemia. *The Lancet* 2:1138.
Saarinen, U. M.
1982 Prolonged breast-feeding as prophylaxis for recurring otitis media. *Acta Paediatrica Scandinavica* 71:567–571.
Sanger, R., and E. B. Bystrom
1982 Breast feeding: Does it affect oral facial growth? *Dental Hygiene* 56:44–47.
Schaefer, O.
1969 Cancer of the breast and lactation. *Canadian Medical Association Journal* 100:625–626.
1971 Otitis media and bottle-feeding. *Canadian Journal of Public Health* 62:478–489.
Schneider, A. P.
1987 Risk factor for ovarian cancer. *New England Journal of Medicine* 317(8):508–509.
Sheard, N. F., and W. A. Walker
1988 The role of breast milk in the development of the gastrointestinal tract. *Nutrition Reviews* 46(1):1–8.
Short, R.
1983 The biological basis for the contraceptive effects of breastfeeding. In *Advances in International Maternal and Child Health,* edited by D. B. Jelliffe and E. F. P. Jelliffe, Vol. 3, pp. 27–39. Oxford: Oxford University Press. Shrestha, M., V. Chandra, and R. Singh
1994 Severe iron deficiency anaemia in Fiji children. *New Zealand Medical Journal* 130–132.
Shrestha, M. V. Chandra, and R. Singh
1994 Severe iron deficiency anemia in Fiji children. *New Zealand Medical Journal* 107:130–132.
Silber, M., B. Larsson, and K. Uvnäs-Moberg
1991 Oxytocin, somatostatin, insulin and gastrin concentrations vis-à-vis late pregnancy, breastfeeding and oral contraceptives. *Acta Obstetricia et Gynecologica Scandinavica* 70:283–289.
Sobrinho, L.
1993 The psychogenic effects of prolactin. *Acta Endrocinologica* 129(1):38–40.
Straub, W. J.
1960 Malfunction and the tongue. Part 1: The abnormal swallowing habit: Its cause and effects, and results in relation to orthodontic treatment and speech therapy. *American Journal of Orthodontics* 46:404–424.
Stuart-Macadam, P. L.
1993 Replacing breasts with bottles: The biological consequences (abstract). *Abstracts: 13th International Congress of Anthropological and Ethnological Sciences. The Cultural and Biological Dimensions of Global Change,* p. 438. IUAES meetings, Mexico City, Mexico, August 1993.
Tao, S. C., M. C. Yu, R. K. Ross, and R. W. Xiu
1988 Risk factors for breast cancer in Chinese women of Beijing. *International Journal of Cancer* 42:495–498.
Temboury, M. C., A. Otero, I. Polanco, and E. Arribas
1994 Influence of breastfeeding on the infant's intellectual development. *Journal of Pediatric Gastroenterology and Nutrition* 18:32–36.

Thapa, S., R. Short, and M. Potts
1988 Breastfeeding, birth spacing and their effects on child survival. *Nature (London)* 355:679–682.

Tyson, J. E.
1977 Neuroendocrine control of lactational infertility. *Journal of Biosocial Sciences Suppl.* 4:23–40.

Udall, J. N., Jr., M. Dixon, A. P. Newman, J. A. Wright, B. James, and K. J. Bloch
1985 Liver disease in alpha-1-antitrypsin deficiency. A retrospective analysis of early breast- versus bottle-feeding. *Journal of the American Medical Association* 253:2679–2682.

United Kingdom National Case-Control Study Group
1993 Breast feeding and risk of breast cancer in young women. *British Medical Journal* 307:17–20.

Uvnäs-Moberg, K., A. -M. Widström, E. Nissen, and H. Björvell
1990 Personality traits in women 4 days post partum and their correlation with plasma levels of oxytocin and prolactin. *Journal of Psychosomatic Obstetrics and Gynaecology* 11:261–273.

Vitzthum, V.
1994 Personal communication.

Weinberg, E. D.
1994 Role of iron in sudden infant death syndrome. *The Journal of Trace Elements in Experimental Medicine* 7:47–51.

Wickes, I. G.
1953 A history of infant feeding. Part 1. Primitive peoples: Ancient works: Renaissance writers. *Archives of Diseases in Childhood* 28:151–158.

Widdowson, E. M.
1976 Changes in the body and its organs during lactation: Nutritional implications. In *Breastfeeding and the Mother*, edited by Ciba Foundation. Elsevier: Amsterdam.

Widström, A. M. J. Winberg, S. Werner, B. Hamberger, P. Eneroth, and K. Uvnäs-Moberg
1984 Suckling in lactating women stimulates the secretion of insulin and prolactin without concomitant effects on gastrin, growth hormone, calcitonin, vasopressin or catecholamines. *Early Human Development* 10:115–122.

Windström, A. M., J. Winberg, S. Werner, B. Svensson, B. Poslocec, and K. Uvnäs-Mobert
1988 Breast feeding-induced effects on plasma gastrin and somatostatin levels and their correlation with milk yield in lactating females. *Early Human Development* 16:293–301.

Wray, J. D.
1990 Breastfeeding: An international and historical review. In *Infant and Child Nutrition Worldwide: Issues and Perspectives*, edited by Frank Falkner, pp. 61–116. Boca Raton, FL: CRC Press.

Yoo, K. Y., K. Tajima, T. Kuroishi, K. Hirose, M. Yoshida, S. Miura, and H. Murai
1992 Independent protective effect of lactation against breast cancer: A case-control study in Japan. *American Journal of Epidemiology* 135:726–733.

Young, H. B., A. Buckley, B. Hamza, and C. Mandarano
1982 Milk and lactation: some social and developmental correlates among 1,000 infants. *Pediatrics* 69(2):169–175.
Yuan, J. M., M. C. Yu, R. K. Ross, Y. T. Gao, and B. E. Henderson
1988 Risk factors for breast cancer in Chinese women in Shanghai. *Cancer Research* 48:1949–1953.

2

A Time to Wean: The Hominid Blueprint for the Natural Age of Weaning in Modern Human Populations

Katherine A. Dettwyler

INTRODUCTION

The primary purpose of this chapter is to attempt to answer one specific question: At what age would human infants be weaned (cease breastfeeding completely) if the process were based only on physiological considerations? That is, acknowledging that humans are primates, and recognizing that lactation and weaning take place according to certain regular patterns in the nonhuman primates, then what do these patterns suggest would be the natural age of weaning in modern humans if these behaviors were not modified by culture? A secondary goal is to put current U.S. weaning practices, and pediatric advice that weaning should take place by 1 year of age, into a broader evolutionary and cross-cultural perspective. In particular, this chapter will evaluate two widespread pediatric "rules of thumb" for determining appropriate weaning age based on biological parameters: tripling of birth weight and equivalence to length of gestation. As will be shown below, both of these rules of thumb are inappropriate. The predictions for a natural age of weaning in modern human populations, based on the nonhuman primate patterns, range between 2.5 and 7.0 years of age. Weaning ages in many traditional[1] societies around the world fall within this range, with most children being weaned between 2 and 4 years of age, while almost all children in the United States are weaned well before 1 year of age. This chapter explicitly does not advocate that children should be nursed for any specific length of time, but merely attempts to establish the biological "hominid blueprint" for weaning in an attempt to illuminate the mismatch between our evolutionary heritage as primates and current pediatric advice and practice in the United States. In the final section of the chapter, the data presented here are considered in terms of their implications for such issues as pediatric advice, child health, child custody, and assessments of maternal motives and competence.

A brief chapter has to limit its discussion of related issues. Several caveats concerning how I have limited the scope of the chapter follow. First, this chapter is written from the perspective of a middle-class, highly educated North American anthropologist of European descent. I have nursed three children of my own, the longest (so far) for 4 years, and have been active in breastfeeding promotion activities for 15 years. I am committed to the evolutionary perspective, and convinced that there are functional consequences to be considered whenever modern humans deviate from the lifestyle to which our hominid ancestors were adapted. When it comes to infant feeding decisions made by parents, I am an advocate of more thorough discussion of the advantages and disadvantages of different infant feeding choices, so that parents can make informed decisions based on what is currently known about the consequences of the different choices for their children and for themselves. I am assuming that the primary audience for this work consists of health care professionals in the United States, including obstetricians, gynecologists, pediatricians, nurses, and lactation consultants, as well as La Leche League leaders and members, again primarily in the United States.

Questions of *why* age at weaning in primates is correlated with various life-history variables, such as multiples of birth weight, fractions of adult body mass, or age at eruption of the first permanent molar, are beyond the scope of this chapter. Nor is it the purpose of this chapter to discuss age at weaning in terms of whether or not it constitutes a biologically meaningful developmental landmark (although I am convinced that it does). Rather, this chapter looks at the *culturally* meaningful—at least in the United States—developmental landmark of weaning, and asks what the correlations discovered among the nonhuman primates suggest might be the biological blueprint for this landmark in modern humans.

Finally, this chapter touches only briefly on a few of the possible implications of an abbreviated duration of lactation on the health of modern human infants. This topic is addressed at some length in the other chapters in this book, and will be illuminated fully only in the future, as the result of further research.

BACKGROUND

Beginning in the 1950s, ethnographic evidence has been accumulating that the systems of beliefs and practices surrounding infant feeding—breastfeeding, the addition of solids, and weaning—vary dramatically from culture to culture, just as systems of kinship and marriage, religious beliefs, subsistence strategies, and political orders vary. Cross-cultural studies of breastfeeding "came of age" in the 1980s, with the publication of a number of books and articles providing detailed descriptions of this most basic of human activities, based on careful, longitudinal field studies by anthropologists. Early on, it became clear that like every other human activity studied from the anthropological perspective, breastfeeding is both a biological process and a heavily *culturized* activity. As a biological process, it is firmly grounded in our mammalian ancestry and absolutely critical to the survival of the species. As a heavily *culturized* activity, it is modified by a wide variety of beliefs, not only about infant health and nutrition, but also about the nature of human infancy and the proper relationships between mother and child, and between mother and father. In addition, breastfeeding practices are affected by such disparate influences as religious beliefs, the structure of the mother's everyday work activities, and seemingly unrelated ideas about personal independence and autonomy.

Understanding of the complex relationships between culture and biology as expressed through the breastfeeding process is only beginning. Beliefs and practices can affect the frequency and length of breastfeeding episodes both during the day and at night; this, in turn, can affect both quality and quantity of milk production. Beliefs and practices can determine the duration of breastfeeding, whether or not the mother nurses into a subsequent pregnancy, and where the child sleeps at night. Beliefs about the appropriate length of time children should nurse affect birth spacing, maternal nutritional status, and children's physical and emotional health and growth.

As primates, humans are members of the class Mammalia, so named for their practice of providing nutrition to their young through the mammary glands of the mother. As members of the order Primates within the class Mammalia, humans have inherited a basic primate pattern of breastfeeding activity. The African Great Apes (gorillas and chimpanzees) are our closest primate relatives, sharing a common ancestor with humans some five to seven million years ago, as well as sharing more than 98% of their genetic material with humans today. It is reasonable to assume that our earliest hominid ancestors followed breastfeeding and weaning patterns similar to those seen among the African Great

Apes today. At the same time, since at least the time of the earliest *Homo* some two and a half million years ago, humans have been modifying the basic primate pattern to conform with beliefs. Indeed, the rise of the infant formula industry in Western industrialized countries during this century and the specifically American (U.S.) practice of solitary infant sleeping represent only the latest in a long line of cultural practices that have led us away from our primate heritage, which was molded by natural selection over millions of years to meet the specific needs of human infants. The enormous costs to children's physical health of *not* breastfeeding have been well documented for both third world and Western industrialized countries (Cunningham, Chapter 9, this volume; Cunningham, Jelliffe and Jelliffe, 1991; McKenna and Bernshaw, Chapter 10; Walker, 1993). The cognitive and emotional costs are more difficult to measure, but evidence is slowly accumulating that these costs may be as profound and far-reaching as the costs to physical health (Rogan and Gladen, 1993; Walker, 1993).

As a first step to understanding how far modern humans have strayed from the hominid blueprint for optimal physical, cognitive and emotional infant health, developed over millions of years of evolution as bipedal hominids foraging on the East African savannah, one can ask the following question: What would modern human breastfeeding and weaning patterns look like if they were not modified by beliefs? What is the "hominid blueprint," the underlying biological basis, for breastfeeding and weaning behavior in modern humans? This seemingly simple question is really quite complex, and includes several components: How often should infants nurse?[2] When should solid foods be added to the diet? Is it normal for infants to wake up often at night to nurse? And, perhaps most critically, at what age should infants be weaned (i.e., stop nursing altogether)? This chapter will be concerned primarily with the last question.

Where can we turn for evidence of this hominid blueprint? Unfortunately, we cannot go back in a time machine to the East African savannah during the Plio-Pleistocene and conduct participant-observation research. We can, however, examine the cross-cultural evidence from low-technology, nondairying human societies, as others have done (Short, 1984). Members of these societies modify the basic primate pattern with beliefs like all humans, but they have fewer options for replacing human breast milk with substitutes than do members of Western industrialized societies, and they still (for the most part) regard women's breasts as body parts designed exclusively for feeding infants, rather than as sexual objects.

A number of early ethnographic sources provide information about weaning age in "traditional" societies before the widespread use of artificial infant formulas. This early cross-cultural literature is fairly consistent in reporting that children are often weaned between 2 and 5 years of age across a wide variety of traditional cultures. For example, in 1931 Shelton reported a weaning range of 3 to 5 years among "so-called primitives and so-called backward-peoples who have no supplies of animal milk with which to supplant mother's milk" [Shelton, 1970:133 (1931)]. In 1945, Clellan Ford published the results of a systematic survey of human reproduction based on data from 64 societies, available from the Human Relations Area Files (Ford, 1964). He reported:

> The length of the nursing period varies markedly from society to society. The average age of weaning in our tribes is between three and four years. In a few societies complete renunciation of the breast is deferred until the age of six or even longer. . . . In the great majority of our tribes other foods are given to the baby, supplementing the breast milk. . . . Quite regardless of the availability and use of other suitable foods, weaning seems to be delayed as long as it is at all possible in the great majority of our primitive societies. (1964:78–79)

Finally, in a review of the literature on "primitive peoples," Wickes reported: "The duration of lactation varies considerably from one tribe to another but the average would appear to be from three to four years" (Wickes, 1953:151).

The data cited above were not collected by ethnographers specifically interested in breastfeeding and weaning patterns, and probably represent ideals or cultural norms, in contrast to the "hard data" on weaning age collected prospectively by modern ethnographers. At the same time, there is no reason to suspect that early ethnographers would have distorted or misrepresented these types of data, and no reason to suspect that informants would have any reason to mislead the ethnographers. The data suggest that prior to the widespread availability and promotion of Western artificial infant feeding products, children across the globe were routinely nursed for 3 to 4 years.

Unfortunately, utilization of the cross-cultural literature on duration of breastfeeding is often dismissed by health professionals because of widespread ethnocentrism—after all, those people are "primitive" and we should not base our modern infant care patterns on what people do in faraway lands (or so they say, as they dismiss years of careful anthropological research). We can, however, look at breastfeeding and weaning behavior among the modern nonhuman primates, our closest relatives in the animal world. Evidence based on the nonhuman primates should carry more weight than the cross-cultural data, as nonhuman primates are commonly presumed not to have beliefs that affect their breastfeeding and weaning behavior. In addition, health professionals routinely cite two "rules of thumb" for what an appropriate weaning age in humans would be, based on age at weaning in other mammals. What, then, *is* the "hominid blueprint" for breastfeeding and weaning behavior?

To answer this question, we can turn to the literature on life history studies of primates. Harvey and Clutton-Brock (1985) provide a compilation of data from studies of 135 primate species, providing information on such variables as length of gestation, age at weaning, and life expectancy, all based on primary field observations by primatologists. In addition to their summary work, there is a small but steadily growing body of literature on primate life history comparisons, which will be summarized below. Surprisingly, to date none of the researchers in this specialized field has made the connection between their studies and modern human behavior. Indeed, one of these researchers was unaware of the controversy in the United States surrounding the question of how long human infants should breastfeed (B. Holly Smith, personal communication).

The purpose of this chapter is to examine the literature on comparative primate life histories and make explicit the implications of this information for our understanding of the hominid blueprint for modern human breastfeeding and weaning behavior, by evaluating the various ways of arriving at a natural age of weaning for humans based on the comparative primate data.

NATURAL AGE AT WEANING IN HUMANS AS DERIVED FROM THE COMPARATIVE NONHUMAN PRIMATE LIFE HISTORY DATA

In this chapter, the term *weaning* refers to the time when the infant is no longer allowed to nurse from its mother's breast, i.e., to the complete cessation of breastfeeding. The use of the term *weaning* to denote complete cessation of breastfeeding recognizes that nonmilk foods will be added to the diet of the infant long before weaning takes place. In all primate species, and in all human cultures studied to date, children receive additional foods from an early age. In most cultures, in addition to various medicines, teas, and "tastes" of other foods given to children in the first few months of life, solid foods are added to the infant's diet gradually from about 6 months. The particular pattern in each culture depends on a number of biological and cultural factors including the baby's size, health, and interest in food, the number of teeth erupted, the kinds of foods available that are thought to be suitable for children (often those that are easy to chew and digest), and beliefs about the appropriate age for solids to be offered. Nonhuman primates and children in traditional cultures worldwide normally experience several years of a transitional diet, with steadily increasing amounts of solid foods in addition to breast milk. The breast milk component of the diet continues to provide an excellent, uncontaminated source of protein as well as of immunological factors, and may be the only food the child desires or can tolerate during illnesses. In addition, the process of breastfeeding itself has consequences for the physical and emotional maturation of the child that cannot be met by other means.

Age at weaning in nonhuman primates and other animals is assumed to be primarily a function of genetics and instinct, with some environmental component relating to child growth thrown in for good measure. The ethnographic literature has revealed great variation in age at weaning among humans, from birth (no breastfeeding at all) to extremes of 15 years (Wickes, 1953), so we know that in humans, beliefs can modify this life history parameter out of all recognition. However, it should be possible to establish a "natural" age at weaning among humans by examining the relevant comparative primate data.

In the sections that follow, I will examine the comparative primate data with reference to the relationship between age at weaning and (1) tripling or quadrupling of birth weight, (2) attainment of one-third adult weight, (3) adult female body weight, (4) length of gestation, and (5) age at eruption of the first permanent molar. Where appropriate, determinations based on data from modern human populations of various adult body sizes are presented.

Researchers who study life history variables have documented a number of general trends among mammals in general, and primates in particular, relating body size to length of the various life stages. Compared to other mammals, primates tend to have longer periods of gestation and infant dependency, and longer life spans. They also tend to have relatively large brains for their body size. Within the order, primate subfamilies that have relatively large neonates (high birth weight to adult weight ratios) have relatively long gestation, late age at weaning, late age at sexual maturity, long life spans, and large neonatal and adult brain sizes, when compared to subfamilies that have relatively small neonates (Harvey and Clutton-Brock, 1985). Finally, "larger primates tend to wean their offspring later relative to their body size than is the case for other mammalian orders" (Harvey and Clutton-Brock, 1985:577). Thus, we would expect humans, as large primates with relatively large neonates, to have among the latest ages at weaning of the order. What, specifically, can we predict from the comparative primate data?

Weaning According to Specific Multiplication of Birth Weight

The idea that mammals generally wean their offspring when the offspring have tripled their birth weight is widely reported in the breastfeeding literature, from medical texts to paraprofessional and lay publications. This "rule" that weaning occurs naturally at tripling of the birth weight is widely accepted and has assumed almost the status of law. For example, Ruth Lawrence's book, *Breastfeeding: A Guide for the Medical Profession*, is consulted by many medical professionals for information on breastfeeding management. Lawrence writes:

> When weaning time is correlated with birth weight in placental mammals, a ratio of 3:1 is noted, that is, *weaning takes place when birth weight has tripled.* (1989:245, emphasis added)

More recent research has reexamined the evidence for linkages between age at 'weaning' and the attainment of "a critical or threshold body weight attained by offspring among large-bodied mammals: the anthropoid primates, ungulates, and pinnipeds" (Lee, Majluf and Gordon, 1991:99).[3] Contrary to earlier reports, which may have been influenced by the inclusion of many small mammals, Lee and colleagues found that 'weaning' occurred when offspring had *quadrupled* their birth weight, regardless of the length of time it took to achieve this milestone of growth. Specifically, they reported:

> Weaning weight appeared to be a relatively constant proportion of neonatal weight such that when a weight of around four times birth weight is reached infants are weaned, irrespective of the *time* taken to achieve weaning. (Lee, Majluf and Gordon, 1991:104)

Thus, a thorough study of the relationship between growth and 'weaning' in large mammals suggests that *tripling* of birth weight, so widely reported in the literature, is not an apparent "weaning trigger" for large mammals, but that *quadrupling* of birth weight may be. When do human infants quadruple their birth weight? Lee, Majluf and Gordon (1991) provide figures for both "captive/food enhanced" and "wild/food limited" human populations to see if the predicted relationship holds. Their data seem to show that weaning takes place in humans when infants reach about 9 kg of body weight, which takes 9 months for their "captive/food enhanced" population, and 36 months for their "wild/food limited" population. Unfortunately, the data they used for this comparison are inappropriate. If 9 kg represents a quadrupling of birth weight, then these populations have very low birth weights (around 5 pounds). In addition, the two populations are assumed to have identical birth weights even though they grow into very different sized adults. The "wild/food limited" population cited is the !Kung, who are light and short as adults. Furthermore, they are not particularly food limited, according to the long-term research of Richard Lee (1993).

In view of the curiously inappropriate data for humans cited by Lee, Majluf and Gordon (1991), we can still ask the question: When would a quadrupling of birth weight typically occur in modern human populations? As they attempted to do, we can divide modern humans into those who come from generally healthy, well-nourished modern industrialized societies (represented by the World Health Organization/ National Center for Health Statistics standards; Hamill, Drizd, Johnson, Reed, Roche and Moore, 1979) and those who live under third world conditions (represented by data collected by the author in a periurban community outside of Bamako, Mali, in West Africa; Dettwyler, 1985).

The WHO/NCHS standards are based on large samples of populations living in the United States. Most of these individuals have access to good medical care, including immunizations, and suffer from few diseases. They live under generally good sanitary conditions, and generally enjoy adequate (often more than adequate) diets. In particular, parents in the United States have easy access to a wide variety of nutrient-rich weaning foods, which come fully prepared in convenient, uncontaminated, individual servings (in the form of several brands of pureed baby foods in glass jars). According to the NCHS standards, the 50th percentile for birth weight for males is 3.27 kg (7 lb 3 oz). A quadrupling of that birth weight, to 13.08 kg (28 lb 12 oz), occurs at around 27 months of age (50th percentile). For females, the figures are 3.23 kg at birth, with a quadrupling of birth weight to 12.92 kg at around 30 months. Thus, for Western industrialized countries, a quadrupling of birth weight is achieved, in general, sometime between 2 and 3 years of age (Table 2.3).

The data from Mali are based on a much smaller sample from a periurban population living in West Africa. Most of these individuals have little or no access to modern medical care, have no access to immunizations, and suffer from many diseases, particularly measles, malaria, and gastrointestinal and upper respiratory infections. They live under generally poor sanitary conditions, and often have inadequate diets, especially for the children. In particular, parents in Mali have mainly nutrient-poor weaning foods, such as bulky carbohydrate-based porridges, to feed their children during the first few years of life. As in many other third world populations, growth in these children is generally good for the first 6 months of life, but falls away sharply from the NCHS standards during the latter part of the first year, and in the second and third years of life. According to data collected by the author in 1981–1983, average birth weight for males is 3.12 kg. A quadrupling of that average, to 12.48 kg, had not been reached by 36 months of age (Dettwyler, 1985:255), at which time the average weight was only 11.58 kg. For females, the figures are 2.78 kg at birth and 11.12 kg at quadrupling, an average value reached between 30 and 36 months. Thus, for one fairly representative periurban third world population, a quadrupling of birth weight is achieved, in general, after a minimum of 2.5 years for girls, and more than 3 years for boys (Table 2.3).[4]

Throughout the foregoing discussion, I have placed the word *weaning* in single quotes, for a specific reason. In their study, Lee, Majluf and Gordon did not use "cessation of breastfeeding" as their definition of weaning for primates and elephants. Rather, they defined weaning for these animals as "the average age of the offspring when reconception took place," noting that "duration of lactation as defined for these species relates to the period when the offspring is highly dependent on milk and is suckling at frequencies likely to inhibit a successful consecutive conception" (Lee, Majluf and Gordon, 1991:101). In other words, and as the authors admit, in many primates species "this time generally does not correspond to 'weaning' defined as the cessation of suckling, since suckling at low levels in many species continues through pregnancy until subsequent parturition" (Lee, Majluf and Gordon, 1991:101). Thus, any estimated age at weaning, if it is defined as complete cessation of breastfeeding, should include the time it takes for quadrupling of birth weight, plus several additional months of "suckling at low levels."

The time it takes to quadruple birth weight in humans is much more than the time it takes to triple birth weight. Growth in weight during the first year of life is relatively rapid. While tripling of birth weight in modern populations usually takes about 1 year, growth slows dramatically during the second year of life, and quadrupling of birth weight does not take place for at least another year. The evidence provided by Lee, Majluf and Gordon (1991) allows us to establish a natural age of weaning (complete cessation of breastfeeding) in humans as *some months after quadrupling of birth weight*, which would be close to 3 years of age for well-nourished, healthy populations, and between 3 and 4 years of age for marginally nourished populations dealing with multiple disease stresses.

While the old "rule of thumb" of weaning when birth weight had tripled was promoted based on knowledge available at the time, more recent examination of the data compels us to revise this estimated age of weaning upward to some months after quadrupling of birth weight.

Weaning According to Attainment of One-third Adult Weight

An alternative to looking at the correlation between weaning (complete cessation of breastfeeding) and multiples of birth weight is to look at weaning and progress toward attaining adult weight. The exact nature of the link between age at weaning and rate of growth is not known, but seems to be strong across a wide variety of mammalian species. According to Charnov and Berrigan: "On average, primates are like other mammals in weaning each offspring when they reach about one-third their adult weight" (Charnov and Berrigan, 1993:192, citing Charnov, 1991 and 1993). What does this mean for humans?

One problem is how to define "adult weight" for humans, since human populations occupy many different ecological niches, and exhibit greater variation in average body weight than nonhuman primate species living within a restricted geographic range. Rather than select one population as representative of all humans, it might be more instructive to use several human populations with a range of adult body sizes, and then examine the range of variation in predicted ages of weaning.

For extralarge Inuit (Eskimo) populations, average adult weight for males is 71.2 kg, and for females is 64.5 kg (Jamison, 1978). On the basis of these data, natural weaning for boys would occur at 23.7 kg, a weight that is reached by most boys between 6 and 7 years of age. Natural weaning for girls would occur at 21.5 kg, around 6 years of age.

For large-bodied human populations (healthy and well-nourished), we can use the WHO-NCHS data for 18 year olds to define "adult weight" and the WHO-NCHS growth data to determine when one-third of this weight is reached in large-bodied populations (Hamill et al., 1979). In this large U.S. sample, average adult weight for males is 69.0 kg, and for females is 57.0 kg. On the basis of these data, natural weaning for boys would occur at 23 kg, at around 7 years of age, and for girls at 19 kg, around 5.75 years of age.

For medium-bodied human populations (not as healthy, not as well-nourished), we can use data from rural Malian (ethnically Bambara) populations. In a rural Bambara sample, adult weight for males averaged 58.8 kg (N=121), and adult weight for females averaged 53.6 kg (N=320) (Dettwyler, 1992:314). Using these adult data, natural weaning for boys would occur at 19.6 kg, at around 7 years of age (Bambara males at 7 years of age have an average weight of 19.52 kg (N=25) (Dettwyler, 1991:452)). In this sample, natural weaning for girls is predicted to occur at 17.9 kg, at around 6 years of age (Bambara females at 6 years of age have an average weight of 17.98 kg (N=20) (Dettwyler, 1991:452).

For small-bodied human populations (similar in health and nutritional status to the Bambara), we can use data from the !Kung. The !Kung adult body weight for males averaged 47.91 kg (N=79), and adult weight for females averaged 40.08 kg (N=74) (Truswell and Hansen, 1976:172). Using these adult data, natural weaning for boys would occur at 16.0 kg, at around 5 to 6 years of age. Natural weaning for girls would occur at 13.4 kg, at around 4 to 5 years of age.

The natural ages at weaning for Inuit, U.S., and Bambara children as determined on the basis of growth patterns and adult body size are remarkably consistent (Table 2.3). Across populations with very different adult body sizes, children reach one-third their adult weight at 7 years of age for males, and 6 years of age for females. In the smaller-bodied !Kung populations, one-third adult body weight is reached earlier, at 5 to 6 years for males, and 4 to 5 years for females. If Charnov and Berrigan (1993) are correct in their assertion that primates wean their offspring when they reach one-third adult weight, then 4 to 7 years of nursing appears to be the appropriate range for *Homo sapiens*, with boys generally being nursed longer than girls.[5]

Weaning According to Adult Body Size

In 1985, Harvey and Clutton-Brock published their compilation of comparative life history data for 135 primate species. They examined the relationships among such variables as adult body weight (by sex), gestation length, birth weight, number in litter, weaning age, age at sexual maturity, interbirth intervals, and neonatal and adult brain weights, as well as others. For humans, they used adult body weights from the !Kung (40.10 kg for females and 47.90 kg for males) as their weight data for representative humans. For weaning age in humans, they used 720 days, a figure that did not come from the !Kung, who generally nurse for much longer than 2 years. Shostak reports that 3 or 4 years is typical for the !Kung (Shostak, 1976), while Howell states that among the Dobe !Kung, "the mother breast-feeds the baby until either the baby dies, the baby outgrows the need or desire for breast milk (*which does not seem to happen before the age of 4 or 5 or even 6* [years]), or the mother becomes pregnant again" (Howell, 1976:145, emphasis added).

Harvey and Clutton-Brock (1985) found that most of the variation in the life history variables they considered occurred between subfamilies, with relatively little variation among species within a genus, or among genera within a subfamily. At the subfamily level in primates, including humans, the correlations between weaning age and the other variables were quite high (Table 2.1).

Harvey and Clutton-Brock also found that many of the life history

Table 2.1. Correlation of Weaning Age with Other Life History Variables in Primates, Analyzed by Subfamily Level Data[a]

Life history variable	*Correlation with weaning age*
Female weight	0.91
Male weight	0.92
Gestation length	0.84
Weight of individual neonates	0.94
Number of offspring per litter	−0.56
Length of estrous cycle	−0.17
Age at first breeding for females	0.90
Age at sexual maturity for females	0.92
Maximum recorded life span	0.70
Interbirth interval	0.89
Age at sexual maturity for males	0.93
Neonatal brain weight	0.89
Adult brain weight	0.91

[a] Data from Harvey and Clutton-Brock (1985).

variables were closely tied to average adult body size within each subfamily. From their data, they derived regression equations for the prediction of the various life history variables as a function of adult female body weight. Their equation for calculation of weaning age is

$$\text{weaning age in days} = 2.71 \times \text{adult female body weight in grams}^{.56}$$

Once again, several different human populations are examined to include the range of variation in adult body size in modern humans. For small-bodied humans such as the !Kung, with an average adult female body weight of 40.10 kg, the regression equation predicts an age at weaning of 1022 days (2.80 years). For medium-bodied humans such as rural Malians (ethnically Bambara), with an average adult female body weight of 53.6 kg, the regression equation predicts an age at weaning of 1205 days (3.30 years). For large-bodied humans such as people in the United States (NCHS data), with an average adult female body weight of 55.35 kg, the regression equation predicts an age at weaning of 1228 days (3.36 years). For extralarge-bodied humans such as the Inuit, with an average adult female body weight of 64.5 kg, the regression equation predicts an age at weaning of 1338 days (3.66 years).

Thus, using Harvey and Clutton-Brock's equation, a natural age at weaning in modern humans might be between 2.8 and 3.7 years, depending on average adult female body weight (Table 2.3). As a final note, it should be pointed out that because Harvey and Clutton-Brock used the relatively young weaning age of 720 days for *Homo sapiens* in developing their overall regression equation for primate subfamilies, all predictions based on that formula will underestimate the weaning age for all primates, including humans. Thus, the numbers derived above for small-, medium-, and large- and extralarge-bodied humans should be considered minimum ages at weaning.

Weaning According to Gestation Length

It is often reported in the breastfeeding literature that weaning age is approximately the same as the length of gestation. For example, Lawrence (1989) writes:

> As a general rule, the smaller the animal, the shorter the time required for both gestation and maturation of the young. *The weaning process is a gradual one, terminating after a time approximately equal to the period of gestation.* The elephant's gestational period is 20 to 21 months, and the young are totally weaned at about 2 years of age. (Lawrence, 1989:245, emphasis added)

The clear implication for humans is that weaning should be expected to take place after only 9 months of breastfeeding, and this relationship is often cited by pediatricians to justify and legitimize their advice to mothers to stop nursing their children. While it is true that the duration of gestation is approximately equal to the time spent nursing for some mammals (e.g., laboratory rats and rabbits, John Bauer, personal communication), the relationship does not hold true across all families and orders. Harvey and Clutton-Brock provide data on life history variables for 135 primate species (1985:562–566, their Table 1); 36 entries include information on both length of gestation and weaning age. The data for weaning age and gestation length in these 36 species are presented in Table 2.2 (extracted from Harvey and Clutton-Brock, 1985), and Figure 2.1, arranged according to increasing adult female body weight.

Overall, the average weaning age/length of gestation ratio for these 36 species is 1.63. That is, on average, primates nurse for just over one and a half times longer than their length of gestation, rather than having weaning age be approximately equal to length of gestation. According to Harvey and Clutton-Brock (1985), the correlation between length of gestation and age at weaning is 0.84. However, a careful examination of Table 2.2 and Figure 2.1 shows that, because the range of variation in primates is extremely wide, the average figure of 1.63 is essentially meaningless.

For many of the small-bodied primates, the weaning age/length of

Table 2.2. Comparison of Gestation Length (in Days) and Age at Weaning (in Days) across Primates Species[a]

Genus and species in order by adult female body weight	*Weaning age*	*Gestation length*	*Weaning/gestation ratio*
Microcebus murinus	40	62	0.65
Cebuella pygmaea	90	136	0.66
Tarsius spectrum	68	157	0.43
Galago senegalensis	75	124	0.60
Callithrix jacchus	63	148	0.43
Arctocebus calabarensis	115	134	0.86
Saguinus fusicollis	90	149	0.60
Saguinus midas	70	127	0.55
Callimico goeldii	65	154	0.42
Leontopithecus rosalia	90	129	0.70
Galago demidovii	45	111	0.41
Lepilemur mustelinus	75	135	0.56
Aotus trivirgatus	75	133	0.56
Perodicticus potto	150	193	0.78
Miopithecus talapoin	180	162	1.11
Nycticebus coucang	90	193	0.47
Galago crassicaudatus	90	135	0.67
Lemur fulvus	135	118	1.14
Lemur catta	105	135	0.78
Varecia variegatus	90	102	0.88
Propithecus vereauxi	180	140	1.29
Macaca fascicularis	420	162	2.59
Hylobates lar	730	205	3.56
Alouatta palliata	630	187	3.37
Lagothrix lagothricha	315	225	1.40
Hylobates klossii	330	210	1.57
Cercocebus albigena	210	177	1.19
Macaca nemestrina	365	167	2.19
Ateles fuscipes	365	226	1.62
Colobus satanas	480	195	2.46
Indri indri	365	160	2.28
Papio anubis	420	180	2.33
Theropithecus gelada	450	170	2.65
Pan troglodytes (chimpanzee)	1460	228	6.40
Pongo pygmaeus (orangutan)	1095	260	4.21
Gorilla gorilla	1583	256	6.18

[a] Data from Harvey and Clutton-Brock (1985).

gestation ratio is less than 1.00 (i.e., duration of breastfeeding is shorter than length of gestation). For example, species of galago, tarsier, callimico, and callithrix all have ratios in the 0.41 to 0.43 range (duration of breastfeeding less than half the length of gestation). *Aotus* is the smallest

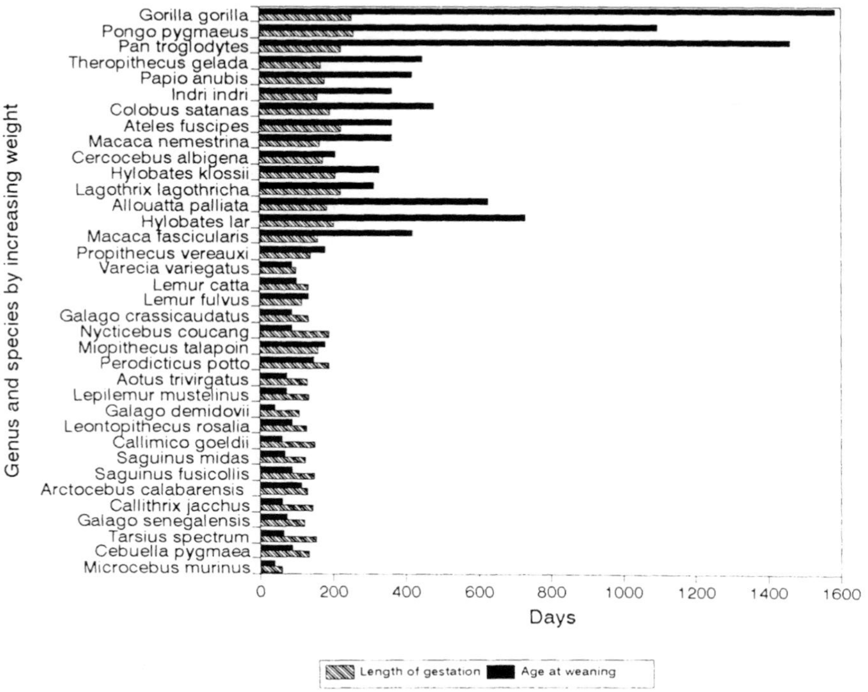

Figure 2.1. Relationship of gestation length to age at weaning in nonhuman primates.

of the New World monkeys, by weight, and has the lowest weaning age/length of gestation ratio (0.56) of the New World monkeys. For all of the larger primates, the weaning age/length of gestation ratio is greater than 1.00 (duration of breastfeeding longer than length of gestation). Among the Old World monkeys, and lesser apes, ratios range from a low of 1.11 for the relatively tiny *Miopithecus talapoin* (monkey) to 3.56 for the medium-sized *Hylobates lar* (gibbon). Among the Great Apes, the closest living relatives of humans, the ratios are 4.21 for *Pongo pygmaeus* (orangutan), 6.18 for *Gorilla gorilla* (gorilla), and 6.40 for *Pan troglodytes* (chimpanzee). Thus, among large-bodied primate species, the average duration of breastfeeding far exceeds the average length of gestation. For humankind's closest relatives, the chimpanzees and gorillas, the duration of breastfeeding is more than six times the length of gestation (Figure 2.1). Humans are among the largest of the primates, and share more than 98% of their genetic material with chimpanzees and gorillas. Interpolating from these comparisons, an estimated natural age at weaning for humans would be a minimum of six times gestation length: 54 months, or 4.5 years (Table 2.3).

The data presented in Table 2.2 and Figure 2.1 provide clear evidence against the commonly held notion that length of breastfeeding is approximately equal to the length of gestation for mammals in general, for primates across the order, and for humans in particular. The fact that laboratory rats, rabbits, and elephants exhibit a weaning age/length of gestation ratio of 1.00 does not mean that humans should also.[6] A more appropriate ratio for humans, based on the comparative primate data, would be close to 6.00.

Weaning According to Timing of Eruption of the First Permanent Molar

In a series of articles, Smith reported a very close correlation between age at first permanent molar eruption (M1) and weaning in 21 different primate species (Smith, 1989, 1991a,b, 1992). She states: "One variable, age at weaning, shows both a high correlation ($r = 0.9$) and isochrony with age of first molar eruption. Indeed, age at weaning is more than isochronic with age at eruption of the first permanent molar; these two variables are, in fact, approximately equal" (Smith, 1992:138). In other words, among many primates, offspring are weaned at the same time that they are erupting their first permanent molars. This relationship estimates a natural age at weaning of 5.5 to 6.0 years for humans (Table 2.3).

The timing of eruption of the teeth in humans is under strict genetic control, with only a small environmental component. Even under conditions of severe dietary and disease stress, children continue to erupt their teeth on schedule (Garn and Bailey, 1978). The isochronous relationship between age at weaning and eruption of the first permanent molar suggests that the factors that underlie age of weaning in nonhuman primates may have a strong genetic basis as well. Smith suggests that "It seems reasonable that weaning to an adult diet might be timed to coincide with appearance of the first permanent molar, for this tooth should enhance a juvenile's ability to process food" (Smith, 1992:138). Thus, Smith implies that eruption of the first permanent molar allows the juvenileto survive *nutritionally* without breast milk. This, in turn, would account for weaning at this time.

On the other hand, juvenile nonhuman primates, like young humans, have a full set of deciduous teeth to help them process food long before they are weaned from the breast. By 24 to 30 months, most human children have a full set of 20 deciduous teeth. It is more likely that reaching a certain developmental age along the pathway to full maturity is marked in the primates both by eruption of the first permanent molar and by complete weaning from the breast.

In humans, achievement of adult immune competence occurs at approximately 6 years of age, the same time as first permanent molar eruption. The fact that children's immune systems do not become mature until 6 years of age is understandable if we assume that the active immunities provided by breast milk were normally available to the child until about this age. Until the age of 6 years, the child's active immune response (both serum and secretory) can be enhanced by the lymphokines in maternal milk (Hahn-Zoric, Fulconis, Minoli, Moro, Carlsson, Böttiger, Räihä and Hanson, 1990; Pabst and Spady, 1990). Children need these lymphokines, even in small amounts, to augment and prime their own immune responses to stress until they achieve adult levels of immune competence (IgA, IgG, IgM) at the age of 6 years (Doren Fredrickson, personal communication). It may be that eruption of the first permanent molar in nonhuman primates is also isochronous with achievement of adult immune competence, which allows the juvenile to survive *immunologically* without breast milk. This, in turn, would account for weaning at this time.[7]

It is possible that both nutritional and immunological benefits from breastfeeding continue to 6 years of age. Finally, it is possible that the conjunction of weaning, first permanent molar eruption, and achievement of adult immune competence is the result of several different and unrelated genetic factors affecting rates of development in primates.

DISCUSSION

Why is it important that we understand the primate biological pattern on which human beliefs have been overlain? The answer to this question is not merely of academic interest, but has implications for a number of issues facing health professionals and parents in the United States today. For example, recent court cases have involved charges of abuse and neglect leveled against women who nursed their children into toddlerhood. Extended nursing has also been used against mothers in court battles over child custody during divorce proceedings, in which the father has requested custody of a nursing child. Judges in such cases have awarded custody of a nursing toddler to the father, ignoring the intense physical and emotional relationship between the nursing child and its mother, in some cases citing the mother's "failure to wean in a timely manner" as evidence of the mother's unsuitability as a parent. In one case, custody of a nursing 4 year old was awarded to the father, in part because a psychologist, testifying on the father's behalf as an expert witness, stated "you have to be crazy to nurse that long" (Lawrence, 1989:253–254; for more examples and discussion of the legal aspects of extended breastfeeding see Baldwin, 1993; Lofton and Gotsch, 1983; Suhler, Bornmann and Scott, 1991; Wilson-Clay, 1990). While anthropologists who conduct cross-cultural research on breastfeeding may shake their heads at the opinions expressed in these cases, and while they may understand the American beliefs that underlie these opinions, they can also ask: "Where can one turn for evidence that nursing a 2 year old (or a 4 year old, or even a 6 year old) *is* both normal and natural for humans?" The nonhuman primate comparisons provide the evidence needed.

Additionally, the relationship between a nursing mother and her child's doctor needs to be one of mutual respect and full access to information for both parties. Physicians should be able to provide parents with complete and accurate information about "normal" breastfeeding and weaning practices in *humans*, not just what is "typical" for women in the United States today. Women should be able to feel free to go to their doctor for problems and issues concerning their nursing children without fear of censure or ridicule, or even fear of being turned over to the authorities on charges of child abuse or neglect. Many pediatricians are openly disapproving of mothers who continue to nurse their infants beyond whatever age the doctor has decided—usually on the basis of personal opinion or bias rather than scientific evidence—is appropriate for weaning. When her pediatrician is known for expressing the view that "Any woman who nurses an infant beyond the age of 6 months is doing it for her own sexual pleasure," how can the mother of a nursing toddler turn to him or her for advice on any aspect of infant feeding? How can she go to him or her for a prescription to treat her 3 year old's thrush, which has infected her breasts as well?

Nursing toddlers in the United States are much more common than most people think. There are many women in the United States who nurse their children for 2, 3, 4 years, or even longer (Avery, 1977; Sugarman and Kendall-Tackett, n.d.). But you do not see or hear about them for several reasons. By the time a child is more than 2 years old, she or he is probably only nursing a few times a day, perhaps first thing in the morning and before a nap or going to sleep at night. People outside the family just assume that the child has been weaned. More importantly, because women know that our society is not supportive of nursing toddlers or older children, rather than spend time defending their actions against the disapproval of friends, grandparents, and even total strangers, it is easier to just tell people that "yes, the child has been weaned." Secretive nursing of this type, sometimes referred to as "closet nursing" or *subrosa* nursing (Avery, 1977; Buckley, 1992; Reamer and Sugarman, 1987; Wrigley and Hutchinson, 1990), is quite common, and mothers and children are very adept at keeping their secret.[8]

Thus, when we do find out that someone is nursing an older child, it seems unusual. Many nursing mothers simply lie to their doctors, and tell them the child has been weaned, thus contributing to the impression among medical professionals that nursing an older child is a rare and unusual behavior.

An additional reason to identify the normal or natural duration of human breastfeeding is to counter the prevailing notion that infants who want or need to nurse for several years are "abnormal," and that mothers who indulge them are simply encouraging dependency. An understanding of our primate heritage should help protect women from misguided charges that they are "infantilizing" their children and preventing their normal development into independent children by prolonging breastfeeding. Overwhelming evidence shows that meeting the dependency needs of children during the first few years of life results in independent, self-sufficient, physically and emotionally healthy children (see Konner, 1976 for a review of this literature). Nevertheless, many developmental psychologists begin from the belief that prolonged nursing is abnormal and unusual, and that women who engage in it must be meeting some need of their own, rather than meeting their infants' needs (Timothy Cavell, personal communication). In this psychological approach, normal human (primate) behavior is made to seem abnormal because it is viewed from the perspective of beliefs that are limited to certain segments of Western, industrialized societies.

Figure 2.2 shows just how "skewed" the pattern of early weaning in the United States is, compared to data from "traditional" societies. The U.S. data come from information presented at a 1993 Ross Laboratories-sponsored seminar on trends in breastfeeding incidence and duration (Ross Labs, 1993). The data for "traditional societies" come from Ford's survey of 64 non-U.S., non-European societies (1964, reprinted from the 1945 edition). The contrasting patterns, U.S. and traditional societies, clearly show that the U.S. pattern of no breastfeeding, or very early weaning, is not "normal" when placed in cross-cultural perspective, just as it is not "normal" when placed in comparative primate perspective. Medical professionals should expand their frame of reference beyond that represented by middle-class Americans if they hope to understand what "normal" human behavior is with respect to breastfeeding and weaning.

Finally, we need to provide empirical evidence to support an alterna-

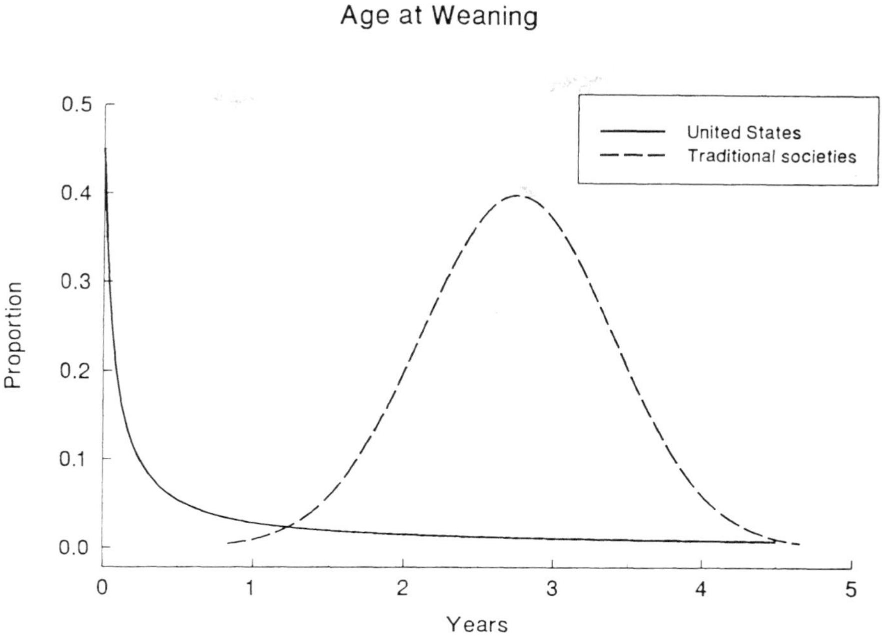

Figure 2.2. A comparison of age at weaning in the United States and in 64 traditional societies.

tive perspective to that offered by scholarly journals and parenting magazines. In 1986, the Jelliffes spoke about the conflict of interest apparent in scholarly publications about breastfeeding:

> It is curiously uncommon for publications of investigations or reviews by those funded by formula companies to be supportive of breastfeeding. Negatively-slanted or 'minimalist' conclusions can, indeed, be predicted by a knowledge of financial support to workshops and/or key contributors. . . . Whatever the results of such studies, the main signals conveyed, especially in summaries, usually emphasize 'difficulties' and/or 'lack of significant differences,' with the over-all inference of 'why bother'? (Jelliffe and Jelliffe, 1986:141).

Most of the time, parenting publications avoid all mention of breastfeeding; this is not surprising in light of the fact that they receive lucrative advertising contracts from the artificial infant formula companies. When they do publish articles about breastfeeding they often "damn with faint praise," by providing inaccurate information about breastfeeding and weaning and making misleading statements. For example, an article in *Working Mother* in 1992 claims that children get primarily emotional gratification from nursing beyond 1 year, and instructs a mother to simply distract the infant who wants to nurse: "bounce her on your knee or show her how to jiggle a box of dried beans" (Conrad, 1992:48). Similarly, an article on 6- to 12-month-old infants in *Parents* magazine (Bernstein, 1993) focuses on weaning, and on the relative merits of weaning from the breast to a bottle or to a cup. This article suggests that infants are easiest to wean before 6 months, ignoring altogether the idea of child-led weaning. Both of these articles assume scheduled nursings.

A final example from the lay literature is provided by the lead story of *Parenting* for October 1993, titled "Breastfeeding: The basics and beyond" (Grady, 1993). Concerning weaning, Grady writes: "The final question of course, is when to stop. Although the American Academy of Pediatrics recommends breastfeeding for 12 months, *not everyone can or wants to continue that long*" (1993:73, emphasis added). Grady goes on to say that one mother weaned her infant at 4 months because she grew tired of lugging a heavy breast pump to work, and was constrained by her "special nursing diet that precluded many of her usual foods" (1993:73). This mother had weaned her two older infants at 9 months and 2.5 months, respectively, and because "both were perfectly healthy, [she] felt confident that four months was adequate" (1993:73).

The very language used in this article ("that long") implies that 1 year is a long time to nurse an infant, when it is, in cross-cultural and evolutionary perspective, not very long at all. There is no evidence that would support Grady's contention that not everyone can continue that long. Many women around the world routinely lactate for 3 or 4 years after each birth. In addition, there is no need to lug a heavy breast pump to and from work. Manual expression works fine for many working women, or they leave their breast pumps (whether a lightweight manual or heavier electric kind) at work because they have no need for them at home. Also, no special diet is required for the breastfeeding mother, as even very poorly nourished women in third world countries produce the same quantity and quality of milk for their infants as well-nourished women (Jelliffe, Jelliffe and Kersey, 1989; Prentice and Prentice, 1988; Prentice, Prentice and Whitehead, 1981a,b). One has to wonder about the quality of this mother's "usual" diet if many of her usual foods are contraindicated simply because she is nursing an infant.[9]

Finally, the *Parenting* article points out that breastfeeding for 4 months *is* much better nutritionally, immunologically, and emotionally for the infant than not breastfeeding at all. However, a wealth of scientific evidence exists documenting the fact that the benefits of breastfeeding (and the risks of artificial feeding) continue for as long as the infant nurses (Cunningham, Chapter 9; Cunningham, Jelliffe and Jelliffe, 1991; McKenna and Bernshaw, Chapter 10; Walker, 1993). The children of the mother referred to above may be "perfectly healthy" at the moment, but statistical data suggest that they are at greater risk for allergies (especially food allergies and eczema, see Cunningham, Chapter 9), and upper respiratory and gastrointestinal illnesses, as well as for chronic health problems such as diabetes and multiple sclerosis. As well, one carefully constructed case-control study reports that artificially fed children have a five- to eightfold greater chance of developing lymphoma before the age of 15 years than children breastfed for longer than 6 months (Davis, Savitz and Graubard, 1988). Aside from health concerns, there is now evidence that the longer a child breastfeeds, the higher that child's IQ score and school grades will be in later years, with a dose effect evident even beyond 2 years of nursing (Rogan and Gladen, 1993). This is not to imply that formula-fed infants will grow up to be "stupid," merely that they will not be as intelligent as they would have been had they been breastfed for 2 years or more.[10]

When the normal and natural duration of breastfeeding cannot be agreed upon by pediatricians, law enforcement and child protective services personnel, psychologists, parenting magazines, and even friends, relatives, and mothers themselves, it becomes clear that we need to take a careful look at the data and try to document what human breastfeeding and weaning patterns would look like if they were not modified by beliefs. Understanding the underlying primate blueprint for age at weaning should go far toward educating health care professionals about a reasonable and appropriate age of weaning for humans, however uncommon it may be in the United States to nurse an infant through toddlerhood and beyond.

What, then, *is* the "hominid blueprint" for breastfeeding and weaning behavior? Table 2.3 and Figure 2.3 compile the various ages for a natural weaning time in humans as calculated from comparative nonhuman primate life history data.

The youngest age is that determined by looking at the relationship between birth weight and growth in the infant: a minimum of 2.3 years for boys and 2.5 years for girls in well-nourished, healthy populations. The oldest ages are those determined by looking at the relationship between adult weight and growth in the infant: 7.0 years for boys and 6.0 years for girls in a variety of populations of different adult body sizes. The majority of determinations fall in the 2.5 to 6.0 year range, suggesting that a natural age at weaning for humans would typically fall between 2.5 and 6.0 years of age. The strong isochronous relationship between age and weaning and first permanent molar eruption in the

Table 2.3. Prediction of "Natural" Weaning Age in Humans from Nonhuman Primate Data

Type of data	*Predicted age of weaning*
Some months after age at quadrupling of birth weight (United States, NCHS data, Hamill et al., 1979)	More than 2.3 years for boys, more than 2.5 years for girls
Some months after age at quadrupling of birth weight (Bambara of Mali, Dettwyler, 1985)	Much more than 3 years for boys; more than 3 years for girls
Age at one-third adult weight (Inuit, Jamison 1978)	6.0–7.0 years for boys; 6.0 years for girls
Age at one-third adult weight (United States, NCHS data, Hamill et al., 1979)	7.0 years for boys; 5.75 years for girls
Age at one-third adult weight (Bambara of Mali, Dettwyler, 1991, 1992)	7.0 years for boys; 6.0 years for girls
Age at one-third adult weight (!Kung of Botswana, Truswell and Hansen, 1976)	5.0–6.0 years for boys; 4.0–5.0 years for girls
Formula based on adult female body weight (Inuit, Jamison, 1978)	3.66 years
Formula based on adult female body weight (United States, NCHS data, Hamill et al., 1979)	3.36 years
Formula based on adult female body weight (Bambara of Mali, Dettwyler, 1992)	3.30 years
Formula based on adult female body weight (!Kung of Botswana, Truswell and Hansen, 1976)	2.80 years
In relation to gestation length; minimum of six times gestation length (Lee, Majluf and Gordon, 1991)	4.5 years
Age at eruption of the first permanent molar (Smith, 1991a)	5.5–6.0 years

nonhuman primates suggests that the maturational equivalent of 6.0 years of age may have been the "original" natural age at weaning for early hominids.

By "maturational equivalent," I mean that early hominids may have nursed their infants until approximately the time of eruption of the infant's first permanent molar. While this occurs at an average chronological age of 6.0 years in modern human populations, the work of B. Holly Smith suggests that this degree of physical and physiological maturity may have been reached at an earlier chronological age among the first hominids (Smith 1991b, 1992, and personal communication).

Why is the range of suggested natural weaning ages so broad in

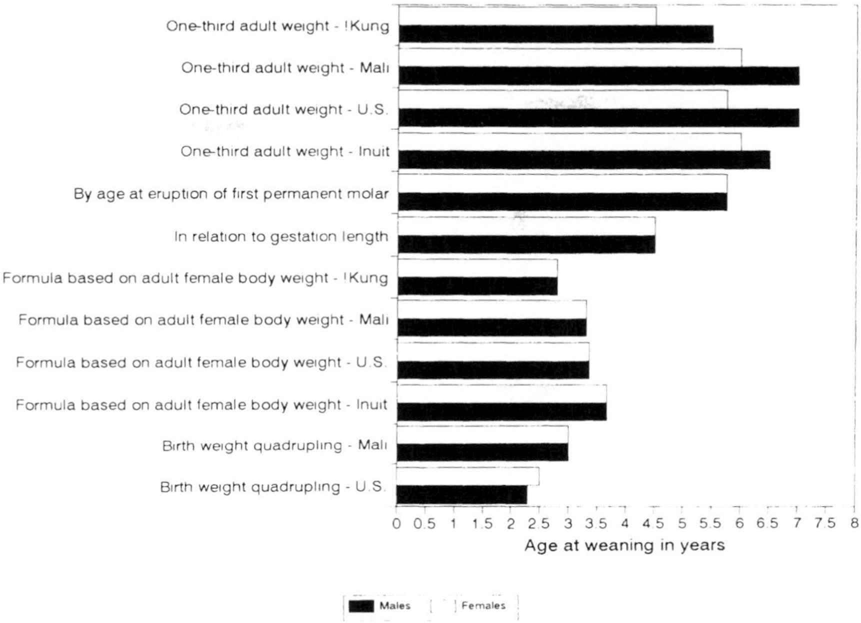

Figure 2.3. Natural age at weaning according to technique used.

humans? Or, to put it another way, why is it the case that the variables—quadrupling of birth weight, attainment of one-third adult weight relationship to adult female body weight, six times the gestation length, and eruption of the first permanent molar—do not fall closer to one another in terms of chronological age of the child? Several factors may account for this relatively large range. First, most primates live their lives in tropical environments. In the tropics, primates face moderate variation in terms of weather, temperature, and food availability from season to season and year to year. In contrast, humans have, relatively late in their evolutionary history, expanded their range out of the tropics to encompass widely varying environmental conditions, with different kinds of dietary resources available, and new diseases with which to cope. Variation in food availability and disease load means variation in growth rates, morbidity, mortality, and fertility. Human populations have had varying success in adapting to these conditions, as well. Flexibility in deciding when to wean may well have been a hallmark of early human cultural adaptation. In some contexts, children could safely be weaned earlier than 6 years because of abundant, appropriate foods and, perhaps more importantly, relatively low levels of disease stress and/or high levels of medical care. The resulting shorter inter-birth intervals would have given humans a competitive edge in reproductive success.

A second important factor has been the uniquely human cultural trait of modifying food texture and nutritional value through both fire (cooking) and the pounding or grinding of plant products, especially once cereals had been domesticated. It is possible that beginning with the earliest use of fire to modify food, perhaps as much as one-half to one million years ago, human populations were able to circumvent the 6-year nursing imperative by providing alternatives to the adult diet of uncooked vegetation and raw animal products (meat, fish, insects, eggs, etc.) consumed by our foraging ancestors for several million years before the use of fire. Additionally, for those populations that domesticated cereal grains and developed food processing techniques involving pounding or grinding, it may have been possible to even further disengage the age of weaning from the age at first molar eruption. Thus, the common modern human pattern of weaning earlier than 6 years may have ancient roots, related to long-standing cultural modifications of the adult diet, which rendered it suitable for young children. At the same time, sedentary life in densely settled villages increases disease stress on human populations, making the immunological benefits of breast milk even more critical for children.

The ethnographic literature reviewed briefly earlier suggests that prior to the widespread use of artificial infant formulas, children were traditionally nursed for 3 to 4 years. Where children are nursed "for as long as they want," parents usually report self-weaning between 3 and 4 years of age. Thus, three to four years may have been the "natural age at weaning" for populations with a relatively steady food supply that could be safely adapted for young children. The steady eroding away of this resource in just a few generations, under the onslaught of Western values and commercial infant formula companies, has resulted in many children today who are allowed to nurse for only 1 or 2 years, even in so-called "traditional" societies. And many, of course, are never allowed to nurse at all. The costs of these changes in terms of rising morbidity and mortality among children has been somewhat hidden in Western, industrialized countries by the development of modern medicine. But antibiotics and vaccines and modern infant formulas can never replace mother's milk, as we are learning. Mother's milk is more than just a product that confers nutritional and immunological advantages to those children who receive it, and breastfeeding is much more than just a process for the transfer of a mother's milk to her child. Breastfeeding is an intricate dance between mother and child, during which the child's physical, cognitive, and emotional well-being are nurtured, and through which they flourish. Further, genetic changes cannot keep pace with cultural changes.

It is reasonable to assume that five to seven million years of evolution as hunting and gathering hominids on the East African savannah have resulted in an organism that relies on nursing to provide the context for physical, cognitive, and emotional development. Natural selection has favored those infants with a strong, genetically-coded blueprint that leads them to expect nursing to continue for a number of years after birth, and that results in the urge to suckle remaining strong for this entire period. Lawrence's statement that "beyond a year, weaning is rarely child-initiated until age four," makes perfect sense in this context (Lawrence, 1989:253).

Most societies today may be able to meet a child's nutritional needs with modified adult foods after the age of 3 or 4 years. Modern, industrialized societies can replace some (but not all) of the immunological benefits of breastfeeding with antibiotics and vaccines.[11] But the physical, cognitive, and emotional needs of the young child persist. Just as infant formula can never match mother's milk, so the rubber nipple of a bottle or pacifier can never replace a warm, soft breast, and a cold, hard, crib mattress is a poor substitute for a warm body to sleep with. When the child's instinctive needs for contact and stimulation are not met by breastfeeding, the child may turn to finger- or thumb-sucking, pacifiers, rocking, hair-twisting, or other self-soothing behaviors in an attempt to assuage these needs.[12] Such behaviors, rather than being viewed as adaptations or accomplishments by independent infants, might be viewed instead as the accommodations of infants to an environment where their primary needs are not being adequately met through the multisensorial contact of extended breastfeeding.

This chapter explicitly does not advocate nursing for any specific length of time. As La Leche League International states: "The length of breastfeeding and the pattern of weaning will differ for each mother-child pair. It is appropriate for the breastfeeding relationship to continue until the child outgrows the need" (La Leche League International, 1992).

This chapter *does* advocate that medical professionals and paraprofessionals, family members, friends, acquaintances, and even strangers, recognize that human children, like their nonhuman primate relatives, are *designed to expect* all the benefits of breast milk and breastfeeding for a minimum of 2.5 years. The information that 3 or 4 years of breastfeeding, or even longer, is both normal and appropriate for human infants, should be disseminated to health care professionals and parents alike. It is to be hoped that people will stop criticizing mothers and suggesting that they need to wean because the child is "too old." Above all, it is to be hoped that people will stop questioning the motives of mothers who nurse their children for several years. It is to be hoped that mothers who follow their own instincts to meet their children's needs—not only their physiological needs for nutrition and immunological protection, but their cognitive and emotional needs for warmth, touching, social contact, and interaction through breastfeeding *as long as the child expresses those needs*—will be encouraged and supported, both by health care professionals and by their families and friends.

SUMMARY

An examination of the relationships between age at weaning and various life-history variables among the nonhuman primates has revealed that, if humans weaned their offspring according to the primate pattern, without regard to beliefs and customs, most children would be weaned somewhere between 2.5 and 7 years of age. The data presented in this chapter reveal that the commonly used pediatric "rules of thumb" suggesting that children should be weaned when they have tripled their birth weight (around 1 year of age) or at the equivalence of their length of gestation (around 9 months of age) are inappropriate. Age at quadrupling of birth weight, and six times the length of gestation, would be more accurate "rules of thumb" to use based on studies of large-bodied nonhuman primates. Substantial evidence is already available, and continues to accumulate, that sharply curtailing the duration of breastfeeding, far below what the human child has evolved to expect, has significant deleterious health consequences for modern humans.

ACKNOWLEDGMENTS

I am heavily indebted to the researchers who compiled the comparative primate data from the primary sources, as well as to the Primate Information Center at the University of Washington, Seattle, for providing me with a bibliographic search on weaning and nursing in nonhuman primates. I also want to thank all the people who provided feedback both on ideas and on earlier drafts of this chapter: Cathy Liles, Betty Crase, Barry Bogin, Roy Stuart, Patty Stuart-Macadam, Steven Dettwyler, Doren Fredrickson, Rowena Tucker, and Mike Lamar. My children Miranda, Peter, and Alexander have provided me with years of hands-on experience both of breastfeeding and nurturing children. I also wish to thank my dear friend Martha Toomey, who first introduced me to the importance and pleasures of breastfeeding, little knowing it would become a lifelong academic interest. Finally, I wish to thank Dr. B. Holly Smith for long and enlightening phone conversations, Joyce Bell for her careful copyediting, and my colleague Dr. David L. Carlson for his generous assistance with formulas and figures.

NOTES

1. "Traditional societies" refer to small-scale societies, usually at the band or tribe level of political organization, which often rely on relatively simple technology (no electricity, no running water, for example). They stand in contrast to modern, Western, industrialized countries.

2. The composition of human milk suggests that human infants are evolved to expect continuous contact with their mothers and "on demand" feeding for the first several years of life (Ben Shaul, 1962; Trevathan, 1987; Wood, Lai, Johnson, Campbell and Maslar, 1985). The iatrogenic problem of "insufficient milk" is often caused by poor lactational management by pediatricians—in particular, infrequent, scheduled feedings and restricted feed duration—who fail to understand the relationships between feed frequency and duration on the one hand, and milk supply and fat content, on the other. See Millard (1990) for an excellent discussion of the cultural history of scheduled breastfeeding.

3. In defense of Lawrence, and the pediatricians who followed her guidelines in recommending weaning at 1 year of age, it should be noted that the apparent link between birth weight tripling and weaning age across all mammals constituted the state-of-the-art in studies of this type for many years. It was an understandable recommendation based on knowledge available at the time. Now, however, we have much more specific and relevant data about primates. Thus, it is time to reevaluate this often repeated, inaccurate characterization of the link between postnatal growth and weaning age.

4. Keep in mind that you cannot extrapolate from data based on population averages to specific individuals. That is, a baby born with a relatively low birth weight of 5 pounds should not necessarily be weaned when she or he reaches 20 pounds, nor should a 10 pound baby necessarily be nursed until she or he weighs 40 pounds. All of the postulated relationships between weaning and quadrupling of birth weight are based on average age at weaning and average birth weight.

5. In addition, this relationship may shed some light on the supposedly purely "cultural" practice of mothers nursing their male infants longer than their female infants, which has been reported from a number of cultures (see McKee, 1984 for citations of this phenomena from Canada, Sweden, Ireland, Ecuador, Brazil, Peru, Guatemala, Taiwan, India, Jordan, Liberia, and Botswana).

6. Once again, in defense of Lawrence, and the pediatricians who followed her guidelines in recommending weaning at 9 month of age, it should be noted that the apparent link between length of gestation and weaning age across all

mammals constituted the state-of-the-art in studies of this type for many years. It was an understandable recommendation based on knowledge available at the time. Now, however, we have much more specific and relevant data about this relationship in primates, and its connection to body size. Thus, it is time to reevaluate this often repeated, inaccurate characterization of the link between length of gestation and weaning age. It should also be noted that Lawrence's example of elephants is also inaccurate, as field studies of elephants have shown lactation to continue for approximately 4 years (more than twice the length of gestation).

7. Identifying and carefully measuring the immunological benefits of breast milk relative to infant formula for children beyond 2 years of age in the United States has been difficult due to both the lower disease risk in the United States—a result of widespread immunization, antibiotics, and good sanitation—and to the lack of women nursing that long who could form the basis of an adequate sample. These difficulties make it impossible currently to state that breastfeeding beyond 2 years of age either *does* or *does not* confer significant immunological benefits to children in general. However, evidence from numerous studies suggests that the longer a child is breastfed, up to the study limits of 24 months, the greater the protection against a variety of illnesses, and the higher the IQ score. There is no reason to suspect that the steady increase in benefits from breastfeeding seen from 0–5 months, 6–11 months, 12–17 months, and 18–24 months, would suddenly stop or reverse the day following the child's second birthday.

8. Reamer and Sugarman (1987:94) write: "This secret nursing is termed 'closet nursing,' and is a protective device for avoiding social criticism while continuing to provide loving nurturing to their growing babies and toddlers. Unfortunately, closet nursing propagates ignorance about long-term breast feeding so that younger mothers, just beginning to nurse, may not realize that experienced long-term breast-feeding mothers are near at hand to give them advice."

9. It is well-known that foods ingested by the mother can affect the breast milk, which then may not agree with the child, leading to fussiness, gas, colic, and even intestinal bleeding. The primary culprit, however, is cows' milk protein, and breastfeeding mothers of sensitive infants are well-advised to omit dairy products from their own diet (see Walker, 1993 for a review of this literature). It has even been suggested that women from families with known cows' milk allergies avoid dairy products during pregnancy. In the case of a baby with sensitivity to cows' milk protein, the worst thing the mother could do is wean the baby onto a cows' milk-based formula. Some children react unfavorably to foods ingested by the mother that produce gas (cabbage, Brussell sprouts, eggplant, etc.), and some children react unfavorably when their mothers consume very spicy foods. Except for these minor dietary adjustments, which are necessary only for a few infants, breastfeeding mothers should be able to eat a wide variety of foods.

10. An important point to remember about relative risk, and reduction of risk, is that some diseases and conditions are very rare. Thus, one might ask "Is it worth changing one's behavior—breastfeeding instead of bottle-feeding—to

reduce the risk of a rare event?" What is abundantly clear from the research comparing the health of breastfed and bottle-fed children is that the reduction in risk for any one disease may be small, and some of the diseases, such as childhood lymphoma, *are* very rare to begin with, but that the accumulated reduction in risk across all the diseases studied to data is substantial. A number of researchers think that the lower risk of many diseases in breastfed infants is due to their stronger immune systems, rather than specific mechanisms of protection for each condition. Thus, lower rates of lymphoma and multiple sclerosis in breastfed infants can probably be attributed to successful defense of the body by a strong immune system. In choosing whether, and for how long, to breastfeed, parents are making decisions that will have long-lasting consequences for their children's health. They need to be fully informed about the risks that may be avoided by breastfeeding, to make informed and responsible decisions. Just as parents today are informed about the risks involved in not using child safety seats, and drinking during pregnancy—dangers unknown a generation ago—parents today need access to information about the risks of infant formula and shortened duration of breastfeeding. No one would suggest that a parent whose child died in a car accident in the 1950s should "feel guilty" for not having used a child safety seat before such seats were invented. Nor should parents feel guilty for having chosen to bottle-feed their children before knowledge of the health consequences has been made widely available.

11. Breastfeeding provides health benefits to children, even first world children, as long as the mother is lactating (Gulick, 1986; Prentice, 1991). Scientific research continues to uncover factors in human breast milk that affect the child's immune system, and that cannot be duplicated in infant formula. Some of these factors may not affect health until the later decades of life. If this is the case, then the next decade should bring more, and more conclusive, evidence of the failure of infant formula to adequately protect children from chronic diseases.

12. Short writes: "Thumb-sucking is almost certainly an abnormal form of behaviour brought about because of inadequate nipple contact. Young monkeys and apes do not suck their thumbs in the wild, but do so if they are artificially reared on the bottle; !Kung babies likewise never suck their thumbs" (Short, 1983:36).

REFERENCES

Avery, J. L.
1977 Closet nursing: A symptom of intolerance and a forerunner of social change? *Keeping Abreast Journal* 2(3):212–227.

Baldwin, E.
1993 Extended breastfeeding and the law. *Mothering* Spring 1993:88–91.

Ben Shaul, D. M.
1962 The composition of the milk of wild animals. *Zoological Yearbook* 4:333–342.

Bernstein, L.
1993 Weaning. *Parents* 68:94–98.
Buckley, K. M.
1992 Beliefs and practices related to extended breastfeeding among La Leche League mothers. *Journal of Perinatal Education* 1(2):45–53.
Charnov, E. L.
1991 Evolution of life history variation among female mammals. *Proceedings of the National Academy of Sciences of the U.S.A.* 88:1134–1137.
1993 *Life History Invariants: Some Explorations of Symmetry in Evolutionary Ecology.* Oxford: Oxford University Press.
Charnov, E. L., and D. Berrigan
1993 Why do female primates have such long lifespans and so few babies? *or* Life in the slow lane. *Evolutionary Anthropology* 1(6):191–194.
Conrad, E.
1992 When to wean. *Working Mother* 15:46–50.
Cunningham, A. S., D. B. Jelliffe, and E. F. P. Jelliffe
1991 Breast-feeding and health in the 1980s: A global epidemiologic review. *The Journal of Pediatrics* 118(5):659–666.
Davis, M. K., D. A. Savitz, and B. I. Graubard
1988 Infant feeding and childhood cancer. *Lancet* 2:365–368.
Dettwyler, K. A.
1985 *Breastfeeding, Weaning, and Other Infant Feeding Practices in Mali and Their Effects on Growth and Development.* Ph.D. dissertation, Department of Anthropology, Indiana University, Bloomington, Indiana.
1991 Growth status of children in rural Mali: Implications for nutrition education programs. *American Journal of Human Biology* 3:447–462.
1992 Nutritional status of adults in rural Mali. *American Journal of Human Biology* 88:309–321.
Ford, C. S.
1964 *A Comparative Study of Human Reproduction.* Yale University Publications in Anthropology, No. 32. New Haven, CT: Human Relations Area Files Press. Reprinted from the 1945 edition.
Garn, S. M., and S. M. Bailey
1978 Genetics of maturational processes. In *Human Growth 1: Principles and Prenatal Growth,* edited by F. Falkner and J. M. Tanner, pp. 307–330. New York: Plenum Press.
Grady, D.
1993 Breastfeeding: The basics and beyond. *Parenting* October, 68–73.
Graham, C. E. (ed.)
1981 *Reproductive Biology of the Great Apes.* New York: Academic Press.
Gulick, E. E.
1986 The effect of breast feeding on toddler health. *Pediatric Nursing* 12(1):51–54.
Hahn-Zoric, M., F. Fulconis, I. Minoli, G. Moro, B. Carlsson, M. Böttiger, N. Räihä, and L. Å. Hanson
1990 Antibody responses to parenteral and oral vaccines are impaired by conventional and low protein formulas as compared to breast-feeding. *Acta Paediatrica Scandinavica* 79:1137–1142.

Hamill, P. V. V., T. A. Drizd, C. L. Johnson, R. B. Reed, A. F. Roche, and W. M. Moore

1979 Physical growth: National Center for Health Statistics percentiles. *American Journal of Clinical Nutrition* 32:607–629.

Harvey, P. H., and T. H. Clutton-Brock

1985 Life history variation in primates. *Evolution* 39(3):559–581.

Howell, N.

1976 The population of the Dobe area !Kung. In *Kalahari Hunter-Gatherers: Studies of the !Kung San and Their Neighbors*, edited by Richard B. Lee and Irven DeVore, pp. 137–151. Cambridge, MA: Harvard University Press.

Jamison, P. L.

1978 Anthropometric variation. In *Eskimos of Northwestern Alaska: A Biological Perspective*, edited by P. L. Jamison, S. L. Zegura, and F. A. Milan, pp. 40–78. US/IBP Synthesis Series No. 8. Stroudsburg, PA: Dowden, Hutchinson & Ross.

Jelliffe, D. B., and E. F. P. Jelliffe

1986 The uniqueness of human milk up-dated: Ranges of evidence and emphases in interpretation. *Advances in International Maternal and Child Health* 6:129–147.

Jelliffe, D. B., E. F. P. Jelliffe, and L. Kersey

1989 *Human Milk in the Modern World*, 2nd ed. Oxford: Oxford University Press.

Konner, M. J.

1976 Maternal care, infant behavior, and development among the !Kung. In *Kalahari Hunter-Gatherers: Studies of the !Kung San and Their Neighbors*, edited by Richard B. Lee and Irven DeVore, pp. 218–245. Cambridge, MA: Harvard University Press.

La Leche League International

1992 *Statement on Weaning*. Franklin Park, IL: La Leche League International.

Lawrence, R. A.

1989 *Breastfeeding: A Guide for the Medical Profession*, 3rd ed. St. Louis: C. V. Mosby

Lee, R. B.

1993 *The Dobe Ju/'hoansi*, 2nd ed. Fort Worth, TX: Harcourt Brace College.

Lee, P. C., P. Majluf, and I. J. Gordon

1991 Growth, weaning and maternal investment from a comparative perspective. *Journal of Zoology London* 225:99–114.

Lofton, M., and G. Gotsch

1983 Legal rights of breast-feeding mothers: USA scene. *Advances in International Maternal and Child Health* 3: 40–55.

McKee, L.

1984 Sex differentials in survivorship and the customary treatment of infants and children. *Medical Anthropology* 8(2):91–103.

Millard, A. V.

1990 The place of the clock in pediatric advice. *Social Science and Medicine* 31(2):211–221.

Pabst, H. F., and D. W. Spady

1990 Effect of breast-feeding on antibody response to conjugate vaccine. *Lancet* 336:269–270.

Prentice, A.
1991 Breast feeding and the older infant. *Acta Paediatrica Scandinavica Supplement* 374:78–88.
Prentice, A. M., and A. Prentice
1988 Energy costs of lactation. *Annual Review of Nutrition* 8:63–79.
Prentice, A., A. M. Prentice, and R. G. Whitehead
1981a Breast-milk fat concentration of rural African women. 1. Short-term variations within individuals. *British Journal of Nutrition* 45:483–494.
1981b Breast-milk fat concentration of rural African women. 2. Long-term variations with a community. *British Journal of Nutrition* 45:495–503.
Reamer, S. B., and M. Sugar
1987 Breast feeding beyond six months: Mothers' perceptions of the positive and negative consequences. *Journal of Tropical Pediatrics* 33:93–97.
Richard, A. F.
1985 *Primates in Nature*. New York: WA Freeman.
Rogan, W. J., and B. C. Gladen
1993 Breast-feeding and cognitive development. *Early Human Development* 31:181–193.
Ross Labs
1993 "Breastfeeding: Trends in Incidence and Duration." Ross Laboratories-sponsored seminar held at the University of Texas School of Nursing on April 21, 1993.
Shelton, H. M.
1970 (originally published 1931) *The Hygienic Care of Children*. Tampa, FL: The American Natural Hygiene Society.
Short, R. V.
1983 The biological basis for the contraceptive effects of breastfeeding. In *Advances in International Maternal and Child Health*, edited by D. B. Jelliffe and E. F. P. Jelliffe, Vol. 3, pp. 27–39. Oxford: Oxford University Press.
1984 Breast feeding. *Scientific American* 250(4):35–41.
Shostak, M.
1976 A !Kung woman's memories of childhood. In *Kalahari Hunter-Gatherers: Studies of the !Kung San and Their Neighbors*, edited by Richard B. Lee and Irven DeVore, pp. 246–278. Cambridge, MA: Harvard University Press.
Smith, B. H.
1989 Dental development as a measure of life history in primates. *Evolution* 43(3):683–688.
1991a Age of weaning approximates age of emergence of the first permanent molar in nonhuman primates (abstract). *American Journal of Physical Anthropology Supplement* 12:163–164.
1991b Dental development and the evolution of life history in the Hominidae. *American Journal of Physical Anthropology* 86:157–174.
1992 Life history and the evolution of human maturation. *Evolutionary Anthropology* 1(4):134–142.
Stewart, K. J.
1988 Suckling and lactational anoestrus in wild gorillas (*Gorilla gorilla*). *Journal of Reproductive Fertility* 83:627–634.

Sugarman, M., and K. Kendall-Tackett
n.d. Age and method of weaning in a sample of La Leche League mothers. Unpublished manuscript.
Suhler, A., P. G. Bornmann, and J. W. Scott
1991 The lactation consultant as expert witness. *Journal Human Lactation* 7(3):129–135.
Trevathan, W.
1987 *Human Birth: An Evolutionary Perspective*. Hawthorne, NY: Aldine de Gruyter.
Truswell, A. S., and J. D. L. Hansen
1976 Medical research among the !Kung. In *Kalahari Hunter-Gatherers: Studies of the !Kung San and Their Neighbors*, edited by Richard B. Lee and Irven DeVore, pp. 166–195. Cambridge, MA: Harvard University Press.
Walker, M.
1993 A fresh look at the risks of artificial infant feeding. *Journal of Human Lactation* 9(2):97–107.
Wickes, I. G.
1953 A history of infant feeding. Part I. Primitive peoples: Ancient works: Renaissance writers. *Archives of Disease in Childhood* 28:151–158.
Wilson-Clay, B.
1990 Extended breastfeeding as a legal issue: An annotated bibliography. *Journal of Human Lactation* 6(2):68–71.
Wood, J. W., D. Lai, P. L. Johnson, K. L. Campbell, and I. A. Maslar
1985 Lactation and birth spacing in highland New Guinea. *Journal of Biosocial Science Supplement* 9:159–173.
Wrigley, E. A., and S. A. Hutchinson
1990 Long-term breastfeeding: The secret bond. *Journal of Nurse-Midwifery* 35(1):35–41.

3

Breastfeeding in Prehistory

Patricia Stuart-Macadam

INTRODUCTION

To breastfeed or not to breastfeed? This is a question confronting modern mothers that never would have occurred to a woman living in prehistory. She had no choice; up until very recent times there was no safe, effective alternative to mother's milk for providing infant nutrition. Even today, in many parts of the world, poor living conditions mean that breast milk substitutes are still not a safe or effective alternative. In fact, for all of our time as hunters and gatherers, more than 99.9% of our existence on earth, all human infants were breastfed. It is important to understand that this has been the method of feeding to which human infants have adapted, and on which human infants have survived, for millions of years. As a result, a complex and unique relationship, which has had profound effects on their psychology, physiology, health, and disease status, has evolved between mothers and infants.

Is it possible to learn about breastfeeding patterns in prehistory? Of course the past will never surrender all of its secrets, but by combining information from sources such as history, ethnology, and demography with archaeology and bone chemistry, it should be possible to develop some ideas about breastfeeding practices in prehistoric times. The implications of prehistoric infant nutrition go far beyond mere curiosity, because a number of studies have shown that different infant feeding practices can have dramatic effects on morbidity and mortality patterns. These studies have shown the impact of the type of feeding (for example, exclusive breastfeeding, partial breastfeeding, or exclusive artificial feeding) on a host of diseases ranging from acute conditions such as otitis media, pneumonia, diarrhea, cholera, meningitis, and sudden infant death syndrome (Cunningham, Jelliffe and Jelliffe, 1991; Walker, 1993) to chronic conditions such as allergies, inflammatory bowel disease, diabetes, atherosclerosis, and even multiple sclerosis and cancer (Cunningham, Chapter 9; Davis, Savitz and Graubard, 1988; Pisacane, Impagliazzo, Russo, Valiani, Mandarini, Florio and Vivo, 1994; Stuart-Macadam, 1993; Walker, 1993). It appears that, particularly in the first 6 months of life, an exclusively breastfed infant suffers less often and less severely from many diseases and has an overall greater chance of survival than a baby fed on any other regime. The more severe the conditions of life for the infant (e.g., poor hygiene, crowding, lack of adequate care, heavy pathogen load, etc.), the greater the disparity there is between the health of the breastfed and the partially or nonbreastfed infant. Even in cultures where breastfeeding is the norm, varying customs or circumstances relating to infant feeding can have an impact on infant health and disease (see Fildes and Quandt, Chapters 4 and 5). This chapter examines the evidence for breastfeeding practices in the window of time between that of our hominid ancestors (see Dettwyler, Chapter 2, for a discussion of the "hominid blueprint" for breastfeeding and weaning behavior) and earliest recorded history (see Fildes, Chapter 4, for a presentation of historical data on breastfeeding), and explores the possibility that varying patterns of infant feeding may have been important determinants of early childhood morbidity and mortality in prehistoric times.

Paleonutrition, or the study of the diet and nutrition of ancient peoples, is a relatively new field in anthropology. There are a number of types of data, both direct and indirect, that can be utilized in our attempts to learn about the diet of our prehistoric ancestors. These include looking at the debris of occupation of a site using techniques such as faunal analysis, paleoethnobotany, coprolite (dried feces) studies, and subsistence technology. The remains of the people themselves can be utilized to provide evidence of diet by evaluation of tooth wear and frequency of caries, skeletal pathology, and bone chemistry. Ethnographic analogy and quantitative modeling techniques can also be used to evaluate quantities and types of food in the diet.

Although paleonutrition studies have provided information on the diet of numerous cultures, traditionally the focus has been on the adult segment of the population (for example, see Sobolik, 1994). The paleonutrition of infants and children has been neglected, for the most part, by anthropologists, or at least has not been considered separately from that of the adults. The fact that for most of our time on earth, human infants and young children have subsisted largely on human breast milk, has been all but ignored in the anthropological literature. This is partly due to the difficulty of obtaining information (for example, it has only been with the recent application of techniques of chemical analysis to archaeological bone that it has been possible to obtain any direct data on this subject), and partly due to male bias in anthropology. A male bias in anthropology has meant that historically there has been a male-centered perspective; a classic example is the evolutionary scenario of "man the hunter" that emphasizes the importance of men or male activities to the neglect of women and their role in evolution. As a result, in anthropological studies in general there has been little consideration of female-related concerns and activities, such as lactation or childbirth, and little awareness of the effects of female physiology on a host of variables.

As with paleonutrition in general, there are both direct and indirect methods available that can provide clues about breastfeeding patterns in prehistory. As it is a subject that has only recently caught the attention of anthropologists, there are very few hard data available at the present time. What there is has been derived from bone chemistry studies on archaeological populations. Since this technique has been applied to prehistoric human populations only recently and infrequently (the earliest study is Sillen and Smith, 1984), it is necessary to turn to other approaches. Consequently this chapter will rely on the synthesis of a number of sources of information, ranging from the highly technical and little known (the bone chemical information) to more general and widely known (ethnographic analogy). Two methods will be introduced that have the potential to provide some useful information on breastfeeding practices, but have not yet been applied to prehistoric populations. These are the use of data on lactose intolerance and demography. A synthesis of information from as many sources as possible should provide a clearer picture of breastfeeding practices in prehistory.

BONE CHEMISTRY

Anthropologists who are interested in paleodietary research have been utilizing bone chemistry since the pioneering work of Brown (1973) and Gilbert (1975). The utility of this technique is based on the fact that food categories differ from each other in certain aspects of their elemental and isotopic composition. For example, corn and fruit differ in the stable carbon isotope ratios of their tissues, and food derived from animal sources differs from that obtained from plants in both strontium concentration and stable nitrogen isotope ratios. These differences are reflected in the tissues and bones of the consumer, and can be determined by analyzing bone collagen and bone mineral using spectrometric and neutron activation techniques. Although many unanswered questions remain in this new area of paleodietary research, there is an enormous potential for advances in knowledge.

Bone chemistry research on prehistoric breastfeeding patterns is in its infancy, but there are two innovative and ground-breaking studies—Fogel, Tuross and Owsley (1989) and Sillen and Smith (1984)—that have provided some useful and provocative data on infant feeding. Fogel et al. (1989) and Sillen and Smith (1984), using different approaches, addressed the question of whether the introduction of agriculture had an effect on breastfeeding practices, therefore birth intervals, in prehistoric peoples. It had been hypothesized that before the development of agriculture, humans nursed their infants longer, and, therefore, because of the contraceptive effect of breastfeeding on the mother, birth intervals were longer. Two other studies—Blakely, 1989, and Price, Swick and Chase, 1986—have provided interesting data on female reproductive status and bone chemistry. Blakely (1989) and Price et al. (1986), also using different approaches, examined the possibility that pregnancy and lactation may affect strontium levels in bone of females. Blakely used prehistoric skeletal remains and Price et al. used a rat model.

Fogel et al. (1989) investigated whether breast milk has a unique isotopic signature that can be used to trace lactation in humans. Knowing that breast milk is a good source of nitrogen, and that nursing infants exist one trophic level (placement of organisms in the food web) up the food chain from their lactating mothers, they hypothesized that protein from infant tissue should be enriched in the stable isotope of nitrogen, ^{15}N, relative to the mother's protein. To develop a modern comparative data base, they sampled one infant and her mother from birth to 15 months in a longitudinal study, and 16 other mother–infant pairs in a cross-sectional study. In all cases, the isotopic composition of the nursing infant's fingernails was enriched in ^{15}N compared to that of the mother. This enrichment of the infant's fingernails occurred from 3 months of age until several months after alternate food sources were introduced (fingernails cut in the first three months of life are synthesized *in utero*). A decrease in infant $\delta^{15}N$ values (a delta value, δ, is defined as the parts per thousand deviation in the abundance ratio of two isotopes—^{15}N and ^{14}N—in a sample relative to that of a standard), toward those of the mothers, correlated with the introduction of alternative food sources, i.e., infant formula, cow's milk, other dairy products or cereals.

To determine whether a "nursing signal" could be detected in prehistoric skeletal remains, bone samples of infants, small children and adults from several pre- and posthorticultural populations were analyzed for age-related differences in $\delta^{15}N$ values of bone collagen. Skeletal remains from three Tennessee Valley Middle and late Archaic period (5500–2000

B.C.) sites and the Sully Site, a protohistoric (A.D. 1650–1700) South Dakota site, were studied. An enrichment in ^{15}N of total collagen was measured in almost all of the bones tested from 1-year-old infants and the $\delta^{15}N$ of bones from both pre- and posthorticultural populations declined sharply at between 18 and 20 months, presumably corresponding with the consumption of food sources other than breast milk. In these populations, all infants, regardless of subsistence pattern, were receiving enough alternative nitrogen food sources by 18 to 20 months of age to decrease their $\delta^{15}N$ values.

In a 1994 publication, Tuross and Fogel focused specifically on data from the Sully Site, South Dakota, one of the sites in their original study. The Sully Site represents one of the largest earthlodge villages on the Missouri River, and was inhabited by the Arikara tribe from 1650 to 1733 A.D. The sample used for bone chemical analysis consisted of 8 adults and 28 children under 5 years of age. The researchers noted that between 3 months and 2 years of age the $\delta^{15}N$ was on average 1.6% enriched relative to the adult population. The $\delta^{15}N$ of bone collagen declined from a high of 12.8% in the 3 month to 2-year-old group to a low of 10.2% in the 2- to 5-year-old group. Tuross and Fogel (1994) concluded that at this site infants were breastfed for 1 year without the introduction of a substantial amount of an alternative nitrogen source. Weaning, defined as complete cessation of breastfeeding, was between 2 and 6 years; weaning age was impossible to determine more precisely, however, mainly because of a lack of knowledge about the relationship between dietary input and subsequent elemental incorporation into bone collagen, especially in infants and children.

Katzenberg (1991, 1992) and Katzenberg, Saunders and Fitzgerald (1993) utilized the information from this innovative work to explore breastfeeding patterns in several historic and prehistoric communities. They have confirmed that there is a significant difference in enrichment of ^{15}N between mothers and infants. In one case (Katzenberg, 1991) the bones of a mother and her infant (documented through historic records) had a $\delta^{15}N$ difference of 2.2% in favor of the infant. In another study, Katzenberg et al. (1993) analyzed stable isotopes of carbon and nitrogen from the bones of 29 individuals buried in an Ontario Iroquoian village site dated A.D. 1530–1580. High $\delta^{15}N$ values in infants relative to adults confirmed the trophic effect found by Fogel et al. (1989). Infants under 2 years were 2–3% higher in $\delta^{15}N$ values than adults. Unfortunately the sample size was not large enough to get a good picture of weaning age; there were no 2–3 year olds and only two 3–4 year olds. Of the 3–4 year olds, one had $\delta^{15}N$ values similar to adults, suggesting a high percentage of non-breast milk foods, and the other had values similar to the younger infants, suggesting a low percentage of non-breast milk foods.

White and Schwarcz (1994) also examined $\delta^{15}N$ values of prehistoric individuals—a sample of 167 Nubians from five cemeteries along the west bank of the Nile River in the Wadi Halfa area of northern Sudan. Combinations of bone, skin, muscle, and hair were available for analysis. The researchers found a significant negative correlation between $\delta^{15}N$ and age, for individuals in the age range between newborn and 6 years. This corresponded to an enrichment of about 3% compared to adult values, confirming the trophic level shift in breastfed infants that Fogel et al. (1989) had first discovered. White and Schwarcz (1994) did not comment on weaning, other than to say that the data show a gradual decrease in $\delta^{15}N$ over the 6-year interval, rather than a discrete shift that would indicate an abrupt change from total reliance on breast milk to total reliance on other foods.

Schurr (1994) collected staple isotope data from the prehistoric Angel site (A.D. 1300–1450), a Middle Mississippian civic-ceremonial center in the lower Ohio River Valley. His sample consisted of 23 juveniles and 47 adults from this group of sedentary maize horticulturalists. Schurr pointed out that previous studies have used simple linear models to demonstrate declines in juvenile $\delta^{15}N$ values, and suggested that nonlinear models would more accurately describe changes related to supplementation and weaning. His data showed that $\delta^{15}N$ values increase after birth, reaching a maximum between the first and third years of life. After age 2, the $\delta^{15}N$ values declined, suggesting that breast milk provided most of the dietary protein until at least 2 years of age. Schurr's use of nonlinear models suggests that weaning was a gradual process that began before the age of 2 years, and that breast milk provided the bulk of dietary protein for at least 6 months after the onset of supplementation. Schurr commented that there is much research to be done before we can understand data obtained from prehistoric bone, particularly since we do not know the collagen source for remodeling and/or growing bone (Schurr, 1994).

Sillen and Smith (1984) demonstrated that the time of dietary supplementation with solid foods can be inferred from the measurement of strontium–calcium (Sr/Ca) ratios of juvenile skeletons. The Sr/Ca ratio of human milk is generally very low because of a discrimination against strontium at the level of the adult gastrointestinal tract and the mammary gland. Therefore calcium is preferentially secreted in human milk with respect to strontium. The Sr/Ca ratio of solid foods is relatively high. As a result, low Sr/Ca ratios in skeletons of prehistoric infants could be interpreted to mean that foods other than breast milk had not yet been introduced to the diet. Sillen and Smith hypothesized that skeletal Sr/Ca ratios would be expected to rise to a peak as the higher-strontium solid foods were introduced. Lower Sr/Ca values in older juveniles and adults would be expected to result from the gastrointestinal discrimination against strontium that occurs with age. Human bones from the medieval (A.D. 800–1300) Arabic cemetery site of Dor, located on the eastern Mediterranean coast about 1 km south of Haifa, were analyzed. The mean Sr/Ca value for the newborn/fetal category was low when compared to the rest of the population, confirming expectations. The Sr/Ca values gradually increased after birth, and individuals in the 1.5 to 3.5 year range were found to have the highest values for the entire population. After this age period, Sr/Ca values declined to the levels seen in adults. The data appeared to be consistent with ethnographic information on traditional Palestinian Arab communities, indicating that most children were weaned between the ages of 2 and 3 years.

Price et al. (1986) examined the effects of pregnancy and lactation on bone strontium levels in laboratory rats. On the basis of their results they concluded that reproductive status is of major consequence with regard to bone strontium. Pregnant and lactating female rats exhibited higher Sr levels than either males or nonpregnant females. They explained this by the fact that there is a discrimination against strontium and in favor of calcium in the transport of ions to the placenta and mammary glands as well as an increased absorption of alkaline earth metals, such as strontium and calcium, from the intestine during pregnancy and lactation.

Blakely (1989) noted that often females from archaeological sites exhibit higher Sr/Ca ratios than males, and that this was usually attributed to lower meat intake among women. However, he emphasized that as Price et al. had discovered, this can also be explained by the effects of female reproductive physiology on the differential absorption of strontium and calcium. Blakely examined bone Sr/Ca ratios and strontium concentrations of reproductive-age females, postmenopausal females, and adult males from two late prehistoric Native American sites in Georgia, the King site and the Etowah site. At the King site, the mean Sr/Ca ratio for females was over 14% greater than that of males. At Etowah, the mean strontium level of reproductive-age females exceeded that of postmenopausal females by almost 25%. He argues that most of these differences are due to pregnancy and lactation, not to dietary factors.

These studies are exciting, because for the first time it is possible to obtain direct data on breastfeeding patterns in past human populations. In the future, as more populations are surveyed, very likely the range and diversity of cultural patterns will be revealed. In the meantime, there are still many unanswered questions with regard to the application of these chemical techniques on modern and, particularly, ancient populations. One important issue is that of weaning versus supplementary feeding. In our contemporary society many people consider weaning, or the complete cessation of breastfeeding, to be an abrupt procedure occurring very shortly after supplementation with other foods, often well before the end of the first year of life. However, in most traditional societies (and very probably in the past), supplementation to the point of complete weaning is a very long, gradual process, occurring over many months as the child becomes accustomed to the family diet. Although bone chemistry studies on prehistoric infants have been able to provide good data on the timing of introduction of supplemental foods, they have been unable to provide data on exact weaning age. This is because there are no contemporary longitudinal data on infants who have been breastfed in the "ancient pattern," that is, for longer than 1 year and with gradual supplementation of additional foods. It is not known how the elemental or stable isotope composition changes in the tissues of such infants. For example, will the $\delta^{15}N$ values of a child who is obtaining most of its nutrition from the family diet but is still breastfeeding occasionally reflect adult values, infant values, or be intermediate? Another problem lies with determining the time lag between the ingestion of a food source and its measurable incorporation into a tissue, such as bone. How long after supplementation of breast milk with other foods will it take for demonstrable changes to occur in the elemental or stable isotope composition of bone? At present this information is not known, which makes it difficult to interpret with confidence the results of bone chemical studies on archaeological bone.

HISTORICAL EVIDENCE

Fildes (1986) has amassed a great deal of historical data on infant feeding and child-rearing practices in antiquity (see Fildes, Chapter 4, for a more detailed discussion). To gain some insight into breastfeeding patterns in antiquity, it may be useful to learn what infant feeding practices were at the time of the earliest known historical records. The earliest known evidence (material, pictorial, and epigraphic) dates back to about 3000 B.C. in the ancient Near East and encompasses the civilizations of Mesopotamia, Egypt, and the Levant. Fildes states "Despite differences of language, culture, and economy, the ways in which these societies regarded young children, and the methods of nurturing them from birth, appear to have been similar, and relatively constant over several millennia." Babies in all these societies were usually breastfed for 2 to 3 years: records from Babylonia specify nursing for 2 to 3 years; 3 years was said to be the common age for weaning for Hebrews as this denoted the transition from infancy to childhood, when the child was old enough to enter the Temple; and an Egyptian papyrus states: "When in due time you were born she still carried you on her neck and for three years she suckled you" (Fildes, 1986).

Information on child care in ancient India comes from medical texts, one of which dates from the Ayurvedic period of 1500 to 800 B.C. This text recommends breast milk as the only food for babies until the end of the first year, then milk and solid food until the second birthday, then gradual weaning after that time. In ancient Greece the first evidence comes from about 1000 B.C., although most of the information comes from the ninth/eighth centuries and the fifth/fourth centuries B.C. Although reference to infants of the nobility being breastfed is made in poems, there is no mention of the duration of breastfeeding. Later in time, wet-nursing contracts from Egypt, in the Greek period, mention suckling from the breast for 6 months and then giving cows' milk for 18 months (Fildes, 1986). In Byzantium, evidence from literary sources between the fourth and seventh centuries B.C. indicates that children should be weaned between the ages of 20 months and 2 years. The Qur'an stipulated that Islamic children be breastfed for at least 2 years. The Talmud, dating from 536 B.C., stated that the child be put to the breast immediately, and suckled for a period of 18 months to 2 years (Davidson, 1953).

It is certainly possible that not all infants in antiquity were breastfed; numbers of feeding vessels have been found in graves of infants from 4000 B.C. (Fildes, 1986). However, it is impossible to determine whether these were used for supplementary feeding, or whether babies were artificially fed from birth. Where there is evidence for artificial feeding (as in later historical records), according to Barness (1987), milk of other mammals was the most widely used replacement. "Dry-nursing" was also used as a feeding method, in which case the infant was given a mixture of some type of grain or bread. For example, in Europe there were two types of dry-nursing preparations, pap and panada. Pap was flour or bread cooked in water and panada was a mixture of flour, cereal, or bread, cooked in broth, and generally combined with butter, or occasionally milk (Davidson, 1953). However, mortality was high, regardless of the source of nutrients, and artificial feeding in the first weeks of life invariably resulted in the death of the infants. After the first month of life, mortality was not so high, with an infant having about a 50% chance of living (Barness, 1987). For example, of 10,272 infants admitted to the Dublin Foundling Hospital between 1775 and 1796 who were dry-nursed, only 45 survived, a mortality rate of 99.6%. "Death from want of breast milk" was the common entry for the cause of death (Davidson, 1953). It is known that in certain areas of Europe from at least the fifteenth century it was the custom not to breastfeed infants at all; these include parts of Germany, Bohemia, Northern Italy, Austrian Tyrol, and parts of Finland, Iceland, Sweden, and Russia (Fildes, 1986). Mortality was not as high as it was in orphanages and foundling hospitals, but even so about 50% of the babies died (Palmer, 1988).

ETHNOGRAPHIC ANALOGY

Data from every known hunter and gatherer society and almost all preindustrial societies indicate that breastfeeding is the method of infant feeding for at least the first months of life (Eaton, Shostak and Konner, 1988). Duration of breastfeeding is variable, but it is likely that many of these groups maintained ancient cultural traditions with respect to infant feeding. In most groups that have been surveyed breastfeeding extends beyond 1 year, and in many cases much longer. A study by Ford (cf. Lawrence, 1989) of 46 nonindustrialized societies from around the world revealed that about 75% weaned between 2 and 3 years of age, 25% at 18 months, and one at 6 months. Wickes (1953), in his survey of various tribes, states that although the duration of the period of lactation varies considerably, the average is 3–4 years. Examples he cited were the Samoans, who weaned at less than 1 year; Australian aborigines, who weaned between 2 and 3 years; Greenlanders at between 3 and 4 years; Hawaiians at 5 years; and Inuit at around 7 years of age. Fildes (1986) collected data on a number of modern rural communities from various countries in Africa and found that the timing of weaning ranged from 21 months (Gambia) to 42 months (Ivory Coast). The mode for the 13 groups surveyed was 24 months and the average was also 24 months. Jelliffe and Jelliffe (1978) provide an extensive survey of weaning times for many groups living in the subtropics and tropics. The timing is variable; examples include northern Sudan, where weaning occurs between 2 and 3 years depending on sex, age, or intervening pregnancy; Morocco and Algeria, where breastfeeding continues into the second year; Pakistan, where 92% of young children are still breastfed at 2 years; and India, where breastfeeding continues into the second or third year of life.

One of the best studied examples of hunter–gatherer society is the !Kung San. Their tradition is to breastfeed frequently and intensively for the first 3 or 4 years of a child's life. This involves giving the breast about four times an hour during the day and several times at night for at least the first 2 years of life (Konner and Worthman, 1980). A cross-sectional study of a group of 78 !Kung infants and children by Konner (1976) showed that the majority were weaned by 3 years of age; 58% were weaned by 2 years, 76% by 3 years, and 90% by 4 years.

The timing of introduction of alternate foods in these societies also varies considerably, but on average 6 months, or the age at which the teeth first start to appear, is when most babies are introduced to semi-solid foods. In some cases this would be items of the family diet that had been prechewed by the mother. For example, the Hadza of Tanzania gradually supplement their babies' diet with foods such as bone marrow, soft fat, and ground baobab berries, and when the baby develops teeth, the mothers prechew meat for them (Palmer, 1988).

Throughout history, as in many societies today, it was common for infants to be given substances other than breast milk in the first few hours or days after birth. For example, as Fildes mentions in her chapter, babies in ancient India were often given a ritual mixture of honey, clarified butter, plant juices, and gold dust. In many societies the first milk, or colostrum, is considered dangerous. For the first few days of life, babies are given to older mothers to be breastfed, or given substances such as honey. Cadogen, an eighteenth century physician, abhorred the British custom of cramming "A Dab of Butter and Sugar down its throat, a little oil, Panada, Caudle, or some such unwholesome Mess so that they set out wrong and the Child stands a fair chance of being made sick from the First Hour" (cited in Wickes, 1953:333). Another eighteenth century physician, William Moss, advocated giving the infant colostrum, instead of withholding it. He felt that the use of colostrum was only natural, especially since the practice of giving pap and panada in the first week of life often led to gripes and even death (Wickes, 1953). These and other substances given to newborns can cause health problems by creating abdominal distress, introducing disease-producing bacteria into the gastrointestinal tract, and/or interfering with the immunological protection provided by breast milk by altering the pH of the stomach and intestines.

LACTOSE INTOLERANCE

Lactose (ß-galactosidase) is a disaccharide, and is the principal carbohydrate of the milk of placental mammals. It occurs in nature only as a specific product of the mammary gland (Johnson, Kretchmer and Simoons, 1974) and is found in higher concentration in human milk than in the milk of any other mammal. It comprises about 7% of the content and about 40% of the calories of human milk (McCracken, 1971). Before disaccharides can be absorbed by the gastrointestinal tract, they must be converted into monosaccharides. In the case of lactose this is achieved by lactase, an enzyme produced in the small bowel. In most mammals lactase production begins before birth (24 weeks of fetal life in humans) and rapidly declines at some point during infancy (Lawrence, 1989; McCracken, 1971). There appears to be a direct relationship between the onset of lactase deficiency and weaning; apart from humans, after the weaning period mammals are unable to hydrolyze lactose efficiently (Kretchmer, Ransome-Kuti, Hurwitz, Dungy and Alakija, 1971). For example, in the rat, rabbit, guinea pig, mouse, cat, and dog, lactase activity is at its highest peak during the perinatal period and decreases to very low values by the time of weaning (Kretchmer et al., 1971). With reference to human populations, Bayless, Paige and Ferry state: "The concept of gradual decrease in lactase activity after infancy would fit with the post-weaning lactase fall seen in most animal species" (1971:605).

Individuals who have insufficient lactase to metabolize the lactose in milk and milk products are considered to be lactase deficient. These individuals can develop various gastric symptoms such as cramps, bloating, borborygmi (rumbling of gas in intestines), flatulence, and diarrhea upon the ingestion of lactose. Studies of numerous human populations have shown that there is a wide variation in levels of lactose tolerance in populations around the world; tolerance levels range from approximately 90% for people of European ancestry to under 10% for most Africans, Orientals, American Indians, and Inuit (Johnson, Cole and Ahem, 1981). Those people who lose the ability to digest lactose after infancy are said to have primary adult hypolactasia, while those people who retain the ability to digest lactose are said to have lactase persistence (Cramer, Xu and Sahi, 1994). According to Cramer et al. (1994) it is now widely accepted that the decline in the activity of human lactase is determined by an autosomal recessive single gene.

The vast majority of humans, with the exception of some European groups, people of European ancestry, and some African cattle-herding groups, are unable to digest lactose beyond childhood (although the evidence for the African cattle-herding groups has been questioned by Scrimshaw and Murray, 1988). Why? McCracken (1971) and others have put forward the hypothesis that there is a relationship between lactose tolerance and the history of domestication of milk-producing animals. It is suggested that as mammal milk is the only natural source of lactose, prior to domestication of animals and the invention of dairying, lactose was not available to adults in significant quantities. Before this time adult humans, like other adult mammals, were naturally lactase deficient. In those groups that became involved in dairying and the consumption of milk products, natural selection favored a genetic adaptation that maintained the ability to digest lactose beyond infancy. However, there have been other hypotheses suggested to account for the patterns of lactase persistence observed around the world including the calcium absorption hypothesis and the gastrointestinal infection hypothesis (Sahi, 1994).

Is there a relationship between lactase deficiency and breastfeeding patterns in prehistory? It is suggested that data on age of onset of lactase deficiency in modern human populations that have not had dairying ancestors or been exposed to substantial gene flow with European populations may provide indirect evidence of our ancient pattern of breastfeeding in terms of weaning age. This approach is speculative and problematic, but it is worth considering. A number of studies have found a strong relationship between age and the onset of lactase deficiency. Although considerable ethnic and regional variation exists in age of onset of lactose maldigestion, there does seem to be a pattern. As Paige, Leonardo, Cordano, Nakashima, Adrianzen and Graham (1972:300) state: "It is clear from published reports that the number of non-Caucasian children in developing areas with normal lactose tolerance declines rapidly after the age of two." Johnson et al. (1974:213) also state that, "It now is generally agreed that those people who are lactose non-digesters as adults actually lose their capacity to digest lactose effectively by 3–5 years of age." And Shwachman and Lebenthal (1975:305) say: "In countries where a high percentage of adults have lactose intolerance, such as India and Thailand, lactose intolerance appears earlier—between two and four years of age." Cautioning about the potential problems associated with the provisioning of disadvantaged groups with milk, Bayless, Paige, Rothfeld and Huang (1975:306) state: "Even the figure of four years as the onset of lactose intolerance in other countries is probably inaccurate because most of these studies, including our own in Peru, have shown that the majority of these children are already intolerant by the age of three years."

After reviewing data on 17 different studies that provide information on onset of lactose maldigestion, Scrimshaw and Murray (1988) concluded that the data are insufficient to determine precisely the relationship between age and prevalence of lactose maldigestion and intolerance in various ethnic groups. However, they do say that "it is clear that the primary (genetic) loss of lactase activity occurs in early childhood and is not progressive throughout life" (1978:1097).

The studies reporting age of onset of lactose maldigestion are variable in quality; some fail to adequately define the population under study, and few include young children. The few studies that surveyed indigenous children in populations with no history of cattle herding show that most children exhibit lactose intolerance by the age of 7 years (Scrimshaw and Murray, 1988). The majority of studies show an age of onset of lactose maldigestion in younger children. For example, a study of 172 children in Thailand (Keusch, Troncale, Miller, Promadhat and

Anderson, 1969) found that by the age of 2 years nearly all children were lactase deficient. Brown, Parry, Khatun and Ahmed (1979) found a 20% prevalence of lactose maldigestion (malabsorption) in well-nourished diarrhea-free Bangladeshi children from 7 to 18 months of age, with a prevalence of 89% in those over 3 years of age. A study in Nigeria (Kretchmer et al., 1971) found that 99% of Yoruba children maldigest (malabsorb) lactose after the age of 1.5–3 years. Other studies have shown similar findings for the Baganda of Uganda and Japanese infants (Kretchmer et al., 1971). Paige et al. (1972) studied a group of 90 Peruvian children from 10 months to 17 years of age and found that 73% of those younger than 3 years were lactose tolerant, and there was a sharp drop in tolerance thereafter. No relationship was apparent between duration of breastfeeding, which ranged from 0 to 48 months, and the individual's subsequent ability to tolerate lactose.

Obviously in a society that has no alternative to breast milk, as most likely was the case until the Neolithic, the ability to digest lactose meant the difference between life and death. Therefore, it must have been vitally important for prehistoric infants to maintain the ability to digest lactose for the normal duration of breastfeeding. It is possible that the imprint of that ancient pattern remains in the timing of the development of lactose intolerance in a number of contemporary human populations. Certainly there is a strong relationship between weaning and the development of lactose intolerance in other mammals. However, there are a number of problems involved in obtaining anything other than a general idea of what the timing of this ancient pattern might have been: problems associated with the type of studies that have been done, the methods used to determine lactose intolerance, and the age, state of health, exposure to dairy products, and genetic composition of the populations that have been sampled. There may have been considerable variability in the duration of breastfeeding among different prehistoric groups that could be reflected in the modern variations in timing of the development of lactose intolerance. However, it does appear that in many lactose-intolerant populations of indigenous peoples who have no history of cattle herding, this intolerance is manifested in the majority of children by the age of 3 years, with a range between 1 and 4 years. From this information it could be deduced that it was common to breastfeed prehistoric infants for at least the first 2 to 3 years of life.

DEMOGRAPHY

Another potential source of information about prehistoric breastfeeding patterns comes from work on infant mortality profiles in historical and modern populations. The biological basis for this demographic approach lies in the fact that the prevalence and duration of breastfeeding significantly influence levels of mortality during the first year of life; breastfed infants experience much lower mortality rates than artificially fed infants. This observation has been borne out in many societies by a number of cross-cultural and diachronic studies (Knodel, 1968; Knodel and Kintner, 1977; Lithell, 1981; Woodbury, 1925). For example, Woodbury (1925) was involved in contemporary research in the 1920s in various North American cities, before the advent of the modern formula industry. He analyzed infant mortality in a sample of 22,422 infants from eight American cities. He found that in the first month, artificially fed infants had a mortality rate of over three times that of breastfed infants, in the second month four times, in the third month six times, and in the fourth, fifth, sixth, and seventh month over five times (Woodbury, 1925).

Lithell (1981) examined the relationship between breastfeeding habits, infant mortality, and marital fertility in three nineteenth century parish groups, two in Sweden and one in Finland. In two of these parish groups custom dictated that infants were not generally breastfed, while in the third, mothers believed in prolonged breastfeeding of infants. After analysis of the data, Lithell concluded that the practice of "horn-feeding" and giving substitutes for breast milk contributed to high infant mortality, particularly in the 1–6 month age group, and to a peak of mortality during the summer. A high frequency of death in the 1–6 month age group was a good indicator of poor infant feeding practices, especially when a low rate of stillbirths and a low infant mortality were found in the neonatal period. Lithell commented that this information could provide a method that might be of use in analyses aimed at establishing the specifics of breastfeeding practices in a population, but that ideally information on three different variables was necessary: (1) patterns of seasonal variation, (2) infant mortality in the age group 1–6 months, and (3) causes of death that can be related to intestinal diseases such as diarrhea and vomiting.

Knodel and Kintner (1977) analyzed data on breastfeeding and infant mortality in detailed surveys on mothers and infants in Bavaria, Germany, in the late nineteenth and early twentieth centuries. They found very striking differences in breastfeeding practices that correlated with levels of infant mortality. The three provinces where breastfeeding was uncommon were characterized by far higher rates of infant mortality than were the three where the large majority of infants had been nursed by their mothers, and the two provinces that were intermediate with respect to breastfeeding were also intermediate with respect to mortality levels. For almost all the areas with little breastfeeding, 30–40% of infants died before the age of 1 year; whereas in most of the areas with extended breastfeeding, less than 20% of infants died by age 1. The data indicated that not only did the level of mortality differ between the breastfed and artificially fed children, but also that the time of death during the first year of life was statistically different for breastfed and artificially fed infants. In populations where breastfeeding was limited, cumulative infant mortality rose particularly steeply during the early months of the first year of life.

Bourgeois-Pichat (1946) developed a widely accepted and utilized technique for the biometric analysis of infant mortality. It provides a simple method of separating infant deaths associated with a prenatal or birth situation (e.g., malformation, obstetrical trauma) from deaths associated with the postnatal environment (such as poor nutrition or disease) (Knodel and Kintner, 1977). Bourgeois-Pichat found that cumulative infant deaths after the first month are usually linearly related to age, and generally fall on a straight line. A major assumption of the biometric analysis of infant mortality, as developed by Bourgeois-Pichat, is that the age structure of infant deaths after the first month of life is virtually constant across time and cultures (Knodel and Kintner, 1977).

However, Bourgeois-Pichat noted that there are exceptions to the linear relationship between mortality after the first month and age, the most common being a situation in which cumulative mortality after several months of life rises more steeply than would be predicted by extrapolation of the line fitting mortality during the first few months. In this case, mortality during the later months fits a second straight line that has a steeper slope than the first (Figure 3.1). This is the result of a break in the relationship at 2, 3, or 4 months, which is generally interpreted to result from "excess mortality" during the remainder of the first year of life. Pressat (1972) also noted that the most common exception to the linear relationship of infant mortality and age described by Bourgeois-Pichat (1952) was a steep rise in the slope of cumulative mortality between several months of age and the end of the first year. Unlike the Bourgeois-Pichat model, where there is a straight line formed by the slope of cumulative mortality between 1 month and 1 year of age, in the case of the exception to the model, mortality in the later months best fits a straight line that has a steeper slope than the line for the first few months (Knodel and Kintner, 1977).

Both Bourgeois-Pichat and Pressat attributed the steeper rise following the early months of life to "excessive" mortality associated with infants who were weaned or artificially fed. Knodel and Kintner (1977) confirmed this observation using data on infant feeding and mortality rates from Bavaria, Germany. Where breastfeeding was nonexistent or restricted, infant mortality rose more steeply during the early months of the first year of life. The difference in the age-structure of mortality was revealed by comparing the slope of the line connecting mortality during

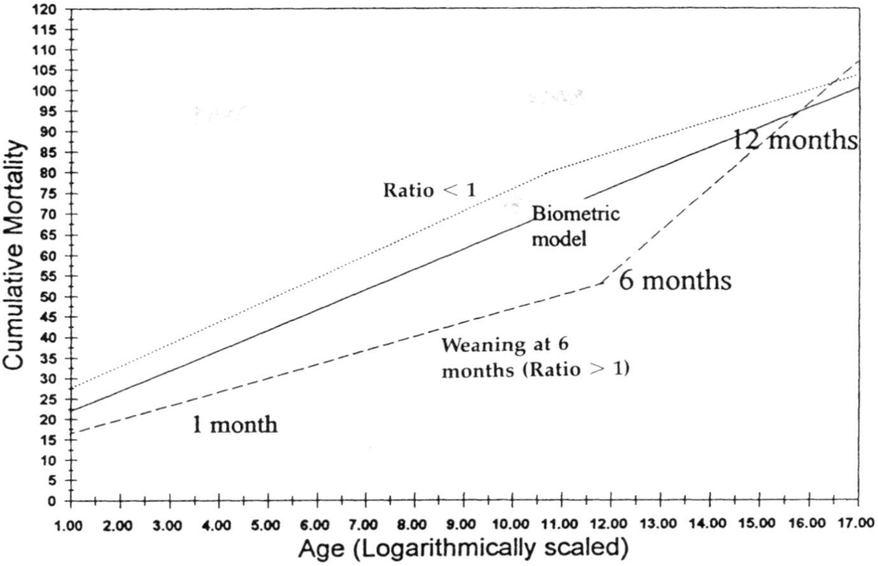

Figure 3.1. Biometric analysis of infant mortailty (courtesy of Henry Choong).

the first half of the year and the one connecting mortality during the second half of the year. A ratio of below one (seen in cases where infants were not breastfed) indicates that mortality rises more steeply than expected during the early months of life compared to mortality during the second half; mortality rises more steeply during the later months of life (ratio above one) for breastfed babies (Choong, 1993). This information could be applied to infant mortality curves obtained from either historic or prehistoric populations to provide clues about breastfeeding practices. For example, Choong (1993) has used this method to interpret breastfeeding customs in various groups living in Gibraltar between 1900 and 1947. Herring, Saunders and Katzenberg (1994) have applied the method to assess breastfeeding and weaning practices of 19th century mothers, based on data from St. Thomas' Anglican Church cemetery in Belleville, Ontario. The method has not, as yet, been applied to prehistoric populations.

As Bocquet-Appel and Masset (1982) have cautioned, there are various problems involved in reconstructing the demographic profiles of prehistoric populations, but the application of this demographic method of reconstructing breastfeeding practices is certainly worth considering, under appropriate circumstances. For example, in the case of prehistoric skeletal populations where the numbers of infant deaths do not appear to be underrepresented, and the sample size from birth to 1 year is large enough, this method should be considered. It may be particularly well suited for ossuary collections where the time period represented by the burials is limited to decades rather than centuries, and/or to collections that are associated with well preserved organic remains that allow for a reconstruction of season of death. In any case, the variables of importance are the patterns of infant mortality in general, seasonal variation in infant mortality, and, particularly, the rate of mortality in the 1–6 month age group, and the difference in slope between the infant mortality profiles for the first and second half of the first year of life. Certainly there appears to be potential for obtaining information about ancient breastfeeding practices by the application of this demographic technique to prehistoric populations.

DISCUSSION

Why is information on prehistoric breastfeeding practices so important? Studies of various researchers, including Fildes (Chapter 4), have shown unequivocally that the impact of feeding practices on infant mortality in historical times was considerable; there is no reason to believe that this was not also the case in the past. For example, Lithell (1981) wanted to determine the impact of living conditions and breastfeeding habits on infant mortality, child mortality, and mortality among women in childbirth. He studied infant mortality rates between 1841 and 1850 in five Finnish parishes, four that were known for encouraging prolonged breastfeeding and one that did not. Mortality in childbirth, infant and child mortality rates in different social and economic groups, and causes of death among children were variables that were considered. As a result of the study, Lithell stated that infant mortality rates alone could not be used as an indicator of living conditions in the past because of the confounding effects of differing breastfeeding practices. He found that prolonged breastfeeding in an area characterized by a low standard of living protects the child, and reduces the impact of the environment. However, both a high infant mortality rate in the neonatal period and a high rate of stillbirth were found to be related to severe living conditions. He also found that child mortality, rather than infant mortality, was more influenced by socioeconomic circumstances and could be a useful indicator of differences in living conditions. In addition, the rate of females dying in childbirth also seemed to be highly correlated with socioeconomic circumstances. He concluded that infant mortality alone cannot be used for verifying the standard of living of past populations, but that the infant mortality rate in the neonatal period, the rate of stillbirths, child mortality, and the rate of females dying in childbirth were all better indicators of socioeconomic status. Lithell stressed that when considering the relationship between mortality and living conditions, it is essential to take into account the role of different breastfeeding practices, as infant mortality is definitely affected by them. DaVanzo (1988) also studied the relationship between socioeconomic factors and infant mortality. He commented that it has been generalized that infant mortality rates tend to vary inversely with the level of socioeconomic development, both over time and across regions. To test this generalization he surveyed groups living in richer and poorer states in Peninsular Malaysia over a time period when socioeconomic conditions improved for all groups, while the duration of breastfeeding decreased in most groups. DaVanzo discovered that in the richer states, the detrimental effects on infant survival of the decline in breastfeeding more than offset the beneficial effects of the improvements in water quality and sanitation. The continued prevalence of extended breastfeeding in the poorer states of Peninsular Malaysia was one of the main factors contributing to the closing of the gap between their infant mortality rate and that of the richer states. It appears then that there is more to the story of infant mortality than socioeconomic development, and that once again it is essential to consider the effects of breastfeeding practices on the morbidity and mortality of prehistoric infants.

Even in times and places where all infants were breastfed, as was probably the case throughout most of prehistory, differing customs or beliefs surrounding infant feeding could affect the health and longevity of infants and young children. As Fildes (Chapter 4) has shown for children in historical times, factors such as beliefs about the dangers of colostrum, the duration of breastfeeding, timing of introduction of supplemental foods, or reasons for weaning could all have affected the health of prehistoric children. For example, modern studies on third world populations indicate that babies who are breastfed exclusively for the first 6 months are healthier than those who are given supplemental foods before this time, and that children who are still receiving breast milk in their second year of life grow better and have fewer infections than their peers who are weaned earlier (Wray, 1990). In cultures where there is a bias for boys, preferential and longer duration of breastfeeding for male infants can produce large discrepancies in morbidity and mortality between boys and girls (Mull, 1992). As mentioned earlier in this chapter, beliefs about the dangers of colostrum and customs such as the giving of ritual substances to the newborn can also have detrimental effects on infant health. In areas of the world today where sanitation is poor and environmental conditions severe, the death rate of infants not fully breastfed is extremely high. For example, it has been said that death among newborns not suckled at the breast in the third world is at least five times more common than among those that receive mother's milk (Lawrence, 1989). Therefore, it may be expected that in times or places in prehistory when environmental conditions were severe, a pattern of unsupplemented breastfeeding for at least the first 6 months, and a long duration of breastfeeding, would have produced less morbidity and mortality in infants and children than early supplementation and weaning.

CONCLUSION

In Chapter 2, Dettwyler argues that based on comparative primate data, the natural age at weaning for our hominid ancestors *could* have been the maturational equivalent of 6.0 years of age. In Chapter 4, Fildes presents a fascinating discussion of infant feeding illustrating the diversity of cultural practices throughout history. What were breastfeeding patterns and practices in prehistory? At present, there are few hard data. However, there are a number of clues that can be assembled from various sources that can at least begin to provide a picture of what may have existed in the past. From these clues it appears that the duration of breastfeeding in many prehistoric populations averaged between 2 and 3 years. Data from bone chemical studies on archaeological populations show that substantial supplementation with foods other than breast milk occurred in 18- to 20-month-old infants in prehistoric Tennessee and South Dakota, and that weaning probably occurred between the ages of 2 and 3 years in children from the medieval Arabic population of Dor (Fogel et al., 1989; Sillen and Smith, 1984). Schurr's (1994) data on a group of prehistoric sedentary maize horticulturalists from Ohio showed that weaning was a gradual process beginning before age 2, with breast milk maintaining its primary importance in the diet for at least 6 months after the addition of other foods to the child's diet. Evidence from historical sources suggests that in the most ancient civilizations, babies were usually breastfed for 2 to 3 years. Ethnographic data indicate that although there is a great deal of cultural diversity, on average weaning occurs at between 2 and 3 years of age. Data on the timing of the development of lactose intolerance in a number of populations suggest that the average duration of substantial breastfeeding in prehistory was at least 2 years, with a range of between 1 and 4 years.

Undoubtedly, there was a great deal of cultural diversity in weaning age of prehistoric populations, as there was in historical times and as exists today, both in traditional and modern societies. Fildes (1986) has shown that historically, there could be enormous differences in weaning age for individual children, even within one family, depending on such factors as the sex and health of the child, the season of the year, phase of the moon, the health of the mother, or an intervening pregnancy. Katzenberg et al.'s (1993) bone chemical data showing differences in the breast milk component of the diet between two 3- to 4-year-old children from the same Ontario Iroquoian village site show that this also occurred in prehistory. As Dettwyler explains, this diversity in weaning age would not have been possible until the cultural innovations of first fire, then later the regular use of cereal grains. These innovations provided the alternatives that allowed a relaxation of the 6-year nursing imperative.

Although reasons for the timing of supplemental feeding and weaning vary among cultures and individuals, it seems that the development of the child's dentition is a major, though not always acknowledged, factor. In many societies, both historical and contemporary traditional, supplemental foods were often given around the time of the eruption of the first teeth at 6 or 7 months, and weaning occurred after the age of 24 months when the dentition had fully erupted. In both cases the child would have the practical apparatus with which to cope with the demands of a new diet. Thus, dentition may have provided the biological basis for the timing of dietary supplementation and weaning, upon which cultural idiosyncracies could then have made their mark.

It is clear that breastfeeding practices vary across cultures and over time (see Quandt and Fildes, Chapters 4 and 5). It is also clear that, as for modern populations, this variation had implications for the health and disease of ancient populations. This fact has not been appreciated by researchers in the field of paleonutrition. To what extent did different breastfeeding practices affect the health of prehistoric infants and children? It is hoped that this chapter will stimulate more research to answer this question, including further bone chemical analyses and the application of the demographic approach. It is fascinating to attempt to delve into the past and, with the help of various clues from a number of sources, to begin to unravel the tangled skeins that make up the story of breastfeeding in prehistory.

REFERENCES

Barness, L. A.
1987 History of infant feeding practices. *American Journal of Clinical Nutrition* 46:168–170.

Bayless, T. M., D. M. Paige, and G. D. Ferry
1971 Lactose intolerance and milk drinking habits. *Gastroenterology* 60(4):605–608.

Bayless, T. M., D. M. Paige, B. Rothfeld, and S-S. Huang
1975 Letter to the editor. *New England Journal of Medicine* 293:306.
Blakely, R. L.
1989 Bone strontium in pregnant and lactating females from archaeological samples. *American Journal of Physical Anthropology* 80:173–185.
Bocquet-Appel, J., and C. Masset
1982 Farewell to paleodemography. *Journal of Human Evolution* 11:321–333.
Bourgeois-Pichat, J.
1946 De la mesure de la mortalitié. *Population* 1:53–68.
1952 Essai sur la mortalite biologique de l'homme. *Population* 7:381–394.
Brown, A. B.
1973 *Bone Strontium Content as a Dietary Indicator in Human Skeletal Populations.* Ph.D. Dissertation, Ann Arbor: University of Michigan.
Brown, K., L. Parry, M. Khatun, and M. G. Ahmed
1979 Lactose malabsorption in Bangladeshi village children: Relation with age, history of recent diarrhea, nutritional status, and breast feeding. *American Journal of Clinical Nutrition* 32:1962–1969.
Choong, H.
1993 Biometric analysis of infant mortality. Research paper written for anthropology course at the University of Toronto.
Cramer, D., H. Xu, and T. Sahi
1994 Adult hypolactasia, milk consumption, and age-specific fertility. *American Journal of Epidemiology* 139(3):282–289.
Cunningham, A. S., D. B. Jelliffe, and E. F. P. Jelliffe
1991 Breastfeeding and health in the 1980s: A global epidemiologic review. *Journal of Pediatrics* 118(5):659–666.
DaVanzo, J.
1988 Infant mortality and socioeconomic development: Evidence from Malaysian household data. *Demography* 25(4):581–595.
Davidson, W. D.
1953 A brief history of infant feeding. *Journal of Pediatrics* 43:74–87.
Davis, M. K., D. A. Savitz, and B. I. Graubard
1988 Infant feeding and childhood cancer. *Lancet* 2:365–368.
Eaton, S. B., M. Shostak, and M. Konner
1988 *The Paleolithic Prescription.* New York: Harper & Row.
Fildes, V. A.
1986 *Breasts, Bottles and Babies.* Edinburgh: Edinburgh University Press.
Fogel, M., N. Tuross, and D. Owsley
1989 Nitrogen isotope tracers of human lactation in modern and archaeological populations. *Annual Report of the Director, Geophysical Laboratory.* 1988–1989, 2150:111–117.
Gilbert, R. I.
1975 *Trace Element Analysis of Three Skeletal Amerindian Populations at Dickson Mounds.* Ph.D. Dissertation, University of Massachusetts.
Herring, D. A., S. R. Saunders, and M. A. Katzenberg
1994 Multiple methods for estimating weaning age in a 19th century cemetery sample from Upper Canada (abstract). *American Journal of Physical Anthropology,* Suppl. 18:106.

Jelliffe, D. B. and E. F. P. Jelliffe
1978 *Infant Nutrition in the Subtropics and Tropics.* Geneva, Switzerland: WHO Monograph No. 29.
Johnson, J. D., N. Kretchmer, and F. J. Simoons
1974 Lactase malabsorption: Its biology and history. *Advances in Pediatrics* 21:197–237.
Johnson, R. C., R. E. Cole, and F. M. Ahem
1981 Genetic interpretation of racial/ethnic differences in lactose absorption and tolerance: A review. *Human Biology* 53(1):1–13.
Katzenberg, M. A.
1991 Isotopic analysis. In *The Links that Bind: The Harvie Family Nineteenth Century Burying Ground,* edited by S. R. Saunders and R. Lazenby, pp. 65–69. Dundas: Copetown Press.
1992 Advances in stable isotope analysis of prehistoric bones. In *Skeletal Biology of Past Peoples: Research Methods,* edited by S. R. Saunders and M. A. Katzenberg, pp. 105–120. New York: Wiley-Liss.
Katzenberg, A., S. Saunders, and W. R. Fitzgerald
1993 Age differences in stable carbon and nitrogen isotope ratios in a population of prehistoric maize horticulturalists. *American Journal of Physical Anthropology* 90(3):267–282.
Keusch, G. T., F. J. Troncale, L. H. Miller, V. Promadhat, and P. R. Anderson
1969 Acquired lactose malabsorption in Thai children. *Pediatrics* 43(4), Part I:540–545.
Knodel, J.
1968 Infant mortality and fertility in three Bavarian villages: An analysis of family histories from the 19th century. *Population Studies* 22:297–318.
Knodel, J., and H. Kintner
1977 The impact of breast feeding patterns on the biometric analysis of infant mortality. *Demography* 14(4):391–409.
Konner, M. J.
1976 Maternal care, infant behavior, and development among the !Kung. In *Kalahari Hunter-Gatherers,* edited by R. B. Lee and I. DeVore, pp. 218–299. Boston: Harvard University Press.
Konner, M., and C. Worthman
1980 Nursing frequency, gonadal function, and birth spacing among !Kung hunter-gatherers. *Science* 207:788–791.
Kretchmer, N., O. Ransome-Kuti, R. Hurwitz, C. Dungy, and W. Alakija
1971 Intestinal absorption of lactose in Nigerian ethnic groups. *Lancet* 2:392–395.
Lawrence, R. A.
1989 *Breastfeeding.* St. Louis: C. V. Mosby.
Lithell, U.
1981 *Breast-feeding and Reproduction.* Stockholm: Almquist and Wiksell.
McCracken, R. D.
1971 Lactase deficiency: An example of dietary evolution. *Current Anthropology* 12(4-5):479–517.
Mull, D. S.
1992 Mothers' milk and pseudoscientific breastmilk testing in Pakistan. *Social Science and Medicine* 34(11):1277–1290.

Paige, D. M., E. Leonardo, A. Cordano, J. Nakashima, B. Adrianzen, and G. G. Graham
1972 Lactose intolerance in Peruvian children: Effect of age and early nutrition. *American Journal of Clinical Nutrition* 25:297–301.
Palmer, G.
1988 *The Politics of Breastfeeding*. London: Pandora Press.
Pisacane, A., N. Impagliazzo, M. Russo, R. Valiani, A. Mandarini, C. Florio, and P. Vivo
1994 Breastfeeding and multiple sclerosis. *British Medical Journal* 308:1411-1412.
Pressat, R.
1972 *Demographic Analysis: Methods, Results, Applications*. Chicago: Aldine-Atherton.
Price, T. D., R. W. Swick, and E. P. Chase
1986 Bone chemistry and prehistoric diet: Strontium studies of laboratory rats. *American Journal of Physical Anthropology* 70:365–375.
Sahi, T.
1994 Genetics and epidemiology of adult-type hypolactasia. *Scandinavian Journal of Gastroenterology* 29 Suppl. 202:7-20.
Schurr, M. R.
1994 Stable-isotopes as evidence for the age of weaning at the Angel site: A comparison of isotopic and demographic measures of weaning age. Conference paper presented at the Visiting Scholar Conference, Center for Archaeological Investigation, Southern Illinois University, Carbondale.
Scrimshaw, N. S., and E. B. Murray
1988 The acceptability of milk and milk products in populations with a high prevalence of lactose intolerance. *American Journal of Clinical Nutrition* 48:1083-1146.
Shwachman, H. and E. Lebenthal
1975 Lactose tolerance in children (letter). *New England Journal of Medicine* 293:305.
Sillen, A., and P. Smith
1984 Weaning patterns are reflected in strontium-calcium ratios of juvenile skeletons. *Journal of Archaeological Sciences* 11:237-245.
Sobolik, K. D., ed.
1994 *Paleonutrition: The Diet and Health of Prehistoric Americans*. Carbondale, IL: Center for Archaeological Investigations. Occasional Paper No. 22.
Stuart-Macadam, P. L.
1993 Replacing breasts with bottles: The biological consequences (abstract). *Abstracts: 13th International Congress of Anthropological and Ethnological Sciences. The Cultural and Biological Dimensions of Global Change*, pp. 438. IUAES meetings, Mexico City, Mexico, August 1993.
Tuross, N., and M. Fogel
1994 Stable isotope analysis and subsistence patterns at the Sully Site. In *Skeletal Biology in the Great Plains: Migration, Warfare, Health, and Subsistence*, edited by D. W. Owsley and R. L. Jantz, pp. 283-289. Washington, D. C.: Smithsonian Institution Press.

Walker, M.
1993 A fresh look at the risks of artificial infant feeding. *Journal of Human Lactation* 9(2):97-107.
White, C., and H. Schwarcz
1994 Temporal trends in stable isotopes for Nubian mummy tissues. *American Journal of Physical Anthropology* 93:165-187.
Wickes, I. G.
1953 A history of infant feeding. *Archives of Diseases of Childhood* Part I, 28:151-158, Part III:332-340.
Woodbury, R. M.
1925 Causal factors in infant mortality. U. S. Dept. of Labor, Children's Bureau Publication No. 142. Washington, D. C.: U. S. Government Printing Office.
Wray, J. D.
1990 Breast-feeding: An international and historical review. In *Infant and Child Nutrition Worldwide: Issues and Perspectives*, edited by F. Falkner, pp. 61-116. Boca Raton: CRC Press.

4

The Culture and Biology of Breastfeeding: An Historical Review of Western Europe

Valerie Fildes

INTRODUCTION

Historical sources indicate that there were many factors that affected maternal and infant health in Western Europe, including social class, religion, nutritional status of the mother, and hygiene of the environment. However, it is clear that infant feeding practices were among the most important determinants of early childhood morbidity and mortality and also had a real impact on maternal health. Like all cultural behaviors, feeding methods had an enormous range, depending on factors such as period in history, geographic locale, and individual preference. This chapter will focus on several variables of infant feeding and the effects of these on health and disease patterns of mothers and infants throughout history in Western Europe. These variables include whether or not an infant was breastfed, the timing and duration of breastfeeding, and the type of supplemental and weaning foods.

BREASTFED OR NOT?

Preindustrial Revolution

Before the Neolithic period, which saw the domestication of plants and animals in some parts of the world, there was probably no effective alternative to human milk. Either an infant was breastfed by its mother, or some other woman, or it died. The question would not have been,

"Was an infant breastfed?" but, "Was an infant breastfed by its own mother or a relative, friend, or wet nurse?" Wet nursing was an ancient, deeply ingrained and widely accepted social custom. It was well-known in ancient civilizations, although it was possibly used less among the Hebrews than in Egypt or Mesopotamia (Fildes, 1988). In ancient Mesopotamia, nurses were carefully chosen, and legal contracts were drawn up to safeguard the arrangements between parents and nurse (Radbill, 1973). The *Code of Laws* of Hammurabi, Amorite King of Babylon (c.1728–1686 B.C.), includes a safeguard against nurses illegally substituting other babies for those who had died in their care. In ancient Egypt the practice of wet nursing was widespread, although at the time of pharaohs wet nurses were used almost exclusively by royalty and the highly born, and for foundlings (Fildes, 1986). In the classical period of Greece (fifth to fourth century B.C.), wet nurses were frequently used, especially by the wealthier classes. Wet nurses were also used extensively in Roman society. The practice spread throughout the Greek colonies and the Roman Empire, and it is possible that wet nursing was introduced into Britain during the Roman occupation (Fildes, 1986, 1988).

Nonmedical sources make it clear that in most of western Europe, from the early second millennium, many wealthy and noble families employed wet nurses to feed their children, while in poorer families the mother nursed her own child (Ruffer, 1921). It has been suggested that this was a reason for the increased "birth rates" among the aristocracy, which also dates from the eleventh century (McLaughlan, 1976). In France, wet nurses were highly organized from the twelfth century onward (Drake, 1935) and by 1715 four employment bureaus existed in Paris for the registration of nurses. By the later medieval period it was well-established for European women of the upper classes to employ wet nurses, although the great majority of infants were probably breastfed at home by their mothers. In some areas during the later Middle Ages it was established practice even for artisans and small shopkeepers to employ wet nurses (Shahar, 1983). Historical evidence shows that throughout the period 1500–1800 wives of the European aristocracy, gentry, wealthy merchants, wealthy farmers, scholars, lawyers, physicians, and some clergymen regularly used wet nurses. It was also essential for foundlings (Fildes, 1986, 1990).

After the mid-eighteenth century it became increasingly fashionable for upper- and middle-class mothers to breastfeed their own children, although young mothers still had to overcome opposition from older women who had been brought up in the tradition of wet nursing. This was a change from the fifteenth and sixteenth centuries when an upper-class woman needed great strength of purpose to go against the cultural norm. This is illustrated by a quote from a 1695 tract: "a lady that will condescend to be a nurse, though to her own child, is become as unfashionable and ungenteel as a gentleman that will not drink, swear, and be profane" (Newcome, 1695). In the same period, a similar movement toward such mothers breastfeeding their own children occurred in France, Holland, Sweden, parts of Germany, and North America (Fildes, 1986; Sussman, 1982; Eekelen, 1986; Badineter, 1981). To some extent it was related to the philosophy of William Locke (1693), William Cadogan (1748), and Jean-Jacques Rousseau (1762), who advocated natural methods of infant nutrition and care, particularly maternal breastfeeding. However, in France and Britain at least, the effectiveness and scale of this change appear to have been neither great nor lasting. In France, only a minority of the Parisian middle classes was affected by the fashion (Sussman, 1982; Badineter, 1981). In Britain it possibly had a greater effect, but both artificial feeding and the employment of wet nurses continued to be common alternatives to maternal breastfeeding throughout the late eighteenth and early nineteenth centuries (Fildes, 1986, 1988).

Early in the history of wet nursing, the wet nurse came into the infant's home to suckle the baby, and there is also evidence from western Europe that from the eleventh century on, when wet nursing began to be established, the wet nurse was usually taken into the child's house where she could be closely supervised by the mother. In that case, the health of the infant was probably not compromised. However, it was when infants were sent away to the home of the wet nurse, often miles away in the country, that problems arose. For example, in many areas of France the quality of care given by wet nurses was very low, and it is probable that even when infants were fostered out to wet nurses, they were at least partially artificially fed or "dry nursed." The mortality of foundlings from Paris who were put out to rural wet nurses in the years 1771–1773 varied according to the province that received the babies. In several regions of France, the mortality of infants breastfed by wet nurses in those years was double that of infants breastfed by their mothers, many of whom were equally poor (Flandrin, 1979; Shorter, 1977).

The earliest known historical documents that refer to infant nutrition record that all infants were either breastfed by their mother or a wet nurse for periods ranging from at least 1 year to 3 or more years (Fildes, 1988). In preindustrial European and colonial society, infant feeding practices remained relatively unchanged for many centuries. In most regions virtually all children were breastfed, either by their mother or by a wet nurse (Fildes, 1986). The duration of breastfeeding varied from 9–12 months in some areas to 2–3 years in others but most children were suckled, usually on demand, for at least a year (Fildes, 1991).

Postindustrial Revolution

Later in history regional and geographic differences in breastfeeding were usually related to long-standing customs (in certain areas) of infants not being breastfed at all, but being raised on animal milks and/or cereal paps. Examples include parts of Germany, Bohemia, Northern Italy, the Austrian Tyrol, Finland, Sweden, Iceland, and Russia. In some areas of Europe, the tradition of artificially feeding all or most infants dated at least from the fifteenth century (Knodel and van der Waale, 1967). All the nonbreastfeeding regions so far identified were in Northern Europe, had a cold dry climate, and many were in mountainous terrain. The climate was an important factor in the success of artificial feeding, especially when the substitute foods contained milk. In warmer countries, milk and other foods rapidly become sour and contaminated, making infants more susceptible to gastrointestinal disease. However, even in colder climates infant mortality must have been high, as Knodel and Kintner (1977) discovered when they examined the statistics from the nineteenth century for provinces in Germany, three of which had traditionally low levels of breastfeeding and two in which breastfeeding was more common. For almost all the areas with little breastfeeding, 30–40% of infants died by age one, compared with a 20% mortality in most of the areas with extended breastfeeding. As would be expected in places where mothers did not breastfeed, wet nursing was virtually nonexistent in these areas (Knodel, personal communication). Given these traditions, the expected result would be that women would have more children, closer together, than where breastfeeding rates were higher. Some research on nineteenth-century populations in German, Swedish, and Finnish nonbreastfeeding areas has confirmed that this was indeed the case (Knodel, 1968; Lithell, 1981; Brandstrom, Brostrom and Persson, 1984).

Effects on Mother and Child

This tour through history makes it clear that whether or not an infant was breastfed had an enormous impact on its health and survival. Artificial feeding was universally accepted as dangerous to life and was normally employed only in cases of necessity, such as where prematurity or congenital deformities made suckling impossible, in institutions, or when a wet nurse could not be employed because the infant had syphilis (Fildes, 1986, 1988). There were some clearly defined regions in northern Europe where, by tradition, children were rarely or never breastfed although the original reasons for this were lost in time. As well, some infants were artificially fed when certain socially privileged groups fleetingly experimented with feeding methods, but the vast majority of infants were not affected by these exceptions (Fildes, 1986).

By at least the medieval period it was generally known that in addition to maintaining general good health, a child breastfed by its mother was less likely to develop rickets, would have less trouble when he or she began teething, would avoid numerous ailments and stunted growth, and was less likely to die in childhood than a child deprived of breastfeeding (Anonymous, 1739; Gouge, 1622; Smith, 1774).

Not breastfeeding was also known to have health consequences for the mother. For example, it has commonly been assumed that women in preindustrial Britain were unaware of the contraceptive function of breastfeeding. However, it is very unlikely that women in general, and midwives in particular, were unaware that if they breastfed the return of menstruation would be delayed. It is the kind of information that mothers would pass on to their daughters, and for this reason would not necessarily appear in written records. References to the relationship between breastfeeding and temporary infertility are infrequent, but a sufficient number have been found in the medical and religious literature to make it clear that the significance of lactational amenorrhea was known, not only to women but also to men. The recorded comments relating to this subject between 1500 and 1800 were of three types: (1) that the wish to have more children quickly was a valid reason for a woman not to breastfeed; (2) that women who breastfed had fewer pregnancies; and (3) that women should breastfeed to avoid pregnancy (Fildes, 1986). For example, the English clergyman, Henry Newcome, said in 1695:

> So vain is that popular pretense that nursing is an impediment to fruitfulness, and to be declin'd by great persons for the better securing of succession, by a numerous posterity: for if those bear faster who dry up their breasts, they that nurse their children commonly bear longer, and bring more up to maturity. (Newcome, 1695)

The surgeon-midwife, Pierre Dionis (1719), speaking of France, where maternal breastfeeding was less common than in Britain (and incidentally the average family size was greater) noted that wealthier married women usually had a child every year, but those that suckled had only two or three at most. He advised women who wished to avoid pregnancy to breastfeed. The Devon physician Hugh Downman (1788) promoted suckling as a means of protecting mothers from the exhausting effects of repeated child-bearing as "the nursing time was meant by wisest Nature, as a stay." With respect to fertility, two clear facts emerge.

First, the women of status in society, who used wet nurses to feed their babies, commonly had large numbers of children, and relatively short birth intervals (McLaren, 1978). Second, the women who became wet nurses had a smaller number of children and longer birth intervals (McLaren, 1978).

Suckling was said to benefit the mother in several ways: (1) by ensuring her health and recovery after childbirth, (2) by preventing women's diseases, (3) by making mothers happier, (4) by giving them pleasure and satisfaction, and (5) by reducing the likelihood of her dying.

So, when maternal breastfeeding was undertaken, the benefits for the mother were said to be pleasure and enjoyment, beauty, good health, and fewer children. The mother–child relationship would be closer and last into adult life, and the child would benefit by being more resistant to disease and death. Adverse consequences for mothers who did not suckle were said to include (1) poor health or disease, (2) an early death, (3) loss of beauty, (4) repeated childbirth, (5) missed pleasures of seeing her children grow and develop, and (6) higher likelihood of infant death.

The main reasons for recommending maternal breastfeeding, therefore, were the health of the mother and the child and the benefits to the maternal–child relationship. The major consequence of mothers not feeding their children was the lack of formation or breakdown of the maternal–child bond during infancy and in later life (wet nursed infants commonly bonded with their nurse and not their mother), with the other main effect being on the health and well-being of the mother and child.

ARTIFICIAL FEEDING

Preindustrial Revolution

By the late fifteenth and sixteenth century, many types of artificial feeding had come into fashion. Children were fed cow's or goat's milk from sucking horns, sucking cans or pots with cloth nipples, bottles, and spoons (Davidson, 1953; Fildes, 1986). Sometimes sugar lumps and bread were held for sucking in a piece of linen that had been pulled into the shape of a nipple (Davidson, 1953). The eighteenth century saw several changes in infant feeding methods, some related to the early industrialization in Britain at this time. The most significant change was the increasing use of artificial feeding, particularly among the very wealthy and the very poor. Dry nursing (the use of substances such as flour, bread, or cereal, usually cooked in broth or water) became fashionable among the aristocracy and some gentry beginning in the last two decades of the seventeenth century (Trumbach, 1978). In the same period, parish and foundling infants were hand fed, partly from necessity but also because it was cheaper to employ a dry nurse than a wet nurse. By the mid-eighteenth century, hand feeding was relatively common, and was being used for infants admitted to the London Foundling Hospital in 1741.

Postindustrial Revolution

The immense changes in lifestyle that occurred during the industrial revolution had a significant influence on infant feeding practices. Although some regions retained traditional habits until the mid-twentieth century, by the 1920s the feeding of most children in Europe, North America, and Australia was radically different from that of babies born 100 years earlier (Fildes, 1991). There were major differences in practice between rural and urban areas, with most rural women continuing to breastfeed as their mothers had done and for a similar length of time, while women who moved to the new manufacturing towns were more likely to supplement their breast milk with other foods early on, or to handfeed. However, breastfeeding practice also depended on the type of work in which a woman was employed, how close she lived to her place of work, whether a creche was available, whether she had relatives nearby who could help with childcare, and whether there was a tradition either of sending infants to be nursed in the country or of employing caretakers during the day (Fildes, 1991).

In the textile towns of Northern England women worked in the mills until shortly before childbirth and went back to work within a few days of delivery. The hours were long and in many places it was common to use very young girls or old women to care for infants during the day. Although some women breastfed their babies in the morning and evening, the infants were fed with a variety of other foods during the day and frequently were also dosed with opiates that made suckling difficult in the evening. In the 1890s and 1900s when statistics on feeding began to be compiled, the incidence of maternal breastfeeding (0–3 months) in some of these areas was as low as 50% (Jones, 1894; Newman, 1906). Although reliable figures for the earlier period are not available, observations by medical and lay writers suggest that the working mothers often did not breastfeed at all, or supplemented it with other foods from soon after birth so that the duration was short. These towns had some of highest infant mortality rates in the country, and this was attributed principally to mothers not breastfeeding because they worked in the mills (Fildes, 1988; Garrison, 1965; Hewitt, 1958; Newman, 1906). Evidence that backed up these assertions was the dramatic fall in infant mortality during the Manchester Cotton Famine in the early 1860s. Because of the fall in raw cotton supplies due to the American Civil War, work in the mills was greatly reduced; women were forced to stay at home and were able to suckle their babies. When production resumed after the war, women went back to work, were no longer able to breastfeed, and the infant mortality rate immediately rose again (Newman, 1906). This phenomenon was noted repeatedly by contemporaries. Where there was high infant mortality due to low breastfeeding rates, any social disruption that enabled urban mothers to remain at home and suckle their babies led to an immediate reduction in infant mortality, even though child and adult mortality might increase (Garrison, 1965; Jones, 1894; Newman, 1906; Vincent, 1904).

There seems to have been considerable variation in the prevalence of breastfeeding in different towns, and also between different districts within towns (Drake, 1908; Newman, 1906; Thompson, 1984; Vincent, 1904; Woods, Watterson and Woodward, 1989). Figures show that this was primarily related to the type of work in which women were employed. In some places it was feasible for mothers at least to partially breastfeed their children because they lived close to their place of work, or were able to leave their infants sufficiently close by (often with a relative), to breastfeed in the middle of the day in addition to before and after work (Drake, 1908; Newman, 1906; Vincent, 1904). Provision of creches by employers and municipal authorities was not common in Britain, but in France, Austria, Italy, and several other parts of Europe these were established from the 1840s onward and enabled women to breastfeed during breaks in their work if they wished to (Garrison, 1965).

From the 1890s, infant feeding data, collected principally by medical officers of health, health visitors, and infant welfare clinics, showed that in many urban areas over 80% of mothers did breastfeed, wholly or partially, especially during the first 3 months, although in certain communities, such as parts of Liverpool, Manchester, and Birmingham, 40–50% of infants were completely weaned onto other foods by the age of 6 months (Jones, 1894; Newman, 1906; Woods et al., 1989). In less industrialized towns, such as Brighton, only 30% of children aged 6–12 months were totally fed on foods other than breast milk (Newsholme, 1906). In rural areas almost all mothers were reported to breastfeed during the first 3 months and the majority of infants were still partly breastfed at 9–12 months (Newman, 1906; Vincent, 1904).

Surveys in the United States showed a similar picture. In Manchester, New Hampshire, where a high percentage of mothers worked in textile mills, 82% initiated breastfeeding, but 47% had completely weaned their infants by 6 months (Apple, 1987; Garrison, 1965). In other urban areas 88% of mothers initiated breastfeeding and three-quarters of their infants were still wholly or partially breastfed at 6 months. In rural areas over 90% of mothers initiated breastfeeding and most were still suckling at 6 months (Apple, 1987; Woodbury, 1926).

In Germany, where details about infant feeding were included in the census, there was a decline in both the incidence and duration of breastfeeding in urban areas after the Industrial Revolution (Kintner, 1985). In Berlin between 1885 and 1910 there was a 27% decline in the proportion of infants receiving breast milk at the time of the census, and the median duration of suckling fell from 8.48 to 2.11 months. In France, an increasing proportion of the thousands of children put out to country nurses was not breastfed. In 1898, in 23 departments only 0–25% of nurslings were breastfed (Sussman, 1982). In some industrial areas of Northern France in 1907–1910 less than 40% of infants were breastfed compared to over 60% throughout the rural south. The figure for the whole country was 55% (Rollet, 1981).

Apart from the urban/rural differences in suckling practices a consistent observation was that of the importance of traditional infant feeding customs in families that migrated to foreign cities. Where breastfeeding was the norm in their home country, immigrant mothers continued to suckle their babies and, often despite poorer living conditions, had a lower infant mortality rate than indigenous mothers in the same area who did not breastfeed. Examples are Irish and Scottish mothers in Liverpool and London, eastern and southern European mothers in North American cities, and Jewish mothers in London, Manchester, Amsterdam, and New York (Garrison, 1965; Newman, 1906).

Although the use of wet nurses declined in English-speaking countries in favor of artificial feeding, this did not happen to the same degree in much of continental Europe. Wealthy mothers who did not wish to breastfeed, particularly in Catholic countries, paid other, poorer, mothers to suckle their children, until the custom was irretrievably disrupted by the first world war, when poor women had the option of working in factories for higher wages instead. In France, where huge numbers of urban children of all classes were customarily placed out to country wet nurses, the incidence of breastfeeding by these nurses declined in favor of bottle feeding. Still, the wealthy could afford to pay the higher rates to employ a healthy wet nurse who did breastfeed. Poorer urban mothers who sent out their children could not afford these rates and their infants were usually bottlefed by equally poor rural nurses. Similarly, the many European foundling hospitals that every year employed thousands of relatively poor wet nurses to feed their charges found that with the increased availability and desirability of artificial feeding, their infants were less likely to be wholly or even partially breastfed than in previous centuries (Fildes, 1986, 1988).

In most of continental Europe, therefore, the decline in breastfeeding was likely to have been confined to the infants of the poor since those of the wealthy continued to receive breast milk from paid wet nurses. In English-speaking countries the decline in breastfeeding affected both the children of the wealthy and the urban poor, but the latter group suffered disproportionately because of their poverty and unsanitary living conditions. In the growing cities, where mills and factories were beginning to employ increasing numbers of women away from their previously home-based work, the poor were no longer able either to fully breastfeed their own children or wet nurse those of others (Fildes, 1988).

Effects on Mother and Child

The decline of wet-nursing meant that women from lower classes, who formerly had small families of 3 to 5, and who used wet nursing to limit their families, lost any contraceptive benefits of breastfeeding. In the industrial cities this was to lead in the nineteenth century to such women having child after child with short birth intervals (Szreter, 1983; Hewitt, 1958). In contrast, those wealthy women who breastfed their own children had relatively fewer pregnancies than when such women used wet nurses or artificial feeding. Women of the middle classes who continued to use either hired wet nurses or artificial feeding to rear their babies tended to have more children, more frequently, than those who breastfed their own offspring (Sussman, 1982; Fildes, 1988; Tilly, Scott and Cohen, 1980).

The mortality of dry-nursed infants generally was much higher than that of breastfed infants, because of unsuitable foods and feeding vessels and lack of a clean water supply (Fildes, 1986). The usual mortality of dry-nursed infants was put at two-thirds by some contemporary authors, five in six by others, and, in the case of some London parish infants, 90–100% (Nihell, 1760; Hanway, 1766). A letter written by Sir Hans Sloane to the vice president of the Foundling Hospital stated that the mortality of dry nursed infants was 53.9% compared with 19.2% for those suckled at the breast (Wickes, 1953). In France there are mortality records for infants who were either wet or dry nursed. At Lyons, foundlings were boarded out to wet nurses within 1 week of reception; the mortality in the first year of life was 33.7%. At Rheims, foundlings were boarded out early but were mainly hand reared; the mortality was 63.9%

(Wickes, 1953). This high mortality of dry-nursed infants led to medical and lay writers urgently advocating maternal breastfeeding as safer than both hand feeding and wet nursing.

In several industrializing countries, concern about high infant mortality (accompanied in some places by falling birth rates) during the late nineteenth and early twentieth centuries led many physicians and administrators to carry out surveys to determine exactly how infants were being fed (Brandstrom et al., 1984; Public Record Office, 1904; Woods et al., 1989). Some of these, as in Germany, were extremely detailed and, in some provinces, included virtually all infants born or living in the region (Kintner, 1985). Others, as in France, covered only infants sent out to nurse and subject to laws protecting such children (Sussman, 1982; Rollet, 1981). In Britain, local surveys were carried out mainly by health visitors, who were responsible for visiting newborn babies and recording the method of feeding on the first visit, and on subsequent visits made at three-monthly intervals (Newman, 1906; Public Record Office, 1904; Vincent, 1904). Infant welfare clinics also kept records of feeding methods (Newman, 1906; Vincent, 1904). The results of these local surveys are less satisfactory because, in many instances, not all the children born in a district were necessarily visited, or attended a clinic. Another problem is that some infant feeding surveys reported the method of feeding only of babies who had died, particularly if the cause of death was diarrheal disease. Others reported the findings for all children, living or dead. It is important, therefore, to discriminate between these, so as to compare like with like. Tables 4.1–4.6 show some results of these breastfeeding surveys.

As a result of this increased interest in the relationship between infant feeding and mortality, milk kitchens and infant welfare clinics were established; health visiting was extended; teaching of infant care to mothers and, in some countries, schoolgirls was instigated; and a campaign was mounted to promote maternal breastfeeding and, if this was not possible, to publicize the dangers of bottle feeding in unhygienic conditions (McCleary, 1933; Dwork, 1987; U.S. Department of Labour, 1913, 1922; Reiger, 1985; Fildes, 1991; Fildes, Marks and Marlard, 1992).

TIMING OF WEANING

The time of complete weaning from the breast varied according to period in history, nationality, local custom, and individual circumstance. An Egyptian papyrus referred to an infant being breastfed for 3 years (Montet, 1958), and records from Babylonia contain agreements with

Table 4.1. Mode of Feeding of Infants in the First Month of Life: British Towns 1903–1916

Place	Date	*Breastmilk* (%)	*Bottle fed* (%)	*Mixed* (%)
Brighton	1903–5	84.4	6.9	8.7
Paddington	1904	77.0	12.0	11.0
St. Pancras	1904	70.0	18.0	12.0
Finsbury	1905	82.5	7.8	9.7
Salford	1907	85.2	9.7	5.4
Salford	1908–10	85.1	7.4	7.4
Rhondda	1910	68.5	19.5	12.1
Rhondda	1911	75.1	21.7	3.2
Middlesbrough	1914	92.9	4.2	2.9
Middlesbrough	1915	98.0	—	—
Birmingham	1916	87.0	—	—

Sources: Medical Officer of Health, *Annual Reports;* G. Newman (1906) *Infant Mortality,* pp. 237–255. London; I. Buchanan (1985) Infant feeding, sanitation and diarrhoea in colliery communities, 1880–1911. In *Diet and Health in Modern Britain,* edited by D. J. Oddy and D. S. Miller, pp. 148–177. London: Croom Helm.

Table 4.2. Mode of Feeding of Infants Who Died from Diarrhoa: British Towns 1899–1911

Place	Date	*Breastfed* (%)	*Bottle fed* (%)	*Mixed* (%)
Rhondda	1899	15.0	—	—
Wigan	1900–1	17.4	77.7	4.9
Finsbury	1901–4	18.3	56.3	25.3
Preston	1903	7.4	72.8	19.8
Birmingham	1903	10.0	80.0	10.0
Brighton	1903–5	6.5	88.5	5.0
Ince	1905	20.7	72.4	6.9
Wigan	1906	23.0	72.7	4.3
Aberdare	1907	12.5	79.2	8.3
Wigan	1908	21.8	75.9	2.3
Wigan	1909	13.7	80.4	5.9
Wigan	1910	9.8	80.4	9.8
Preston	1911	7.3	87.3	5.4

Sources: Medical Officer of Health, *Annual Reports;* G. Newman (1906) *Infant Mortality,* pp. 237–255. London; R. Vincent (1904) *The Nutrition of the Infant,* pp. 266–288 London; I. Buchanan (1985) Infant feeding, sanitation and diarrhoea in colliery communities, 1880–1911. In *Diet and Health in Modern Britain,* edited by D. J. Oddy and D. S. Miller, pp. 148–177. London: Croom Helm.

Table 4.3. Mode of Feeding of Infants Who Died from Any Cause: British Towns 1891–1914

Place	*Date*	*Breastfed (%)*	*Bottle fed (%)*	*Mixed (%)*
Birmingham	1891	—	39.0	—
York	1905	11.0	84.0	5.0
Rhondda	1910	37.2	43.8	19.0
Rhondda	1911	30.5	58.8	10.7
Wigan	1914	34.0	51.3	14.7

Sources: Medical Officer of Health, *Annual Reports;* G. Newman (1906) *Infant Mortality,* pp. 254. London; R. Vincent (1904) *The Nutrition of the Infant,* p. 273, London; I. Buchanan (1985) Infant feeding, sanitation and diarrhoea in colliery communities, 1880–1911. In *Diet and Health in Modern Britain,* edited by D. J. Oddy and D. S. Miller, pp. 148–177. London: Croom Helm.

wet nurses that specified nursing for 2 or 3 years (Wallis-Budge, 1925). Three years was said to be common age of weaning for the Hebrews (Brim, 1936). An early Ayurvedic text from India recommends weaning from the breast only after the second birthday (Pal, 1973). Sources from Byzantium indicate the recommended age of weaning to be between 20 months and 2 years (Fildes, 1986). The Koran states that a child should be breastfed for at least 2 years. Soranus, in the first to second century A.D., felt that a child should be weaned once he was taking cereal food readily, and had teeth to chew more solid foods "which in the majority of cases takes place around the third or fourth half-year." Galen said that the child should be weaned completely after the age of 3 years. Fildes (1986) summarizes medical opinions on infant feeding from the Graeco-

Table 4.4. Mode of Feeding of Infants in the First Month of Life: United States 1917–1919

Place	*Breastfed (%)*	*Bottle fed (%)*	*Mixed (%)*
Rural Kansas	92.0	2.00	6.0
Rural southern Wisconsin	92.0	6.00	2.0
Rural northern Wisconsin	89.0	6.0	6.0
Saginaw, Michigan	88.0	9.0	3.0
Akron, Ohio	88.0	8.0	4.0
New Bedford, Massachusetts	83.0	12.0	5.0
Manchester, New Hampshire	82.0	15.0	3.0

Source: Adapted from R. Apple (1987) *Mothers and Medicine: A Social History of Infant Feeding 1890–1950,* p. 153. Madison, WI: University of Wisconsin Press.

Table 4.5. Mode of Feeding of Infants in the First Month of Life: New South Wales 1904–1914

Place	*Date*	*Breastfed (%)*	*Bottle fed (%)*	*Mixed (%)*
City of Sydney	1904	72.2	6.50	21.3
City of Sydney	1909	82.8	2.2	15.0
City and suburbs, Sydney	1912	85.9	4.6	9.5
City of Sydney	1913	92.1	2.4	5.4
New South Wales	1913	90.2	2.6	7.3
Newcastle	1914	62.6	1.0	27.4
City and suburbs, Sydney	1914	94.1	2.4	3.5

Sources: Medical Journal of Australia (1915), 1. 112, 364; (1917) 1. 45–46; (1939) 2. 643; C. K. Mackellar (1917) *The Mother, the Baby, and the State*, p. 11. Syndey.

Roman, Byzantine, and Arabian periods between 98 A.D. and 1036 A.D. and notes that the recommended age of weaning varies between 18 months and 3 years.

During the medieval period of Europe weaning age varied between 1 and 2 years. During the Renaissance the normal duration of nursing was usually 2 years (Fildes, 1988) although by the late fifteenth and sixteenth centuries several types of artificial feeding had come into fashion (Davidson, 1953). Children were given cows' milk or goats' milk from sucking horns, sucking cans with cloth nipples, bottles, and spoons (Davidson, 1953). Even as late as the 1740s, medical authorities were basing their advice on the length of breastfeeding on the ancient physicians such as Soranus, Galen and Avicenna (Fildes, 1986). In the six-

Table 4.6. Mode of Feeding of Infants Who Died from Diarrhea in the City of Sydney 1903–1906

Year	*Breastfed (%)*	*Wholly or partially bottle fed (%)*
1903	4.3	95.7
1904	3.0	94.0
1906	11.5	88.5

Source: Adapted from M. Lewis (1980) The problem of infant feeding: The Australian experience from the mid-nineteenth century to the 1920's. *Journal of Historical Medicine* 35:174–187.

Table 4.7. Median Weaning Age in Two Countries

Country	*City*	*Period*	*Weaning age (months)*
Britain		Early sixteenth century	18
Britain		Mid sixteenth to seventeenth century	12–17
Britain		Late eighteenth century	7–9
Italy	Florence	Early nineteenth century	12
	Rome	Early nineteenth century	14
	Brescia	Early nineteenth century	18
	Perugia	Early nineteenth century	24

teenth and seventeenth centuries this ranged from 21 to 24 months, although the age at which children were actually weaned appeared to be somewhat less, between 11 and 12 months. The reason for the recommendation, from antiquity until the early eighteenth century, that weaning occur at 18–24 months was because this was the age by which most children possessed all their teeth.

In Britain, the median weaning age changed from 12 to 17 months in the sixteenth and seventeenth centuries to between 7 and 9 months in the late eighteenth century (Table 4.7). In Italy in the early nineteenth century, different regions weaned their infants at different ages ranging from 12 to 24 months (Table 4.7) (Livi Bacci, 1977). The weaning age for an area can often be deduced from the length of time allowed for the wet nursing of infants in foundling institutions. In the Italian survey mentioned above, the city foundling hospitals followed the local custom for weaning. Children of the London Foundling Hospital in the eighteenth century were apparently weaned at about 12 months of age. Variation in weaning age could depend on a variety of factors, for example, some physicians recommended that boys be weaned 6 to 12 months later than girls (Jones, 1579). This was the practice in some parts of France, where girls were weaned at 1 year and boys at 2 years (Fildes, 1986). Weaning age also varied from child to child and family to family depending on various factors including the health of the child, the season of year, phase of the moon, and circumstance of the mother (Fildes, 1986).

The benefits of breastfeeding and the dangers of weaning were understood even in historical times. For example, in medieval times it was recommended that sickly children be breastfed longer than normal, as well as twins and male infants, and that weaning not occur in the hot days of summer (Fildes, 1988). It is now known that the immunological and health benefits of breastfeeding can extend even into the second and third year of a breastfed child's life (Wray, 1990). It is very possible that differences in timing of weaning could have had a recognized impact on the health and disease patterns of infants in different times and cultures.

SUPPLEMENTAL FOODS

Feeding vessels have been found in infant graves from 4000 B.C. onward, and analysis has shown some to contain residues of milk (Lacaille, 1950). Illustrations record the use to which such vessels were put, and descriptions in the literature range from artificial nipples in the Roman Empire to animal horns in the dry-nursing of some medieval saints (McLaughlan, 1976), sucking-bottles in fifteenth-century Germany, to the widespread custom of handfeeding in nineteenth-century Europe and North America (Fildes, 1981). Whether such utensils were used for supplementary feeding only or whether—and how often—babies were artificially fed from birth is impossible to determine.

There is evidence that early in recorded history ritual substances and/or the milk of a woman other than the infant's own mother were often given to a newborn infant. For example, Indian texts from the fourth century B.C. to the first century A.D. advocate giving a newborn an electuary of honey, clarified butter, and the expressed juice of Brahmi leaves and Anata, mixed with a little gold dust (Susruta Samhita, fourth–second centuries B.C.) For the first few days the infant was not fed milk, but was fed three times (morning, noon, and evening) on the first day with clarified butter and honey, mixed with Anata roots that had been sanctified with a mantra. On the second and third days the infant was to be fed on clarified butter prepared with Lakshana root. It was advised that mother's milk and honey both be given from the fourth day on. In the first century A.D. Soranus of Ephesus, a physician, recommended that the first food given a newborn child be boiled honey, or honey and goats' milk. He felt that for the first 20 days the maternal milk was unwholesome, so the child should be fed by a wet nurse. Women did a number of things to maintain their milk supply, including being suckled by other animals. Between 1550 and the end of the eighteenth century many medical writers made recommendations about the first food of neonates, or described the common practice (Fildes, 1988). The recommendations include colostrum, breast milk from another woman, a purge, food, medicinal substances, and combinations of these (Fildes, 1982). The most popular and enduring purge was butter/oil of sweet almonds combined with sugar/honey/syrup. This combination is very ancient; it is mentioned in the Old Testament (*Isaiah*, 7, 15) and was recommended by Soranus in the first/second century A.D. (Soranus, first/second century A.D.) There was a slow change in medical ideas about colostrum (i.e., putting the baby to the mother's breast within the first few days of birth) dating from the end of the seventeenth century. Before this time, mothers were often advised not to breastfeed their child for up to a month after delivery.

The idea that the mother's first milk or colostrum is a "bad" substance that should be expressed and discarded before the child is allowed to suck was a belief of a number of cultures throughout history. However, this first milk has important protective and nutritive functions. It aids the evacuation of the sticky, black contents (meconium) of the neonate's intestine, and contains several antibodies and other proteins that protect the newborn infant from bacterial infections. It also has concentrated amounts of nutrients, including zinc, which have been shown to be very important in protecting against neonatal infections. About the third or fourth day after delivery, colostrum is gradually replaced by more normal-looking milk, but this retains certain properties until the infant is several weeks of age. Clearly, the newborn infant who is breastfed from the first day by its mother, and receives these important substances, will stand a better chance of fighting infections than one who is fed with "older" breast milk or substitute foods. Cultural differences in ideas and/or practice in the feeding of the newborn could have significantly affected the health and survival of infants in the first weeks of life.

Some of the earliest information about supplementary foods comes from Greek and Roman Egypt. This information stipulates that once a child is several months old, it should be fed other foods than breastmilk, particularly animal milk and eggs, and that even after weaning its principal food be the milk of animals such as camels, goats, sheep and cows (Herodotus, fifth century B.C.; Montet, 1958; Radbill, 1973). Additional foods were introduced into the child's diet quite late, and these were almost exclusively of fruit and vegetable origin. The physician Soranus, writing of Rome in the first and second centuries, strongly recommended that infants should be fed only on breast milk until about 6 months old, but makes it clear that this was not necessarily general practice:

> Those women are too hasty who, after only 40 days, try to give cereal food (as do those for the most part who find nursing a burden). (Soranus, first/second century A.D.)

Once the infant could digest it, he suggested crumbs of bread that had been softened with hydromel or milk, sweet wine, or honey wine. For later he suggested soup made from spelt (a grain), a very moist porridge, and an egg that could be sipped.

The Lives of the Saints (Shahar, 1983) records that during the first millennium in Britain some 3-month-old babies were drinking fluids other than breast milk, and that slightly older children were being given solid foods long before weaning. The age at which supplementary foods were introduced varied according to local custom, but there is a considerable body of evidence that in preindustrial Europe, some mothers administered extra nourishment in the form of cereal pap (a mixture of flour or bread cooked in water) or animal milk from soon after birth (Fildes, 1986). In country areas, especially in France and Italy, when mothers or wet nurses had insufficient breast milk, infants were suckled by animals such as goats, sheep, and asses (Fildes, 1986). According to Wickes (1953), in eighteenth-century Europe the differentiation between hand and breastfeeding became progressively more meaningless since it was probably customary to give pap and panada in addition to the breast. In 1783, De Claubry, a French physician, described pap as "the most dangerous of all foods for infants" in that "it has caused to perish a great number, or has rendered them infirm and diseased all their lives" (Wickes, 1953).

It is now known that the ideal situation for maintaining and preserving the immunological benefits of breastfeeding is for the infant to receive breast milk alone for at least the first 6 months (Gerrard, 1974). The high-lactose, low-phosphate, and low-protein content of breast milk produces a low pH in the gastrointestinal tract that is inimical to the growth of bacteria. The introduction of cow's milk, or any other food, elevates the pH of the intestine and stool and provides a medium for the colonization of bacteria, including *Escherichia coli*. Therefore, throughout history, a young infant who had not been supplemented with animal's milk or other foods would have had an immunological advantage over infants who had been fed a supplemented diet.

WEANING FOODS

There is little reference to foods being given to infants as supplements or during weaning from the breast in ancient Greece, although the simple milk and cereal dishes later mentioned by Soranus (first/second century A.D.) and Galen (the second-century physician), were probably employed. After weaning, children were said to have been fed on milk and honey and apparently young children thrived on the shoots of fig trees (Rosaria, 1917). There are references to nurses chewing food before giving it to the child, and Atheneus told of a man who had his nurse chew his food for him all his life (Rosaria, 1917). Foods to be eaten during weaning from the breast were discussed by numerous medical writers through the centuries. Weaning foods usually differed from those suggested for mixed feeding, with fewer milk foods and increased use of meat broths and other meat dishes, which were not usually advised for children until they had teeth with which to chew them. Specific foods recommended by most authors included chicken broth, prechewed meat, meat broths, bread and butter, pap and panada, and porridge.

At the beginning of the seventeenth century the French obstetrician Guillemeau wrote a text on infant nutrition in which he advocated that weaning begin when the upper and lower incisors have erupted, with the giving of sops, bread, panada (a mixture of flour, cereal, or bread, cooked in a broth, and combined with butter or milk), or gruel. Later (at about 15 months) minced poultry was to be added, with meat after the age of 2 (Wickes, 1953). Advice about pre- and postweaning diet was confined mainly to the eighteenth century, and, especially after 1750, most relates to the earlier age of weaning in that century. Before then, children were assumed by medical authors to be at least a year old, probably well into their second year of life, and in possession of several teeth, before weaning was considered; they were expected to continue until then on the paps and panadas used for mixed feeding. This implies that by the time it was ready to be weaned, a child was able to sit up at table, had some ability to feed itself, had teeth with which to chew a variety of hard foods, including meat, and generally behaved more like a child than an infant.

The description given by the physician John Jones (1579) of the food given to the children of the French king after weaning would probably apply to most wealthy English households in the same period:

> Bread of fine wheate floure, of fine starch, also of almonds, of barley, or bigge, of wheat, which we call furmentie, of rye, of pease and suchlike, or soft bread steeped in the broath of fleshe of kiddes, tuppes, calves, hennes, etc. And sometimes a capon's wing minced in small pieces, or the breast of a pheasant rosted, cut in pieces.

Milk foods, and milk as a drink, were not a normal part of the adult diet of the wealthier sections of society. Milk was held to be a food for infants (i.e., children who were not weaned), the very old, and the sick, which explains its absence in the suggested weaning diets of this era.

If such a diet—devoid of fresh fruits, vegetables, and dairy products—were given to richer children regularly, over a long period, then diseases such as scurvy, rickets, bladderstone, and some degree of night blindness, accompanied by a lowered resistance to infection, would have been common among young children after weaning because, in a mainly meat and cereal diet that excludes fresh fruits, vegetables, and dairy foods, vitamins A, D, and C are absent and the amount of calcium may be insufficient for a growing child. Children of poorer families, whose diet consisted mainly of bread, cheese, salt meat (predominantly pork), and pulses may have fared better in nutritional terms (provided they received a sufficient quantity) than richer children. In the sixteenth century white meats or dairy foods, including eggs, were eaten by the poor and, as many cottagers kept a cow, milk was more likely to be consumed by these people than by the wealthy.

By the eighteenth century the situation had changed. Infants were considered ready for weaning before they could sit up at a table. They had few or no teeth, little ability to feed themselves, and were more vulnerable to diseases, especially of the gastrointestinal tract, than children of 1 to 2 years. Medical writers recognized an association between weaning and rickets. Young (1780) reported that rickets was rare before weaning. The "weaning illness" or "weaning brash" was a gastrointestinal disorder that occurred when children were weaned from the breast. The Scottish surgeon John Aitken described one of the causes as early weaning. Leanness, wasting (a gradual loss of weight), and poor growth were particularly associated with early weaning and with improper foods and too sudden change of the milk for solid foods at weaning. Wasting was part of the weaning illness described by Aitken (1786) and would have been associated with symptoms such as diarrhea and vomiting.

Weaning is known to be a precarious time for a young child, particularly when weaning foods are inappropriate or the environment of the child is generally unhygienic, resulting in contaminated foods. Throughout most of history, for most children, weaning was a slow, gradual process that was initiated only after a number of teeth had erupted. However, in Europe, by the eighteenth century, children began to be weaned before they had teeth or could sit up at a table. The result was an increase in diseases of the gastrointestinal tract, rickets, and growth disorders.

CONCLUSIONS

Historical data provide a window into the past through which the customs, living conditions, and health and disease of ancient populations can be viewed. They make it possible to see how mothers and infants throughout history have been affected by the style of infant feeding practiced. The data show that there are very complex interactions between the biology and culture of breastfeeding. Customs relating to breastfeeding practices and supplemental and weaning foods have varied immensely depending on the geographic locale and time period. However, it does appear that the beneficial effects of breastfeeding for mother and child have been known since time immemorial. Breastfeeding was known to affect the nutrition, the physical and psychological health of the child, and the health and fertility of the mother. As this chapter has shown, the decision to breastfeed or not and the timing and type of supplemental and weaning foods have had profound effects on maternal and infant health throughout history.

ACKNOWLEDGMENTS

Research for this paper was funded by Nestlé (UK) Ltd. and the Wellcome Trust. I wish to thank one of the editors, Patricia Stuart-Macadam, for her active help and encouragement in completing this paper.

REFERENCES

Aitken, J.
1786 *Principles of Midwifery*, 3rd ed. London.
Anonymous
1739 *Ladies Physical Directory: By a Physician*, 7th ed. London.
Apple, R.
1987 *Mothers and Medicine: A Social History of Infant Feeding 1890–1950*, p. 153. Madison: University of Wisconsin Press.
Badineter, E.
1981 *The Myth of Motherhood: An Historical View of the Maternal Instinct*, translated by R. DeGaris. London: Souvenir Press.
Brandstrom, A., G. Brostrom, and L. A. Persson
1984 The impact of feeding patterns on infant mortality in a nineteenth century Swedish parish. *Journal of Tropical Pediatrics* 30:154–159.
Brim, C. J.
1936 Medicine in the Bible. *The Pentateuch.* New York: Torah.
Buchanan, I.
1985 Infant feeding, sanitation and diarrhoea in colliery communities, 1880–1911. In *Diet and Health in Modern Britain*, edited by D. J. Oddy and D. S. Miller, pp. 148–177. London: Croom Helm.
Cadogan, W.
1748 *An Essay Upon Nursing and the Management of Children from Their Birth to Three Years of Age*. London.
Davidson, W. D.
1953 A brief history of infant feeding. *Journal of Pediatrics* 43:74–87.

Dionis, P.
1719 *A General Treatise on Midwifery*. Trans., anon. London.
Downman, H.
1788 *Infancy or, The Management of Children. A Didactic Poem in Six Books*, 4th ed. London: printed for G. Kearsly. Drake, Mrs.
1908 A study of infant life in Westminster. *Journal of the Royal Statistical Society* 71:678–686. Drake, T. G. H. 1935 Infant welfare laws in France in the 18th century, *Annals of Medical History* 7 (N. S.), 49–61.
Dwork, D.
1987 *War Is Good for Babies and Other Young Children: A History of the Infant and Child Welfare Movement in England 1898–1918*. London: Tavistock.
Eekelen, A. K.
1986 Towards a rational infant feeding. The science of nutrition and paediatrics in Netherlands (1840–1914). In *Childcare through the Centuries*, edited by J. Cole and E. Turner, pp. 153–164. Cardiff: British Society for the History of Medicine.
Fildes, V. A.
1981 The early history of the infant feeding bottle. *Nursing Times* 77:128–129 and 168–170.
1982 *The History of Infant Feeding* 1500–1800. Unpublished Ph.D. thesis, Department of Human Biology and Health, University of Surrey.
1986 *Breasts, Bottles and Babies: A History of Infant Feeding*. Edinburgh: Edinburgh University Press.
1988 *Wet Nursing: A History from Antiquity to the Present*. Oxford: Basil Blackwell.
1990 *Women as Mothers in Pre-Industrial England*. London: Routledge.
1991 Breast-feeding practices during industrialization 1800–1919. In *Infant and Child Nutrition Worldwide: Issues and Perspectives*, edited by Frank Falkner, pp. 1–20. Boca Raton, FL: CRC Press.
Fildes, V. A., L. Marks, and H. Marlard
1992 *Women and Children First: International Maternal and Infant Welfare, 1870–1945*. London: Routledge.
Flandrin, J-L.
1979 *Families in Former Times: Kinship, Household and Sexuality*, translated by R. Southern. Cambridge: Cambridge University Press.
Garrison, F. H.
1965 *History of Pediatrics*. Philadelphia, PA: W. B. Saunders.
Gerrard, J. W.
1974 Breast-feeding: Second thoughts. *Pediatrics* 54(6):757–763.
Gouge, W.
1622 *Of Domestical Duties. Eight Treatises*. London: printed by John Haviland for William Bladen.
Hanway, J.
1766 *An Earnest Appeal For Mercy to the Children of the Poor*. London: J. Dodsley.
Herodotus
Fifth century B.C. *The Famous History of Herodotus*, translated B. R. 1584, in the Tudor translations, second series, 6, London, 1924.

Hewitt, M.
1958 *Wives and Mothers in Victorian Industry*. London: Rockliff.
Jones, H. R.
1894 The perils and protection of infant life. *Journal of the Royal Statistical Society* 57:1–103.
Jones, J.
1579 *The Arte and Science of Preserving Bodie and Soule in Health, Wisedome, and Catholicke Religion: Physically, Philosophically and Devinely Devised*. London.
Kintner, H. J.
1985 Trends and regional differences in breastfeeding in Germany from 1871 to 1937. *Journal of Family History* 10:161–182.
Knecht-van Eekelen, A.
1986 Towards a rational infant feeding. The science of nutrition and paediatrics in the Netherlands (1840–1914). In *Childcare Throughout the Centuries*, edited by J. Cule and E. Turner, pp. 153–164. Cardiff: British Society for the History of Medicine. Also personal communication.
Knodel, J.
1968 Infant mortality and fertility in three Bavarian villages: An analysis of family histories from the nineteenth century. *Population Studies* 22:297–318.
Knodel, J., and H. Kinter
1977 The impact of breast feeding patterns on the biometric analysis of infant mortality. *Demography* 14(4):391–409.
Knodel, J., and E. van der Waale
1967 Breastfeeding, fertility and infant mortality: An analysis of some early German data. *Population Studies* 21:109–131.
Lacaille, A. D.
1950 Infant feeding bottles in prehistoric times. *Proceedings of the Royal Society of Medicine* 43:565–568.
Lewis, M.
1980 The problem of infant feeding: The Australian experience from the mid-nineteenth century to the 1920s. *Journal of Historical Medicine* 35:174–187.
Lithell, U. B.
1981 Breastfeeding habits and their relation to infant mortality and marital fertility. *Journal of Family History* 6:182–194.
Livi Bacci, M.
1977 *A History of Italian Fertility During the Last Two Centuries*. Princeton, NJ: Princeton University Press.
Locke, W.
1693 *Some Thoughts Concerning Education*. London.
Mackellar, C. K.
1917 *The Mother, the Baby, and the State*, p. 11. Sydney.
McClaren, D.
1978 Fertility, infant mortality, and breastfeeding in the seventeenth century. *Medical History* 22:378–396.
McCleary, G. F.
1933 *The Early History of the Infant Welfare Movement*. London: H. K. Lewis.

Mclaughlan, M. M.
1976 Survivors and surrogates: Children and parents from the ninth to the thirteenth centuries. In *The History of Childhood*, edited by L. De Mause, pp. 101–181.
Montet, P.
1958 *Everyday Life in Egypt in the Days of Rameses the Great*. Translated by A. R. Maxwell-Hyslop and M. S. Drower. London: E. Arnold.
Newcome, H.
1695 *The Compleat Mother or, An Earnest Persuasive to all Mothers (especially those of Rank and Quality) to Nurse Their Own Children*. London.
Newman, G.
1906 *Infant Mortality: A Social Problem*. London: Methuen.
Newsholme, A.
1906 Domestic infection in relation to epidemic diarrhoea. *Journal of Hygiene* 6:139–148.
Nihell, E.
1760 *A Treatise on the Art of Midwifery*. London: A. Morley.
Pal, M. N.
1973 The Ayurvedic tradition of child care. Pediatric wisdom of Ancient India. *Clinical Pediatrics* 12:122–123.
Public Record Office
1904 Report of the Royal Commission of the decline of the birthrate and on the mortality of infants in New South Wales, 904. London, Maternal and Child Welfare files, MH 48.
Radbill, S. X.
1963 Pediatrics in the Bible. *Clinical Pediatrics* 2:199–212.
1973 Mesopotamian pediatrics. *Episteme* 7:283–288.
Reiger, K. M.
1985 *The Disenchantment of the Home: Modernizing the Australian family 1880–1940*, pp. 128–152. Melbourne: Oxford University Press.
Rollet, C.
1981 Infant feeding, fosterage and infant mortality in France at the end of the nineteenth century. *Population*. Selected papers 7:1–14.
Rosaria, Sister M.
1917 *The Nurse in Greek Life*. Unpublished Ph.D. dissertation. Catholic University of America, Boston.
Rousseau, J. L.
1762 *Émile*, Translated by Emile B. Foxley. London, 1911.
Ruffer, M. A.
1921 *Studies in the Paleopathology of Egypt*, edited by R. L. Moodie. Chicago: University of Chicago Press.
Shahar, S.
1983 Infants, infant care, and attitudes towards infancy in the medieval lives of the saints. *Journal of Psychohistory* 10(3):81–309.
Shorter, E.
1977 *The Making of the Modern Family*. New York: Basic Books.

Smith, H.
1774 *Letters to Married Women on Nursing and the Management of Children*, 3rd ed. London.
Soranus of Ephesus
1956 First/second century A.D. *Soranus' Gynecology*. Translation by O. Temkin with the assistance of J. Nicholson. Baltimore: Johns Hopkins University Press.
Sussman, G. D.
1982 *Selling Mothers' Milk: The Wet-nursing Business in France 715–1914*. Chicago: University of Illinois Press.
Susruta Samhita
Fourth–second centuries B.C. An English translation of the Susruta Samhita, Translated by K. K. L. Bishagratna, Vol. 2, Calcutta, 1911.
Szreter, S. R. S.
1983 *The Decline of Marital Fertility in England and Wales c. 870–1914: A Critique of the Theory of Social Class Differentials*. Unpublished Ph.D. Dissertation, University of Cambridge.
Thompson, B.
1984 Infant mortality in nineteenth-century Bradford. In *Urban Disease and Mortality in Nineteenth-Century England*, edited by R. Woods and J. Woodward, pp. 120–147. London: Batsford.
Tilly, L. A., and J. W. Scott
1978 *Women, Work, and Family*. New York: Holt, Rinehart & Winston.
Tilly, L. A., J. W. Scott, and M. Cohen
1980 Women's work and European fertility patterns. In *Marriage and Fertility: Studies in Interdisciplinary History*, edited by R. I. Rotberg and T. K. Rabb, pp. 219–248. Princeton: Princeton University Press.
Trumbach, R.
1978 *The Rise of the Egalitarian Family*. New York: Academic Press.
U. S. Department of Labor
1913 Children's Bureau Baby-saving campaigns. A preliminary report on what American cities are doing to prevent infant mortality. Washington, DC: U. S. Government Printing Office.
1922 Children's Bureau Infant Mortality and Preventative Work in New Zealand. Washington, DC: U. S. Government Printing Office.
Vincent, R.
1904 *The Nutrition of the Infant*, pp. 266–288. London: Religious Tract Society
Wallis Budge, E. A.
1925 *Babylonian Life and History*. London: Religious Tract Society.
Wickes, I. G.
1953 A history of infant feeding. *Archives of Diseases in Childhood* 28:151–158, 232–240, 332–340, 416–422, 495–502.
Woodbury, R. M.
1926 *Infant Mortality and its Causes*. Baltimore, MD: Williams & Wilkins.
Woods, R. I., P. A. Watterson, and J. H. Woodward
1989 The causes of rapid infant mortality decline in England and Wales, 1861–1921. *Population Studies*.

Wray, J. D.
1990 Breast-feeding: An international and historical review. In *Infant and Child Nutrition Worldwide: Issues and Perspectives,* edited by F. Falkner, pp. 61–116. Boca Raton, FL: CRC Press.
Young, G.
1780 *A Treatise on Opium.* London.

5

Sociocultural Aspects of the Lactation Process

Sara A. Quandt

INTRODUCTION

Breastfeeding is better viewed as a behavioral domain than as a single feeding behavior. This domain consists of a number of dimensions that can be isolated and described to characterize the breastfeeding individual woman or the modal patterns of breastfeeding by groups. The most important of these dimensions of breastfeeding include (1) whether and when breastfeeding is initiated, (2) the frequency, duration, and timing of breastfeeding episodes, and (3) the duration of exclusive breastfeeding.

Breastfeeding is similar to other forms of eating in that the variation in its component behaviors is regulated by the social and cultural milieu in which the participants interact. And as with other types of eating behavior, variants of breastfeeding behaviors have meanings and values ascribed to them that are consistent with other aspects of the culture of which the mother–infant dyad is a part.

Yet breastfeeding is distinct from other domains of feeding behaviors in one critical aspect. Variations in its component behaviors have clear biological ramifications for the entire lactation process, affecting everything from the amount of milk available to the child, to the nutrient content of the milk, to the nutritional and reproductive status of the mother. This chapter will review the biobehavioral interactions of breastfeeding. It will then use historical and cross-cultural data to demonstrate how these biobehavioral interactions have been shaped by social and cultural factors into the wide variety of infant feeding practices extant today.

BIOBEHAVIORAL INTERACTIONS OF BREASTFEEDING

Breastfeeding of any kind depends on early initiation of suckling. This early initiation triggers the production and ejection of milk through hormonally regulated processes that have been described only in the last several decades. The preparation of the breast to respond to the infant's stimulation is part of the total reproductive cycle that commences at conception and ends at the resumption of regular ovulatory cycles postpartum in the mother. While reports of lactation without pregnancy (Waletzky and Herman, 1976) and of relactation (Phillips, 1993) exist, they are few, and indicate that lactation in women whose bodies have not been prepared during pregnancy requires both specific knowledge and a lot of effort to achieve. Thus, unlike other modes of feeding for infants or adults, there is a specific "window of opportunity" within which breastfeeding must be initiated; failure to do so greatly reduces the possibility of maternal lactation serving as a nutrient source for an infant.

At parturition, the rapid and abrupt fall in progesterone triggers the production of milk, lactogenesis (see Glasier and McNeilly, 1990, for a recent review). Once breastfeeding is initiated, the frequency of suckling and its duration regulate the volume and nutrient content of the milk. The primary hormonal process at work is the production of prolactin, which promotes the synthesis of milk. The mechanisms through which prolactin influences milk production are not well understood (Institute of Medicine, 1991). As a reflex to the infant suckling at the breast, prolactin is released from the anterior pituitary almost immediately. Elevations in prolactin cause milk to be synthesized in the breast within 2 to 3 hours of the prolactin release. Prolactin levels begin to fall immediately after its release, so that within 2 hours of a suckling event, serum concentrations are back to baseline. Its lactogenic activity is thus limited to a short period immediately following its release unless suckling occurs so frequently that prolactin levels remain elevated. There appears to be a greater prolactin release in response to suckling in the afternoon than in the morning (Glasier, McNeilly and Howie, 1984). Such findings need to be validated cross-culturally, as prolactin patterns may be different among women who have a more continuous feeding style, with co-sleeping and frequent night feeds. However, this daily variation in prolactin secretion is also seen in nonlactating women. Research on nonhumans suggests that the basal level of prolactin may vary with suckling intensity, but this has been difficult to quantify for humans. It has been suggested that Lunn, Watkinson, Prentice, Morrell, Austin and Whitehead's (1981) finding that malnourished women have elevated basal prolactin levels is the result of stronger sucking required by the infants to obtain adequate milk supplies (Glasier and McNeilly, 1990).

The volume of milk varies as a function of suckling frequency, and this is probably related to prolactin levels. Both experimental manipulation of nursing frequency and observations of normal variation in frequency have confirmed this supply and demand feature of lactation (Egli, Egli and Newton, 1961; Rattigan, Ghisalberti and Hartmann, 1981). The more frequent the nursing episodes, the greater the volume of milk. Conversely, as the number of nursing episodes is decreased and the time between them increases, the volume of milk produced declines. This relationship is most pronounced in the early stages of lactation.

Milk production may be controlled by a negative feedback system, as well as by prolactin levels. Wilde, Addey, Casey, Blatchford and Peaker (1988) report that a constituent of the whey protein in milk inhibits milk secretion in a dose-dependent manner. The accumulation of milk in the breast presumably inhibits the production of more milk through the increased concentration of this inhibitor. Without the emptying of the breast, lactogenesis eventually stops. This may be the mechanism through which the decrease in milk production with engorgement observed in animals occurs (Neville and Neifert, 1983). Similarly, this may explain why mothers report differences in milk production between breasts associated with infants' preference for one side over the other.

The actual ejection of milk from the breast is regulated by oxytocin. Its release from the posterior pituitary is stimulated by nerve impulses sent to the hypothalamus as a result of suckling. Oxytocin causes the myoepithelial cells in the breast to contract. This reflex ejects milk from the storage alveoli to the lacteal sinuses. The infant can then easily remove it during nursing (Woolridge and Baum, 1988). This reflex differs from the lactogenic reflex in that it is under psychosomatic control (Newton and Newton, 1967). Psychological factors such as anxiety or fear can lead to an increased level of epinephrine, which causes constriction of blood vessels around the alveoli and decreased circulation of the oxytocin necessary for milk ejection (Jelliffe and Jelliffe, 1978).

Nutrient composition of breast milk is also under the biobehavioral control of nursing frequency, though composition is generally regarded as less labile than milk volume. Prolactin has a number of metabolic effects. In particular, its level is linked to fat. Higher levels of serum prolactin result in increased lipoprotein lipase (LPL) activity in mammary tissue and decreased LPL activity in other fat tissue (Scow, Mendelson, Zinder, Hamosh and Blanchette-Mackie, 1973; Zinder, Hamosh, Fleck and Scow, 1974). This has the effect of mobilizing fat stores in peripheral tissues and increasing the uptake of fatty acids in the breast for incorporation into breast milk (Hamosh, 1980). Quandt (1983) found that women who nursed more frequently showed greater decreases in upper arm fat (measured as upper arm fat area) than women practicing a less frequent nursing pattern. Kramer, Stunkard, Marshall, McKinney and Liebschutz (1993) have shown site-specific differences in fat patterns related to nursing. Prolactin has also been linked to casein synthesis and lactose levels in animals (Horrobin, 1979).

Thus, breastfeeding constitutes an infant feeding mode in which the amount and composition of the food are biologically regulated by both maternal behaviors and infant behaviors. These behaviors vary widely, influenced by biological, social, and cultural forces. It is important to realize that the patterns of breastfeeding produced by these factors are highly varied, and that the common approach of classifying breastfeeding as "restricted" versus "on demand," or "mother-led" versus "baby-led" (Woolridge, Ingram and Baum, 1990) conveys a false simplicity.

BREASTFEEDING BEHAVIORS AND BIRTH-SPACING

In addition to regulating aspects of milk production directly, maternal breastfeeding behaviors affect infant nutrition *indirectly* through their impact on ovulation and, thus, on birth-spacing. The connection between breastfeeding and birth-spacing is well established in the demographic literature, with the duration of postpartum infecundability considered a function of the duration and intensity of suckling (Bongaarts, 1978; Bongaarts and Potter, 1983; Wood, 1990). Knauer (1985) was able to demonstrate this connection in a prospective study of Canadian women. However, competing explanations for fecundity regulation also exist, because the actual mechanisms by which fecundity is regulated are not entirely clear.

The major competing explanation centers on maternal nutritional status. In view of the apparently longer duration of postpartum amenorrhea in malnourished mothers, poor maternal nutritional status, particularly low percent body fat, has been suggested as a factor delaying the return of ovulation postpartum. This follows from the work of Rose Frisch and colleagues who have argued that fecundity, in a range of circumstances from menarche to amenorrhea in athletes to lactational amenorrhea, depends on a critical minimum percentage of body fat (Frisch, 1990; Frisch and Revelle, 1971; Frisch, Revelle and Cook, 1973; Frisch, Snow, Gerard, Johnson, Kennedy, Barbieri and Rosen, 1992; Frisch, Snow, Johnson, Gerard, Barbieri and Rosen, 1993).

This explanation is a logical extension of the evolutionary concept of "nutritional thriftiness," which argues that morphological forms and physiological processes that conserve energy should have been selected in the course of human evolution (James and Trayhurn, 1976; Stini, 1975). The investment of energy in reproduction only when the maternal resources necessary to guarantee success (infant survival) are present is a logical outcome of such selective pressures (Quandt, 1984b). Early criticisms of Frisch's explanation focused on her supporting data, particularly measurement and statistical issues (Johnston, Roche, Schell and Wettenhall, 1975; Scott and Johnston, 1982), and conflicting studies (Billewicz, Fellowes and Hytten, 1976; Cameron, 1976; Huffman, Chowdhury and Mosley, 1978) without considering the physiological processes and breastfeeding behaviors that might support her general argument for reproductive nutritional thriftiness.

In an attempt to integrate the nutritional and lactational explanations for fecundity regulation, Quandt (1984b) proposed a model that emphasized existing knowledge of the behavioral regulation of lactation physiology. She proposed that frequent breastfeeding should be associated with anovulation and decreasing or stable adipose stores, both being hormonally induced. Infrequent feeding, conversely, should be associated with the return of ovulation and *either* increasing or decreasing adiposity, depending upon the dietary intake of the mother. More recent work using advances in nutritional assessment and endocrinology supports this model, and provides evidence for the direct link originally proposed between fatness and fecundity (e.g., Frisch, 1990; Frisch et al., 1992, 1993; Maclure, Travis, Willett and MacMahon, 1991). The issue is by no means settled.

BREASTFEEDING STYLE: A KEY CONCEPT

Research on breastfeeding suggests that the manner in which social and cultural factors affect infant well-being is in the regulation of those breastfeeding behaviors that affect milk volume, milk composition, and maternal reproductive status. Those key behaviors have been patterned into what has been called "breastfeeding style" (Quandt, 1985, 1986). Figure 5.1 shows the pathways by which these breastfeeding styles lead to different infant health outcomes. Social and cultural factors will have their greatest effect if they influence the initiation and duration of breastfeeding, the spacing and frequency of breastfeeding episodes, and the role other foods play in the infant's diet.

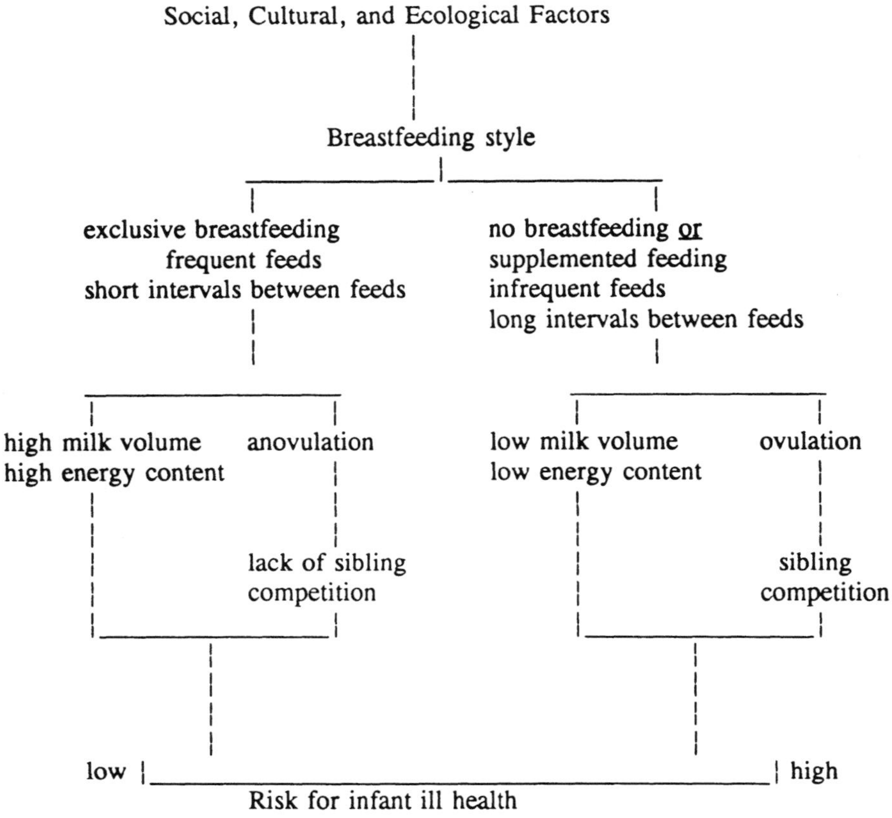

Figure 5.1. Model for the impact of breastfeeding style on infant health.

IMPACT OF SOCIAL AND CULTURAL FACTORS ON BREASTFEEDING STYLE

Recent research on infants stresses the active role infants can take in meeting their own needs and demanding responses from their caregivers. McKenna and Mosko (1993), for example, report co-sleeping infants actively "positioning and repositioning themselves with respect to their mothers," mostly to achieve a position that facilitates nursing. In addition, a variety of studies have found that infants can regulate their intake volume and fat intake by infant-led variation in degree of breast-emptying, length of feeding episodes, and between-feed intervals (Matheny, Birch and Picciano, 1990; Tyson, Burchfield, Sentance, Mize,

Uauy and Eastburn, 1992; Woolridge et al., 1990). The following discussion concentrates on the ways social and cultural factors compete with infant control by altering the extent to which mothers can or do respond to infant demands.

The Physical Environment

The location of activities in space exerts a strong influence on mother–infant interactions. In many cultures dwellings are not partitioned, allowing occupants engaged in activity in one area to observe or interact with those engaged in other activities elsewhere (Kent, 1984). This facilitates mothers hearing or seeing infant hunger cues such as rooting or crying. Partitioned space, such as that found in most western homes, reduces this communication when coupled with the belief that infants should occupy space separate from mothers, sleeping in cradle or crib and occupying a separate room at night and for naps. Most of the work on the impact of use of space on infant feeding has relied on research in different cultures. For example, Konner and Worthman's (1980) report of co-sleeping and extremely frequent feedings among the !Kung San has been contrasted with Western breastfeeding styles. More definitive information will come with a focus on intracultural variations, where at least some of the other parameters influencing feeding style can be held constant. In one such study, Quandt (1981) noted that breastfeeding styles differed between compact and spread-out dwellings of Euro-American mothers in the United States. Mothers in compact dwellings breastfed more times per day, with shorter intervals between feedings. This was independent of socioeconomic status, all mothers claimed to be breastfeeding on demand, and the study predated the use of "infant intercoms." Quandt concluded that with the prevailing custom of infants sleeping in a separate crib, mothers in compact dwellings became aware of their infants' waking sooner than those in more spread-out dwellings, thus perceiving the "demand" sooner and shortening the times between feedings. Naggan, Forman, Sarov, Lewando-Hundt, Zangwill, Chang and Berendes (1991) found house type to be a predictor of exclusive breastfeeding duration among Bedouin Arabs in the Negev, Israel, but related it to differences in traditional vs. modern values rather than any effect of the physical structure on breastfeeding.

Other aspects of material culture can influence the interaction of mothers and infants. The traditional use of slings to carry and hold infants in many cultures permits more rapid communication of hunger and easier access to the breast than the array of items currently available to western mothers: strollers, prams, swings, bouncers, and recliners.

Beliefs and Values

Infant feeding practices, including whether and how to breastfeed, are supported in all cultures by a web of meanings and values. This is particularly evident when one looks at trends in infant feeding in recent history. In the United States, breastfeeding has undergone dramatic shifts in and out of fashion, reflecting changes in values and attitudes of U.S. society as a whole. Although alternatives to breastfeeding (e.g., use of wet nurses or milk substitutes) have been available throughout recorded human history (Fildes, 1986 and Chapter 4, this volume), in the twentieth century there was an unprecedented decline in breastfeeding. The first to turn to artificial feeding were middle- and upper-class women, those who could afford to purchase breast milk substitutes. Recognizing the infant mortality associated with artificial feeding, physicians such as Thomas Morgan Rotch (1907) began to promote the scientific composition of infant "formulas" prescribed by physicians for individual infants. With the general perception of great value of things scientific held in the twentieth century (Rosenberg, 1976; Starr, 1982), the notion of superiority of artificial milks was established in the general public, if not completely within the medical profession (Apple, 1987). Disaggregation of breastfeeding rates by ethnic and socioeconomic groups shows that the rejection of breastfeeding among white middle-class women was soon followed by that of African-American women and those with lower incomes and less education (Institute of Medicine, 1991).

These changes in breastfeeding rates were not entirely the result of mothers failing to initiate breastfeeding with their newborns. They also resulted from beliefs about the way in which breastfeeding should be practiced. Increasing numbers of births took place in hospitals, where mothers were frequently anesthetized for births and where infants were kept in separate nurseries. Infants were nursed on set schedules, with feedings several hours apart, rather than in response to infant demand. This was consistent with the medical advice given mothers even after hospital discharge.

Millard (1990) has traced the use of the clock and scheduling in pediatric advice appearing in pediatric texts through the 1900s. She notes a factory-like approach to infant care and feeding during this time, with an emphasis on efficiency in child care and a hierarchical approach to feeding, with the pediatrician issuing a schedule and the mother imposing it on the infant. Advice was provided on the length of time an infant should be allowed to nurse and the interval between feedings. The latter increased from 2 to 4 or 5 hours from early to mid century. There was also a focus on "irregular" schedules as a source of infant morbidity.

Journals read by practitioners urged feeding practices in line with the textbooks. Sackett (1953), for example, promoted "a new concept of baby feeding" that consisted of feeding the infant on the same schedule followed by older members of the household. This approach reflected the importance given to training a child to fit into family life at the earliest possible age. Clein (1943) proposed a "streamlined infant feeding," urging mothers to add solids earlier and reduce the number of feedings. The implied benefit was greater efficiency for the mother in carrying out domestic tasks.

The ramifications for breastfeeding of following such advice are obvious. Even mothers who wished to breastfeed found their milk supply dwindling as between-feeding intervals were long and supplementary foods diminished infant demand for breast milk.

This emphasis on schedules and scientific childrearing is not strictly an American phenomenon. Whitaker (1993) reports equally severe pressure on mothers in Italy, coincident with the rise of fascism. Mothers were instructed to weigh the infant before and after nursing at each breast to regulate the amount of milk consumed by the infant. Elaborate scales dominated nurseries, and (not surprisingly) few mothers reported feeling the sensation of "let-down" generally noted by mothers as the oxytocin-induced ejection reflex pushes milk from the alveoli to the lacteal sinuses. Breastfeeding rates plummeted.

The resurgence of breastfeeding in the 1960s and 1970s in the United States can also be linked to changes in social values. With the women's movement and the rise in environmental awareness, middle- and upper-class women began to advocate "natural mothering," which included breastfeeding on demand (Mead, 1979). This was accompanied by demands for unmedicated "natural" childbirth and rooming-in of newborns with mothers in hospitals, and by use of baby carriers that encouraged closer mother–infant contact. The result was a breastfeeding style more conducive to adequate milk production and infant satiety. As with the infant feeding trends away from breastfeeding in the early twentieth century, this more recent trend has been led by those best able to afford it: middle class, well-educated, higher income, and predominantly white. Change has been slower in other parts of the population.

The Social Environment

Students of the history of infant feeding have been quick to point out that the social environment in which a woman mothers her newborn has a profound effect on her behavior. Raphael (1966, 1981) proposed the term "doula" for what was regarded as a near universal—the person or persons culturally prescribed to assist the new mother, offering instrumental support and advice as she cares for her infant. In terms of breastfeeding, the doula teaches the mother specific techniques necessary for successful breastfeeding, and also relieves her of other domestic responsibilities.

The importance of a supportive social environment is shown by a number of other studies, in which the attitude toward breastfeeding of the infant's father is related to the mother's decision whether or not to breastfeed, as is the mother's own feeding history (Gabriel, Gabriel and Lawrence, 1986). In recent years, much attention has also been focused on the role of health care workers in supporting breastfeeding, both in international (Forman, 1984) and domestic contexts.

Working Mothers

Mothers have always combined infant care with other tasks, but considerable attention has focused recently on problems encountered as women seek to combine breastfeeding with employment outside the home (e.g., Carballo and Pelto, 1991). Early contributions to the debate alleged that women's entry into the labor force was a key to the decline in rates of breastfeeding. More comprehensive reviews have not supported this (Van Esterik and Greiner, 1981; Winikoff and Baer, 1980). It is clear from these reviews that when interviewed in survey format, most women do not attribute decisions to not breastfeed or to wean early to working outside the home. However, when more detailed examination of the relationship of work and infant feeding is carried out, there is often a complex relationship in which certain features of work may lead to lower rates of breastfeeding. For example, Wright, Clark and Bauer (1993) found that among unemployed women and those without maternity leave, the need to be ready to return to work with little or no notice led to a choice of bottle feeding among the Navajo. This was complicated by distance from home to work (mothers living close by thought they would be able to take nursing breaks) and childcare arrangements. Van Esterik (1989) also cites distance from work, as well as work conditions, as factors entering into mothers' decisions about breastfeeding in a large-scale study of breastfeeding in Columbia, Indonesia, Kenya, and Thailand.

These studies have led to more general study of women's work roles and infant feeding. For example, Levine (1988) and Panter-Brick (1991, 1992a,b), working in different parts of Nepal, have provided extensive analyses of the ways women in different types of occupations accommodate infant feeding. They note that women frequently blend breastfeeding into their daily routine in such a way that work productivity is unaffected. Moreover, the choice to add semisolid paps rather than to bottle feed results in a situation where the food *supplements* rather than *replaces* breast milk. Duration of breastfeeding is therefore not compromised. Quandt has shown that among U.S. mothers, when other foods are added to the breast milk diet early, they do indeed replace breast milk, with measurable impacts on growth and breastfeeding duration, whereas later addition results in supplementation of breast milk, rather than replacement (Quandt, 1984a).

It is important in the study of maternal employment and breastfeeding to appreciate the considerable time depth of some feeding practices, and not to assume that some "natural" pattern of intensive, prolonged exclusive breastfeeding has existed until quite recently. King and Ashworth (1987, 1991) compare contemporary feeding practices in several developing countries. They note that in some places such as the Caribbean, the impact of slavery and forced women's work resulted in the adoption of European practices of early feeding of paps and porridges. Gussler reports that mixed feeding from a few weeks of age has been traditional on St. Kitts (Gussler, 1979). Quandt (1988), studying infant feeding practices in Guyana, found recipes for porridges in 1988 virtually identical to those reported by Fildes (1986) for eighteenth-century Europe.

THE INSUFFICIENT MILK CONTROVERSY

This controversy provides a focus for the interaction of behavioral and biological factors in breastfeeding, and the impact of social and cultural forces. The first round in this debate began with the publication of a paper by Gussler and Briesemeister (1980) that attempted to explain the high frequency of reports by mothers that they had terminated breastfeeding early or supplemented early because they perceived that their breast milk was not satisfying their infant. Gussler and Briesemeister pointed out that this syndrome was associated with urbanization, and cited characteristics of urban life that might lead to either the perception or reality of insufficient milk. Based on an evolutionary argument that evidence indicates that humans evolved as frequent feeders with close mother–infant contact, they postulated a traditional style of breastfeeding disrupted by factors in urban living. In particular, they claimed that those claiming insufficient milk had, for a variety of reasons, adopted a pattern of widely spaced feedings that led to declines in milk volume, fretful babies, anxiety, and therefore, insufficient milk.

In response, Greiner, Van Esterik and Latham (1981) took a slightly different approach, criticizing what they considered an overly pessimistic view of the compatibility of breastfeeding with urban life. They pointed out that breastfeeding exists in a variety of circumstances, not all of which entails constant contact between mother and child. They suggested that attention should be focused not on early termination of breastfeeding, but on why mothers increase the feeding of breast milk substitutes. To investigate this, they turn away from the more biobehavioral approach of Gussler and Briesemeister and examine the influence of infant food company promotions in leading women to choose bottle-feeding.

Together, these articles call for examining *why* so many women in widely varying cultural and economic circumstances around the world claim that they have insufficient milk to satisfactorily breastfeed their infants. Like the other researchers cited elsewhere in this chapter, they point to the complex interplay between the biology of lactation and the culturally embedded behavioral domain of breastfeeding.

There is no simple answer to the question of what factors determine whether and how women in any particular population will breastfeed their infants, and this chapter has not attempted to present a comprehensive review of the voluminous research literature on the topic. What it *has* done is propose a model linking the biology of lactation and social and cultural factors through specific breastfeeding behaviors. This model suggests that research into the determinants of breastfeeding, and efforts to relate infant feeding and infant well-being should examine the way in which breastfeeding is practiced. Researchers who maintain a dual emphasis on qualitative participant observation and quantitative survey design are particularly well-suited to produce such integrated analyses of breastfeeding.

REFERENCES

Apple, R. D.

1987 *Mothers and Medicine: A Social History of Infant Feeding 1890–1950*. Madison, WI: University of Wisconsin Press.

Billewicz, W. Z., H. M. Fellowes, and C. A. Hytten

1976 Comments on the critical metabolic mass and the age of menarche. *Annals of Human Biology* 3:51–59.

Bongaarts, J.

1978 A framework for analyzing the proximate determinants of fertility. *Population and Development Review* 4:105–132.

Bongaarts, J., and R. G. Potter

1983 *Fertility, Biology, and Behavior: An Analysis of the Proximate Determinants*. New York: Academic Press.

Cameron, N.
1976 Weight and skinfold variation at menarche and the critical body weight hypothesis. *Annals of Human Biology* 4:279–280.
Carballo, M., and G. H. Pelto
1991 Social and psychological factors in breast-feeding. In *Infant and Child Nutrition Worldwide*, edited by F. Falkner, pp. 175–190. Boca Raton, FL: CRC Press.
Clein, N. W.
1943 Streamlined infant feeding: A feeding routine utilizing earlier addition of solid foods and fewer feedings. *Journal of Pediatrics* 23:224–228.
Egli, G. E., N. S. Egli, and M. Newton
1961 The influence of number of feedings per day on milk production. *Pediatrics* 27:314–317.
Fildes, V.
1986 *Breasts, Bottles and Babies: A History of Infant Feeding*. Edinburgh: University of Edinburgh.
Forman, M. R.
1984 Review of research on the factors associated with choice and duration of infant feeding in less-developed countries. *Pediatrics* 74:667–694.
Frisch, R. E.
1990 The right weight: Body fat, menarche and ovulation. *Bailliere's Clinical Obstetrics and Gynecology* 4:419–439.
Frisch, R. E., and R. Revelle
1971 Height and weight at menarche and a hypothesis of menarche. *Archives of Diseases of Children* 46:695–701.
Frisch, R. E., R. Revelle, and S. Cook
1973 Components of the critical weight at menarche and at initiation of the adolescent growth spurt: Estimated total water, lean body mass, and fat. *Human Biology* 48:469–483.
Frisch, R. E., R. Snow, E. L. Gerard, L. Johnson, D. Kennedy, R. Barbieri, and B. R. Rosen
1992 Magnetic resonance imaging of body fat of athletes compared with controls, and the oxidative metabolism of estradiol. *Metabolism* 41:191–193.
Frisch, R. E., R. C. Snow, L. A. Johnson, B. Gerard, R. Barbieri, and B. Rosen
1993 Magnetic resonance imaging of overall and regional body fat, estrogen metabolism, and ovulation of athletes compared to controls. *Journal of Clinical Endocrinology and Metabolism* 77:471–477.
Gabriel, A., K. R. Gabriel, and R. A. Lawrence
1986 Cultural values and biomedical knowledge: Choices in infant feeding. *Social Science and Medicine* 23:501–509.
Glasier, A., and A. S. McNeilly
1990 Anatomy and development of the breast. *Bailliere's Clinical Endocrinology and Metabolism* 4:379–395.
Glasier, A., A. S. McNeilly, and P. W. Howie
1984 The prolactin response to suckling. *Clinical Endrocrinology* 21:109–116.
Greiner, T., P. Van Esterik, and M. C. Latham
1981 The insufficient milk syndrome: An alternative explanation. *Medical Anthropology* 5:233–247.

Gussler, J. D.
1979 Village women of St. Kitts. In *Breastfeeding and Food Policy in a Hungry World*, edited by D. Raphael, pp. 59–65. New York: Academic Press.
Gussler, J. D., and L. H. Briesemeister
1980 The insufficient milk syndrome: A biocultural explanation. *Medical Anthropology* 4:145–174.
Hamosh, M.
1980 Breast milk fat: Origin and digestion. In *Human Milk: Its Biological and Social Value*, edited by S. Freier and A. I. Eidelman, pp. 62–67. Amsterdam: Excerpta Medica.
Horrobin, D.
1979 Prolactin. *Annual Research Reviews*, X, Volume 7. St. Albans, VT: Eden Press.
Huffman, S. L., A. K. M. A. Chowdhury, and W. H. Mosley
1978 Postpartum amenorrhea: How is it affected by maternal nutritional status? *Science* 200:1155–1157.
Institute of Medicine
1991 *Nutrition During Lactation.* Washington, DC: National Academy of Sciences.
James, W. P. T., and P. Trayhurn
1976 An integrated view of the metabolic and genetic basis of obesity. *Lancet* 2:770–772.
Jelliffe, D. B., and E. F. P. Jelliffe
1978 *Human Milk in the Modern World.* Oxford: Oxford University Press.
Johnston, F. E., A. F. Roche, L. M. Schell, and H. N. B. Wettenhall
1975 Critical weight at menarche: Critique of a hypothesis. *American Journal of Diseases of Children* 129:19–23.
Kent, S.
1984 *Analyzing Activity Areas: An Ethnoarchaeological Study of the Use of Space.* Albuquerque, NM: University of New Mexico Press.
King, J., and A. Ashworth
1987 Historical review of the changing patterns of infant feeding in developing countries: The case of Malaysia, the Caribbean, Nigeria and Zaire. *Social Science and Medicine* 25:1307–1320.
1991 Contemporary feeding practices in infancy and early childhood in developing countries. In *Infant and Child Nutrition*, edited by F. Falkner, pp. 141–174. Boca Raton, FL: CRC Press.
Knauer, M.
1985 Breastfeeding and the return of menstruation in urban Canadian mothers practising "natural mothering." In *Breastfeeding, Child Health and Child Spacing*, edited by V. Hull and M. Simpson, pp. 187–211. London: Croom-Helm.
Konner, M., and C. Worthman
1980 Nursing frequency, gonadal function, and birth spacing among !Kung hunter-gatherers. *Science* 207:788–791.
Kramer, F. M., A. J. Stunkard, K. A. Marshall, S. McKinney, and J. Liebschutz
1993 Breast-feeding reduces maternal lower-body fat. *Journal of the American Dietetics Association* 93:429–433.

Levine, N. E.
1988 Women's work and infant feeding: A case from rural Nepal. *Ethnology* 27:231–251.
Lunn, P. G., M. Watkinson, A. M. Prentice, P. Morrell, S. Austin, and R. G. Whitehead
1981 Maternal nutrition and lactational amenorrhoea. *Lancet* 1:1428–1429.
Maclure, M, L. B. Travis, W. Willett, and B. MacMahon
1991 A prospective cohort study of nutrient intake and age at menarche. *American Journal of Clinical Nutrition* 54:649–656.
Matheny, R. J., L. L. Birch, and M. F. Picciano
1990 Control of intake by human-milk-fed infants: Relationships between feeding size and interval. *Developmental Psychobiology* 23:511–518.
McKenna, J. J., and S. Mosko
1993 Evolution and infant sleep: An experimental study of infant-parent co-sleeping and its implications for SIDS. *Acta Paediatrica Supplement* 389:31–36.
Mead, M.
1979 Family contexts of breast feeding. In *Breastfeeding and Food Policy in a Hungry World,* edited by D. Raphael, pp. 3–23. New York: Academic Press.
Millard, A. V.
1990 The place of the clock in pediatric advice: Rationales, cultural themes, and impediments to breastfeeding. *Social Science and Medicine* 31:211–221.
Naggan, L., M. R. Forman, B. Sarov, G. Lewando-Hundt, L. Zangwill, D. Chang, and H. W. Berendes
1991 The Bedouin Infant Feeding Study: Study design and factors influencing the duration of breast feeding. *Paediatric Perinatal Epidemiology* 5:428–444.
Neville, M. C., and M. R. Neifert, eds.
1983 *Lactation: Physiology, Nutrition, and Breast-Feeding.* New York: Plenum Press.
Newton, N., and M. Newton
1967 Psychological aspects of lactation. *New England Journal of Medicine* 277:1179.
Panter-Brick, C.
1991 Lactation, birth spacing and maternal work-loads among two castes in rural Nepal. *Journal of Biosocial Science* 23:137–154.
1992a Working mothers in rural Nepal. In *The Anthropology of Breast-Feeding,* edited by V. Maher, pp. 133–150. Oxford: Berg Publishers.
1992b Women's work and child nutrition: The food intake of 0–4 year old children in rural Nepal. *Ecology of Food and Nutrition* 29:11–24.
Phillips, V.
1993 Relactation in mothers of children over 12 months. *Journal of Tropical Pediatrics* 39:45–48.
Quandt, S. A.
1981 *The Biobehavioral Dynamics of the Infant Feeding Process.* Ph.D. Dissertation, Michigan State University. Ann Arbor: University Microfilms.
1983 Changes in maternal postpartum adiposity and infant feeding patterns. *American Journal of Physical Anthropology* 60:455–461.

1984a The effect of beikost on the diet of breast-fed infants. *Journal of the American Dietetic Association* 84:47–51.
1984b Nutritional thriftiness and human reproduction: Beyond the critical body composition hypothesis. *Social Science and Medicine* 19:177–182.
1985 Biological and behavioral predictors of exclusive breastfeeding duration. *Medical Anthropology* 9:139–151.
1986 Patterns of variation in breast feeding behaviors. *Social Science and Medicine* 23:445–453.
1988 *Guyana Food Marketing and Nutrition Education Project*, consultant report, Education Development Center, Inc., Newton, MA.

Raphael, D.
1966 *The Lactation-Suckling Process in the Matrix of Supportive Behavior*. Ph.D. Dissertation, Columbia University. Ann Arbor: University Microfilms.
1981 The midwife as doula: A guide to mothering the mother. *Journal of Nurse-Midwifery* November/December:13–15.

Rattigan, S., A. V. Ghisalberti, and P. E. Hartmann
1981 Breast-milk production in Australian women. *British Journal of Nutrition* 45:243–249.

Rosenberg, C. E.
1976 *No Other Gods: On Science and American Social Thought*. Baltimore: Johns Hopkins University Press.

Rotch, T.M.
1907 An historical sketch of the development of percentage feeding. *New York Medical Journal* 85:532–537.

Sackett, W. W., Jr.
1953 Results of three years experience with a new concept of baby feeding. *Southern Medical Journal* 46:358–363.

Scott, E. C., and F. E. Johnston
1982 Critical fat, menarche, and the maintenance of menstrual cycles: A critical review. *Journal of Adolescent Health Care* 2:249–260.

Scow, R. O., C. R. Mendelson, O. Zinder, M. Hamosh, and E. J. Blanchette-Mackie
1973 Role of lipoprotein lipase in the delivery of dietary fatty acids to lactating mammary tissue. In *Dietary Lipids and Postnatal Development*, edited by C. Galli, G. Jacini, and A. Pecile, pp. 91–114. New York: Raven Press.

Starr, P.
1982 *The Social Transformation of American Medicine*. New York: Basic Books.

Stini, W. A.
1975 Adaptive strategies of human populations under nutritional stress. In *Biosocial Interrelations in Population Adaptation*, edited by E. S. Watts, F. E. Johnston, and G. W. Lasker, pp. 19–41. The Hague: Mouton.

Tyson, J., J. Burchfield, F. Sentance, C. Mize, R. Uauy, and J. Eastburn
1992 Adaptation of feeding to a low fat yield in breast milk. *Pediatrics* 89:215–220.

Van Esterik, P.
1989 *Beyond the Breast-Bottle Controversy*. New Brunswick, NJ: Rutgers University Press.

Van Esterik, P., and T. Greiner
1981 Breastfeeding and women's work: Constraints and opportunities. *Studies in Family Planning* 12:182–195.
Waletzky, L. R., and E. C. Herman
1976 Relactation. *American Journal of Family Physicians* 14(2):69–74.
Whitaker, E. D.
1993 Italian fascism and the regimentation of infant feeding practices: Changing concepts of work and time in the evolution of scientific mothering. Paper presented at the 92nd Annual Meeting, American Anthropological Association, Washington, DC.
Wilde, C. J., C. V. P. Addey, M. J. Casey, D. R. Blatchford, and M. Peaker
1988 Feed-back inhibition of milk secretion: The effect of a fraction of goat milk on milk yield and composition. *Quarterly Journal of Experimental Physiology* 73:391–397.
Winikoff, B., and E. Baer
1980 The obstetrician's opportunity: Translating 'Breast is Best' from theory to practice. *American Journal of Obstetrics and Gynecology* 138:105–117.
Wood, J. W.
1990 Fertility in anthropological populations. *Annual Reviews in Anthropology* 19:211–242.
Woolridge, M. W., and J. D. Baum
1988 The regulation of human milk flow. In *Perinatal Nutrition*, edited by B. S. Lindblad, pp. 243–257. Bristol-Myers Nutrition Symposia, Vol. 6. New York: Plenum Press.
Woolridge, M. W., J. C. Ingram, and J. D. Baum
1990 Do changes in pattern of breast usage alter the baby's nutrient intake? *Lancet* 336:395–397.
Wright, A. L., C. Clark, and M. Bauer
1993 Maternal employment and infant feeding practices among the Navajo. *Medical Anthropology Quarterly* 7:260–280.
Zinder, A., M. Hamosh, T. R. C. Fleck, and R. O. Scow
1974 Effects of prolactin on lipoprotein lipase in mammary gland and adipose tissue of rats. *American Journal of Physiology* 266:744–748.

6

The Politics of Breastfeeding: An Advocacy Perspective

Penny Van Esterik

INTRODUCTION[1]

Politics may be defined as the practice of prudent, shrewd, and judicious policy. Politics is about power. How, then, can politics have anything to do with breastfeeding? When health, profits, and the empowerment of women are at stake, how could politics not be involved? Extraordinary changes in the way power is allocated in the world would be necessary for breastfeeding to flourish in this world. Many people believe such changes are impossible to make, that we have "advanced" too far into industrial capitalism to ever retreat into natural infant feeding regimes not based on profits. But even state policies influencing infant feeding practices can change, particularly when people begin to ask some very basic questions about child survival.

Advocacy on behalf of breastfeeding is incomplete and probably ineffective unless accompanied by a politically informed analysis of the obstacles to breastfeeding. These obstacles include the marketing practices of infant formula manufacturers, physician-dominated medical systems, and the relationship between industry and health professionals. This relationship has resulted in widespread misinformation about breastfeeding, including false claims of the equivalence between breast milk and artificial substitutes, and the devaluing of women's knowledge about the management of breastfeeding.

The purpose of this chapter is to trace the development of infant feeding as a public policy issue over the last few decades, to examine the role of nongovernmental groups (NGOs) in influencing public policy, and to place breastfeeding within the advocacy debates on the promotion of commercial breast milk substitutes, with the modest goal of putting the voices of industry critics more directly into discussions of the politics of breastfeeding. The chapter concludes with a call for anthropologists to include advocacy discourses as a valid addition to other modes of understanding and interpretation.

A brief chapter has to limit coverage. Three caveats concerning how I have limited the scope of the chapter follow. This chapter is written from a North American perspective. While what I am describing was and remains a worldwide movement, the strategies employed and their impacts vary in different national contexts. Although involved in international work on infant feeding, my position is that of a participant observer in the Canadian and American advocacy groups even when the action is taking place in Switzerland or Nairobi or Bangkok. This positionality is important because other reviews of the controversy emerge from European, Australian and British perspectives and experiences (cf. Allain, 1991; Chetley, 1986; Minchin, 1985; Palmer, 1993).

Second, it is impossible to place breastfeeding in its complete political context in a brief chapter because this would require analysis of the politics of transnational corporations, international trade agreements, poverty, the media, the status of women, and the power of industrial capitalism, to name but a few of the political contexts relevant to this discussion. Thus, the political context discussed here refers only to the immediate context of infant feeding policy rather than the broader political context within which infant feeding decisions are made.

Finally, the work of advocacy groups documented here is only one factor influencing changes in infant feeding policy. Granted, it is the factor that is most often omitted from discussions of health policy. The parallel work of international bureaucrats in the United Nations system, the legal initiatives to limit the power of transnational corporations, and the support of related consumer movements are not documented here.

ANCIENT HISTORY

Alternatives to maternal breastfeeding have a long history. Reflecting Eurocentric biases, we often turn to the ancient Near East, the "cradle of civilization"—the civilizations of Mesopotamia, Sumer, Babylon, Egypt—to find the roots of current Euro-American practices. Here we find texts and objects reflecting beliefs that "the ability to bear and suckle children is a gift from God" (Fildes, 1986:3), and evidence of the high regard for lactating women in the form of images of mother goddesses suckling infants, and advice to mothers to ensure that the process of breastfeeding will be successful. Sixteenth-century B.C. texts recommend potions and treatments to protect breast milk:

> To get a supply of milk in a woman's breast for suckling a child, warm the bones of a Xra-fish in oil and rub her back with it.
>
> Let the woman sit cross-legged and eat fragrant bread of soured *Dourra* while rubbing the parts with a poppy plant.
>
> Remedy for a breast (mamma) which is ill: Calamine, gall of ox, fly's dirt, yellow ochre are mixed together, and the breast is rubbed therewith for four days. (Fildes, 1986:5)

These images and words from three thousand years ago, from civilizations we understand only partially, are comprehensible to women today. They touch us across time, whereas a papyrus text about the lives and work of men in the third millennium B.C. might not touch men in the same way because there would be so few points of connection to link men across time. But concerns with maintaining milk supply and reducing engorgement resonate with current concerns of breastfeeding women.

However, these earliest references to breastfeeding exist side by side with evidence of alternatives to maternal breastfeeding. A Sumerian lullaby from the third millennium B.C. describes the wife of the ruler of Ur promising for her son "the nursemaid, joyous of heart, will suckle him." The Code of Laws of Hammurabi of Babylon (1728–1686 B.C.) includes laws to regulate and safeguard wet nursing (Fildes, 1986:6). Infants who were not breastfed were probably fed animal milk, possibly suckling directly from animals. By 1500 B.C., terra cotta feeding bottles often depicting breastfeeding attest to the existence of artificial feeding with cow's milk or other products (Fildes, 1986:18).

It seems that the cradle of civilization harbored women who chose or were forced to choose between bottle feeding and breastfeeding. The point of this historical note is to remind us that women have always had choices about infant feeding methods; the difference is that in the past, choices that did not involve breastfeeding probably resulted in sickness and death of their children. Today, in modern, industrialized contexts, choices that do not involve breastfeeding still result in sickness and death for some children, but the advent of modern antibiotics and sanitation and improved infant formula has narrowed the difference between breastfed and bottle-fed children, or postponed the ill-effects of bottle feeding until later in life.

Then, as today, external forces influenced the choice of infant feeding method. These external forces included the state, which regulated the choice of wet nurses in ancient Babylon, religious texts, which admonished women to breastfeed for at least 2 years, and working conditions for women.

Another historical detour to contextualize infant feeding choices takes us to France during the eighteenth and nineteenth centuries, where the predominant pattern of infant care was rural wet nursing. As young women found low-paid work in industrial factories or domestic service in the cities of France, conditions for breastfeeding were far from ideal. But artificial feeding remained expensive, difficult, and dangerous. Women solved the problem by providing modest wages for rural women to breastfeed their infants for them (Sussman, 1982:10). At the same time, wealthy, elite women were choosing not to breastfeed because they had the power and money to coerce other women to do this work for them. Lower middle- and working-class families, then, sent their newborns to rural peasant women, who took babies from the cities into their cottages for the nursing period, while well-to-do families recruited rural women as live-in nurses. By the end of the nineteenth century, these city babies did not even receive breast milk from their rural nurses but were "dry-nursed" with inadequate breast milk substitutes (Sussman, 1982:2), resulting in the death of thousands of infants in the industrial cities of France.

The French example demonstrates that changing patterns of work result in changes in infant feeding practices. Wet nursing is a reminder that class is an important dimension of infant-feeding practices. The explanations for this historical pattern in France are not well understood, but they clearly reflect attitudes toward children as expendable creatures, adaptations to changing socioeconomic conditions of urban industrialization, and the lack of safe alternatives to breastfeeding.

The point of these historical detours is to stress that today is not the first time in history that women have found substitutes for maternal breastfeeding. This is, however, the first time in history when infants lived through these experiments long enough for others to measure the impacts on their health. This is also the first time that huge industries have promoted certain options for women, and profited from mothers' decisions not to breastfeed or to supplement breast milk with a commercial product. It is this historical and economic fact that requires us to place breastfeeding in a broad political context.

NOT SO ANCIENT HISTORY

An early presentation on the problem of bottle feeding may be traced to a Rotary Club address made by Dr. Cicely Williams in Singapore in 1939 entitled "Milk and Murder." She argued that the increased morbidity and mortality seen in Singapore infants were directly attributable to the increase in bottle feeding with inappropriate breast milk substitutes, and the decline of breastfeeding. And she dared to call this murder—not something that happens to poor people over there, but murder. Her words:

> If you are legal purists, you may wish me to change the title of this address to *Milk and Manslaughter*. But if your lives were embittered as mine is, by seeing day after day this massacre of the innocents by unsuitable feeding, then I believe you would feel as I do that misguided propaganda on infant feeding should be punished as the most criminal form of sedition, and that these deaths should be regarded as murder. (Williams, 1986:70)

Although conditions in other cities in the developing world may have been similar or worse than in Singapore, the voices of warning and reproach were hesitant, isolated, and easily ignored. Conditions in many inner city and Native communities in North America today may be little improved over the conditions Williams found in Singapore in 1939.

Occasionally, reports from missionaries and health workers would confirm the devastating effects of bottle feeding on infant morbidity and mortality. But these were single voices and never stimulated a social movement. And it was easy to assume that the "problem" was "over there" and thus was irrelevant to promotional practices of infant food manufacturers in developed industrial countries. Only recently has the full extent of the dangers of commercial infant formula been acknowledged or publicized (Cunningham, Jelliffe, and Jelliffe, 1991; Palmer, 1993:306–312; Walker, 1993).

From the 1930s, the promotion of breast milk substitutes steadily increased, particularly in developed countries. In North America, competition between American pharmaceutical companies and the depression reduced the number of companies producing infant formula to three large firms—Abbott (Ross), Bristol-Myers (Mead-Johnson), and American Home Products (Wyeth) (cf. Apple, 1980). Food companies like Nestlé were already producing baby foods before the turn of the century. Both food- and drug-based companies producing infant formula expanded their markets during the post-World War II baby boom, as breastfeeding halved between 1946 and 1956 in America, dropping to 25% at hospital discharge in 1967 (Minchin, 1985:216). By that time, the birth rate in industrialized countries had dropped, and companies sought new markets in the rapidly modernizing cities of developing countries. As industry magazines reported "Bad News in Babyland" as births declined in the 1960s in North America, their sales in developing countries increased, with only isolated and occasional protests from health professionals and consumer groups.

Other points of resistance to the increasing collaboration between infant formula manufacturers and health professions in North America came from mothers who wanted to breastfeed their infants and met with resistance or lack of support from the medical profession. These voices of resistance were not raised against the infant formula industry or against the medical profession per se. Rather, they took the form of mother-to-mother support groups. The prime example is La Leche League, a group founded in 1956 in Chicago by breastfeeding mothers. The founding of Le Leche League represented women's growing dissatisfaction with physician-directed bottle feeding regimes. While mother-to-mother support groups in some countries have lent support to infant food industry critics, it is important to remember that since its inception, La Leche League never directed its energies outward against infant formula companies, but rather inward toward the nursing couple. Only in recent years has the linkage been made between advocacy groups oriented toward consumer protests and mother support groups.

One phrase in a speech in 1968 by Dr. Derrick Jelliffe caught the attention of a much wider audience. He labeled the results of the commercial promotion of artificial infant feeding as "commerciogenic malnutrition." Like "Milk and Murder," this phrase grabbed headlines and became the focus for advocacy writing. By the mid-1970s, publications like the *New Internationalist* (1973) were bringing the problem to public attention. Reports such as Muller's *The Baby Killer* (1974) and the version by a Swiss group called *Nestlé Totet Babys* (Nestlé Kills Babies) prompted responses from Nestlé. In 1974, Nestlé filed libel charges in a Swiss court for five million dollars against the Third World Action Group for their publication *Nestlé Kills Babies*, leading to a widely publicized trial. The judge found the members of the group guilty of libel and fined members a nominal sum, but clearly recognized publicly the immoral and unethical conduct of Nestlé in the promotion of their infant feeding products. The libel suit and these popular publications provided focal points around which public opinion gradually developed, strengthening the efforts of advocacy groups in two complementary directions, the organization of a consumer boycott and drafting a code to regulate the promotion of baby foods (bottles, teats, and all breast milk substitutes, not just infant formula).

STRATEGY FOR CHANGE: CONSUMER BOYCOTTS

Since the mid-1970s, a broad range of people from all walks of life, in many different parts of the world, have participated in a public debate known as the infant formula controversy, the baby food scandal, or the breast–bottle debate. Changes in infant feeding practices do not occur spontaneously, or as a result of health promotion campaigns. In North America, one catalyst for the "back to the breast" movement and a resurgence of interest in breastfeeding was a consumer movement organized by grass roots advocacy groups that drew attention to how the existence and advertising of commercial infant formula affected women's perceptions of their breasts, breast milk, and breastfeeding. They demonstrated that there was a direct and specifiable link between changes in infant feeding practices and the promotion of commercial infant formula in developing countries. The participation of ordinary people in North America in this debate was mostly through the direct action of a consumer boycott. Without the social mobilization of the consumer boycott, the work to promote a code for the marketing of breast milk substitutes would not have been as effective.

Both boycott groups and promoters of a code to regulate the way infant formula was being promoted and marketed argued that the decline in initiation rates and the duration of breastfeeding could be linked to the expanding promotion of breast milk substitutes, usually by multinational food and drug corporations, and to bottle feeding generally. The boycott against Nestlé's products, and eventually those of other infant formula manufacturers, generated the largest support of any grass roots consumer movement in North America, and its impact is still being felt in industry, governments, and citizen's action groups around the world. Women were the primary supporters of the boycott against Nestlé and other manufacturers of infant formula, although the movement in North America was strongly male dominated. Nevertheless, many women gained experience in analyzing the relations between corporate power and public health through their experience of working on the boycott campaign.

The groups that took on the task of challenging the infant formula companies were, for the most part, small and underfunded, and in many cases ran on voluntary labor. While they were not the only people to recognize the problems of bottle feeding, they were the first to effectively mobilize to challenge the industries promoting it. Their success against the forces ranged against them, including powerful governments and multinational corporations, is a study in the power of cooperative networking. The importance of these small, nongovernmental groups cannot be overstressed.[2]

IBFAN (the International Baby Food Action Network) is a single-issue network of extraordinarily dedicated people—flexible, nonhierarchical, decentralized, and international in organization (Allain, 1991). IBFAN works to promote breastfeeding worldwide, eliminate irresponsible marketing of infant foods, bottles, and teats, advocate implementation of the WHO/UNICEF International Code of Marketing of Breast Milk Substitutes, and monitor company compliance with the Code.

In North America and Europe, advocacy groups also formed around the issue—most notably the Interfaith Centre for Corporate Responsibility (ICCR), the Infant Formula Action Coalition (INFACT) in Canada and the United States, the Baby Milk Action Group in Britain, the Geneva Infant Feeding Association (GIFA), and the many groups in developing countries that formed part of the IBFAN network. Throughout the late 1970s and early 1980s, these groups provided evidence of the unethical marketing of infant formula in their communities. This evidence was critically important in convincing delegates to the World Health Assembly (WHA, the meetings of the World Health Organization) that a regulatory code of industry practices was necessary.

The New York-based ICCR, formed in 1974, monitored multinational corporations, provided information to church groups on responsible corporate investments, and publicized cases such as the lawsuit filed by the Sisters of the Precious Blood against Bristol-Myers in 1976 for misleading stockholders about their infant formula marketing practices. Although the lawsuit was dismissed, information about the marketing of breast milk substitutes circulated in church basements among groups interested in third world development and justice issues, bringing a new constituency into the movement. Public education on the promotion of breast milk substitutes often featured the 1975 film, *Bottle Babies*, a vivid portrayal of the tragic effects of bottle feeding in Kenya.

In 1977, several action networks began the campaign to boycott Nestlé products in North America. The American INFACT (now called Action for Corporate Accountability) grew out of a student group at the University of Minnesota, while the Canadian INFACT groups developed around justice ministries of the Anglican and United Churches, first in Victoria, British Columbia. These groups were linked together through IBFAN to represent the views of coalition members at international health policy meetings such as the World Health Assembly.

It was through these groups that the general public in North America was made aware of the infant formula controversy (or the breast–bottle controversy) through an increasingly sophisticated campaign involving public debates, newsletters, radio and T.V. shows, petitions, demonstrations, posters, buttons, and the first consumer boycott of Nestlé's products, which ended in 1984.

The advocacy position as defined by the boycott groups is quite straightforward. It argues that the makers of infant formula should not be promoting infant formula and bottle feeding in developing countries where breastfeeding is prevalent and the technology for adequate use of infant formula is absent. Advocacy groups claim that multinational corporations (like Nestlé), in their search for new markets, launched massive and unethical campaigns directed toward medical personnel and consumers that encouraged mothers in developing countries to abandon breastfeeding for a more expensive, inconvenient, technologically complex, and potentially dangerous method of infant feeding—infant formula from bottles. For poor women who have insufficient cash for infant formula, bottles, sterilization, equipment, fuel, or refrigerators, who have no regular access to safe, pure drinking water, and who may be unable to read and comprehend instructions for infant formula preparation, the results are tragic. Misuse of infant formula is a major cause of malnutrition and the cycles of gastroenteritis, diarrhea, and dehydration that lead eventually to death. Advocacy groups place part of the blame for this "commerciogenic malnutrition" on the multinational companies promoting infant formula.

The boycott groups have never advocated a ban on the sale of infant formula, although some have advocated its "demarketing" (Post, 1985). *Nor were women to be pressured to breastfeed against their will, although their critics represented their aims in this light.* "Better to bottle feed with love than breastfeed with reluctance" is a cliche cited by many different people convinced that protecting mothers from feelings of guilt for not breastfeeding is more important than removing obstacles to breastfeeding. The intentions of INFACT and other boycott groups are clearly stated in their demands:

1. An immediate halt to all promotion of infant formula.
2. An end to direct product promotion to the consumer, including mass media promotion and direct promotion through posters, calendars, baby care literature, baby shows, wrist bands, baby bottles, and other inducements.
3. An end to the use of company "milk nurses."
4. An end to the distribution of free samples and supplies of infant formula to hospitals, clinics, and homes of new mothers.
5. An end to promotion of infant formula to the health professions and through health care institutions.

The infant formula companies responded to the boycott groups by modifying their advertising to the public, but they were slow to meet all INFACT demands and certainly never met the spirit of the demands, namely, to stop promoting their products. They simply promoted new products such as follow-on milks for toddlers, developed new marketing strategies, and hired public relations firms to answer their critics and to improve their corporate image.

Nestlé's efforts were concentrated on trying to improve their tarnished public image by hiring a prestigious public relations firm, sending clergy glossy publications about their contributions to infant health, and generally discrediting their critics as being merely uninformed opponents of the free enterprise system (Chetley, 1986:46,53). Companies such as Nestlé continue their efforts to buy social respectability by sponsoring events at international medical and nutrition conferences, and events celebrating the Canadian Year of the Family, for example, in addition to funding research on infant feeding.

Meanwhile, the boycott campaign against the promotion of infant formula begun in 1977 was very successful as a tool for social mobilization. The Nestlé boycott has become one of the most successful consumer boycotts in history. In Toronto, for example, a market research firm found that 10% of the inhabitants of the city of two million were boycotting Nestlé products (INFACT Canada, February 1982). Toronto City Council not only endorsed the boycott, but urged removal of Nestlé products from all civic premises.

Like all mass action social movements, the rhetoric used by advocacy groups oversimplifies the issue and seldom provides the statistically significant evidence that both the infant formula industry and medical journals call for (cf. Gerlach, 1980). But that is the nature of advocacy communication used by all social mobilization groups. At one level of analysis, the issue is both clear and simple; it is complicated only by the many obstacles ranged against breastfeeding. Nevertheless, the words and sentiments voiced in the original advocacy documents still ring clear today. However, the American boycott groups stressed the problem of baby food marketing in developing countries, rather than the problems growing in the bottle feeding communities at home.

STRATEGY FOR CHANGE: CODE WORK

Another parallel stream of activities for advocacy groups concerned lobbying and attending drafting sessions on the development of a code to regulate the marketing of breast milk substitutes. Health professionals called for establishing policy guidelines on infant feeding through United Nation groups such as the Protein–Calorie Advisory Group. In 1979, WHO and UNICEF hosted an international meeting to develop an international code regulating the marketing of breast milk substitutes. That meeting enabled nine infant formula companies to form the International Council for Infant Food Industries (ICIFI) (Palmer, 1993:237), and to lobby UN agencies for guidelines least damaging to their profits.

The code was drafted with the cooperation and consent of the infant formula industry and is very much a compromise, a minimal standard rather than the ideal.

North American advocacy groups in IBFAN "had to divide their very scarce resources and energy between running a boycott of Nestlé and the expensive periodic visits to Geneva for the Code drafting sessions" (Allain, 1991:10). Work in the United States to document abusive marketing practices of infant formula companies was brought to a head in 1978 by the Congressional Hearings on the Marketing and Promotion of Infant Formula in the Developing Nations chaired by Edward Kennedy. During the hearings, Ballarin, a manager of Nestlé's Brazilian operations, claimed—to the amazement of the hearing—that the boycott and the campaign against the infant formula companies were really an "attack on the free world's economic system," led by "a worldwide church organization with the stated purpose of undermining the free enterprise system" (United State Congress, 1978:127).

In May 1981, the World Health Assembly adopted a nonbinding recommendation in the form of the WHO/UNICEF Code for the Marketing of Breast milk Substitutes with a vote of 118 for, 3 abstentions, and 1 against. The negative vote was cast by the United States, in spite of the fact that it was the United States Senate that had proposed the idea of a Marketing Code and had initiated and actively participated in the drafting process. The American delegate to the WHA had been an enthusiast for the Marketing Code until shortly before the vote, when direct orders from his government ordered him to vote against its adoption. The Reagan White House had responded to direct lobbying from the infant formula industry (Chetley, 1986). The delegate who was ordered to reverse his nation's stance did so, and then resigned his post.

The Marketing Code is not a code of ethics but a set of rules for industry, health workers, and governments to regulate the promotion of baby foods through marketing. It covers bottles, teats, and all breast milk substitutes, not just infant formula. The code includes these provisions:

- No advertising of any of these products to the public.
- No free samples to mothers.
- No promotion of products in health care facilities, including the distribution of free or low-cost supplies.
- No company sales representatives to advise mothers.
- No gifts or personal samples to health workers.
- No words or pictures idealizing artificial feeding, or pictures of infants on labels of infant milk containers.
- Information to health workers should be scientific and factual.

- All information on artificial infant feeding, including that on labels, should explain the benefits of breastfeeding, and the costs and hazards associated with artificial feeding.
- Unsuitable products, such as sweetened condensed milk, should not be promoted for babies.
- Manufacturers and distributors should comply with the Code's provisions even if countries have not adopted laws or other measures. (World Alliance for Breastfeeding Action, 1994)

AFTER THE CODE

Following the establishment of the Code, Nestlé and other infant formula companies publicly released special instructions to its marketing personnel to comply with the Code, and asked the International Boycott Committee, a subgroup of IBFAN groups who were working on the boycott, to call it off. However, the boycott continued until 1984 when some means of monitoring company compliance with the Code could be established, and WHO member countries could draft national codes.

The advocacy groups, in the absence of national machinery, continued their monitoring role, recording and publicizing noncompliance of the Code (IBFAN, 1991). WHO and UNICEF have never monitored Code compliance, although they occasionally have taken individual companies to task. UNICEF's executive board extracted a promise that manufacturers would end all free supplies of infant formula to hospitals by the end of 1992. This was not done.

In the Philippines, a law banning free supplies was passed, but was evaded by the company tactic of invoicing for milk supplies and not bothering to collect payment. In the face of this and other flagrant violations, a second boycott against Nestlé and American Home Products in the United States, and Nestlé and Milupa in Germany was launched in 1988 by groups who were part of the IBFAN network. To date (1995) the second Nestlé boycott has spread to 14 countries and is most active in Europe and Latin America. However, it has never gained momentum in North America, ironically, because it could never live up to the success of the first boycott.

Disagreements about Code interpretations were to be referred to WHO. By the late 1980s, it was clear that Nestlé and other baby food companies had diverted part of their marketing budgets from public promotion into expanding the tactic of placing large quantities of free or low cost milk in maternity facilities. Because of the inadequacy of medical training in breastfeeding management, health officials use these supplies for routine bottle feeding of newborns, which sabotages the successful establishment of breastfeeding.

In 1986, a World Health Resolution was adopted that acknowledged the detrimental effect of free or low cost supplies and clarified the relevant Articles in the Code by banning such supplies. According to the resolution, free or low cost supplies of infant formula were not to be given to hospitals. If supplies were donated to an infant, they were to be continued for as long as the infant required the milk. Hospitals that needed small quantities of infant formula for exceptional cases could buy them through the normal procurement channels. Thus, free supplies could no longer be used as sales inducements. Most of the major companies who were giving free supplies ignored the resolution, arguing that they would stop distributing free supplies only if governments brought in laws against them. However, the Code states that "Independently of other measures" manufacturers and distributors should take steps to ensure their conduct at every level conforms to the principles and aims of the Code.

At the World Health Assembly meeting in May of 1994, advocacy groups' successful lobbying reminded delegates that free and low cost supplies of infant formula are marketing devices pure and simple, and not charity, a point made in 1989 by the Nigerian Minister of Health during the WHA. A few European countries including Ireland and Italy, and most forcefully, the United States delegation tried to defeat the resolution to end free supplies. But their efforts were thwarted by a block of African delegates and a very effective Iranian delegate who made it clear that the American position was the industry position as advocated by the International Association of Infant Food Manufacturers (IFM, the successor to ICIFI). The meeting ended with a consensus to withdraw all amendments and support the original text proposed by WHO's Executive Board to end donations of infant formula to all parts of the health care system worldwide. Once again, the question remains how such resolutions can be implemented and monitored. No doubt the advocacy groups will take up the challenge, or at least ensure that the issue does not quietly disappear from the world's conscience.

For all their rhetoric, and what some have decried their so-called confrontational tactics, the advocacy groups deserve great credit for bringing about what decades of clinical observations alone failed to accomplish: public awareness and concern about the dangers of breast milk substitutes. This struggle for corporate accountability is often recounted in development education workshops as well as marketing classes (Post, 1985). For the first time, nongovernmental organizations like INFACT, IBFAN, and ICCR had a direct role in the deliberations at WHO and UNICEF in 1979 and in subsequent meetings regarding infant feeding policy. Chetley points out that in spite of industry's concerns about the "scientific integrity" of allowing popular organizations, mother's groups, and consumer groups to participate, delegates to the international meetings were impressed with the contributions of the nongovernmental organizations (1986:65–69). It is the NGOs that keep alive the underlying concern about corporate responsibility, human rights, and infant feeding as a justice issue.

THE UNHOLY ALLIANCE

Allain refers to the "unholy alliance" (1991:15) between the medical profession and the baby food companies. Certainly the medical profession and medical associations followed rather than led the advocacy groups in their criticism of industry. Although there was resistance by some doctors to the promotion of commercial baby foods, only occasional voices of protest were heard from health professionals in the 1950s and 1960s, as infant feeding became more completely medicalized.

In the United States, continuing efforts by doctors like Derrick Jelliffe and Michael Latham continually brought the issue of breastfeeding and promotional practices of industry to the attention of health organizations. Internationally, the advocacy groups turned a number of physicians into more outspoken public advocates for breastfeeding, stimulating a medical consensus on the value of breastfeeding. But many university and medical school research projects on infant nutrition are funded by industry money. Doctors are beginning to speak out against practices in their own hospitals, but they may be criticized by the medical establishment for doing so. As researchers are increasingly being warned (Margolis, 1991), there is no such thing as a free lunch, nor do people bite the hand that feeds them.

In 1986, an international group of doctors at an IBFAN Conference in Thailand drafted and endorsed the "Doctors' Declaration on Breastfeeding." Among several statements of commitment to probreastfeeding practices the Declaration promises not to permit the use of feeding bottles, teats, or pacifiers in hospitals or to accept personal funding from an infant food company. UNICEF's Physician's Pledge simply asks doctors to do their part "to protect, promote and support breastfeeding and to work to end the free and low-cost distribution of breast milk substitutes in our health care systems" (UNICEF news release, July 22, 1994). While individual health professionals around the world work to change practices in their hospitals, hospitals and medical research still depend on industry support.

BREASTFEEDING IN THE NINETIES

In 1990, a global initiative sponsored by a number of bilateral and multilateral agencies resulted in the adoption of the Innocenti Declaration, which reads in part:

> As a global goal for optimal maternal and child health and nutrition, all women should be enabled to practice exclusive breastfeeding and all infants should be fed exclusively on breast milk from birth to 4–6 months of age. Thereafter, children should continue to be breastfed, while receiving appropriate and adequate complementary foods, for up to two years of age or beyond. . . . Efforts should be made to increase women's confidence in their ability to breastfeed. Such empowerment involves the removal of constraints and influences that manipulate perceptions and behavior towards breastfeeding, often by subtle and indirect means. This requires sensitivity, continued vigilance, and a responsive and comprehensive communications strategy involving all media and addressed to all levels of society. Furthermore, obstacles to breastfeeding within the health system, the workplace and the community must be eliminated. (Innocenti Declaration, 1991:271–272)[3]

This carefully worded statement is nothing less than a challenge to change the priorities of the modern world. The language stresses the empowerment of women rather than their duty to breastfeed, a change that should bring more advocates for women's health to support breastfeeding.

Later in 1990, UNICEF convened a meeting to review progress on breastfeeding programs and concluded that if the Innocenti Declaration were ever to be implemented, work would have to be done by NGOs rather than governments alone. This led to the formation of an umbrella group called the World Alliance for Breastfeeding Action (WABA). WABA is a global network of organizations and individuals who are actively working to eliminate obstacles to breastfeeding and to act on the Innocenti Declaration. The groups include those who approach problems of breastfeeding from different perspectives—from consumer advocates to mother support groups and lactation consultants.

As part of their social mobilization efforts to gain public support for implementing the Innocenti Declaration, WABA sponsors World Breastfeeding Week (August 1–7) to pull together the efforts of all breastfeeding advocates, governments, and the public. The first campaign, in 1992, focused on hospital practices, and was called the Baby Friendly Hospital Initiative (BFHI). This campaign established steps that hospitals should take to support breastfeeding and to implement the Innocenti Declaration, and was based on the WHO/UNICEF statement, Ten Steps to Successful Breastfeeding. By 1994, over 1000 hospitals worldwide had been approved as baby-friendly (BFHI Progress Report, April, 1994). The second campaign, in 1993, tackled the problem of developing Mother-Friendly Workplaces, where breastfeeding and work could be combined. The complexity of the integration of women's productive and reproductive work, and the relevant cultural and policy issues have been explored elsewhere (Van Esterik, 1992). In 1994, attention returned to implementing the Code for the Marketing of Breast milk Substitutes in all countries to meet the goals of the Innocenti Declaration. The 1995 theme of Breastfeeding: Empowering Women provided a link with the 4th International World Conference of Women in Bejing.

BROADENING SUPPORT FOR BREASTFEEDING

The public appeal of the infant formula controversy was that it was presented as a simple, solvable problem. People in North America were attracted to the campaign because it put many of their unspoken concerns about the power of multinational corporations into a clear, concrete example of exploitative behavior that could be acted upon. For some boycott groups, the solution to the problem of bottle feeding with infant formula was for multinational infant formula manufacturers to stop promoting infant formula in developing countries. When the companies agreed to abide by the conditions of the WHO/UNICEF Code and the boycott was lifted, this marked the end of the campaign, a victory of small grass roots organizations over huge corporations. As with other social movements, it was hard to sustain interest in the issue after a "victory" had been declared. But the advocacy groups and most breastfeeding supporters recognized that infant feeding decisions are not related to marketing abuse alone; rather, the issue was embedded in a set of problems that requires rethinking broader questions about the status of women, corporate power over the food supply, poverty, and environmental issues.

For example, the implications of bottle feeding have not been explored from an environmental perspective with the exception of the position paper by Radford (1992). The ecology and environmental justice movements have been slow to recognize breastfeeding as part of sustainable development and breast milk as a unique underutilized natural resource. The report of the World Commission on the Environment and

Development, *Our Common Future* (1987), made no reference to nurturance or infant feeding, although economy, population, human resources, food security, energy, and industry are all discussed as part of sustainable development.

Sustainability refers to courses of action that continue without damaging the environment and causing their own obsolescence. A sustainable infant feeding policy must consider the impact of decisions a number of years in the future, rather than simply examining conditions at the present. If we compare breastfeeding and bottle feeding as modes of infant feeding, each has very different implications for sustainability; breast milk is a renewable resource, a living product that increases in supply as demand increases. It reinforces continuity with women's natural reproductive phases and is a highly individualized process, adapting itself to the needs of infant and mother. The infant is actively empowered and "controls" its food supply.

By contrast, the bottle feeding mode—most commonly associated with infant formula even in developing countries—is a prime example of using a nonrenewable resource that uses even more nonrenewable resources to produce and to prepare. It puts demands on fuel supplies and produces solid wastes—for every 3 million bottle fed babies, 450 million tins are discarded. It is a standardized product that does not take into consideration individual needs (although in practice it is not really standardized; it is commonly adulterated in its industrial production with insect parts, rat hairs, iron filings, and accidental excesses of chlorine and aluminum, or adjusted by the preparer to individualize it by the addition of herbs and sugar). The bottle-fed infant is passive, controlled by others, and becomes a dependent consumer from birth.

The issue of environmental pollution is critically important. A sustainable development policy for infant feeding must take careful note of the fact that women's capacity to breastfeed successfully is often a gauge for judging when our capacity to adapt to environmental stresses—air and water pollution, environmental toxins, radiation—has been overstrained. But women are not canaries or cows or machines. Breastfeeding promotion that treats women as merely milk producers is bound to fail, and the issue itself will be rejected by women's groups. Hence, an ongoing task for advocacy groups is to reposition breastfeeding so that it can be productively placed within the agendas of other advocacy groups, particularly environmental and feminist groups (cf. Van Esterik, 1994).

ADVOCACY AND ANTHROPOLOGY

Advocacy activism is tiring work, and many authors in this book are full time anthropologists working in academic settings, not full time activists or breastfeeding counselors. Yet many of us have been drawn to research on breastfeeding by our personal experiences of mothering or by witnessing the commercial exploitation of women in different countries. Advocacy lessons are personal lessons because they require each of us to put our values on the line—even occasionally to suspend academic canons of reserve and noninvolvement, and respond emotionally to things we feel strongly about. In the study of breastfeeding, there is a convergence of different ways of knowing—a convergence of scientific knowledge, experimental knowledge, and experiential knowledge of generations of women, with moral and emotional values that all support action to support, protect, and promote breastfeeding. Few areas of research in anthropology encourage such integration. Further, advocacy lessons are never far from us, as advocacy action permeates different parts of our lives and links diverse causes—from the women's movement to environmental concerns.

In this climate of reflexive anthropology, and the increasing responsibility that the profession as a whole is taking in human rights debates, it is important that we clarify our relation to advocacy discourse and action as professional anthropologists and as citizens. Anthropology has a long history of applied work, but more recent and more problematic is the commitment of individual anthropologists to advocacy work (cf. Harries-Jones, 1985). But advocacy anthropology is still suspect to some in the profession. Advocacy refers to the act of interceding for or speaking on behalf of another person or group (Van Esterik, 1986), or promoting one course of action over another. This takes us beyond presentations, analyses, and discussion of evidence to recommend particular alternatives. Advocacy work draws some anthropologists into taking action with regard to well-defined goals that may best be implemented outside of academic settings. What has made this position acceptable in anthropology? First, the increasing numbers of anthropologists who have become involved in "causes" such as the rights of indigenous peoples, famine, AIDS, and women's rights have made such commitment more visible within the profession. At the same time, the increasing involvement of indigenous peoples and special interest groups in advocating on their own behalf has resulted in anthropologists working with or for these groups.

Second, these individual and collective initiatives occurred at the same time as theoretical work arguing that there is no such thing as "scientific objectivity," and that many past examples of applied anthropology were both paternalistic and supportive of the status quo.

Third, feminist anthropology's epistemological stance on the lack of separation between theory and action justifies and even requires advocacy stances. Feminist methodology calls for explicit statements of the positionality of the author. The feminist axiom "the personal is political" breaks down past opposition between "emotional advocacy action" and "cool, detached scientific reasoning," and accepts experience and emotion as valid guides to moral stands. As this volume attests, *research results following the most stringent canons of experimental method also confirm what advocacy groups have argued for years regarding breastfeeding*. But as advocacy groups remind us, it is politics that determine whose truth is heard.

Finally, the recent involvement of all branches of anthropology in human rights debates, the theme of the 1994 meetings of the American Anthropological Association, requires rethinking the relation between advocacy and anthropology.

Advocacy for breastfeeding is one enormous anthropology lesson. Breastfeeding is simultaneously biologically and culturally constructed, deeply embedded in social relations, and yet cannot be understood without reference to varying levels of analysis including individual, household, community, institutional, and world industrial capitalism. As much a part of self and identity as political economy; as personal as skin and as impersonal as the audit sheets of international multinational corporations, breastfeeding research requires a synthesis of multiple methods and theoretical approaches. At a time when anthropology hovers on the brink of self-reflexive nihilism and fragmentation on the one hand, and greater involvement in studying global change, internationalism, and public policy on the other (cf. Givens and Tucker, 1994), breastfeeding provides a challenging focus for holistic, biocultural, interdisciplinary research.

NOTES

1. The most comprehensive history of the controversy is Andrew Chetley's *The Politics of Baby Foods* (1986) and *Baby Milk: Destruction of a World Resource* from the Catholic Institute for International Relations (1993). I also review the history in my book *Beyond the Breast-Bottle Controversy* (1989), and am using this opportunity to update that discussion. Here, I trace the development of the controversy highlighting the focal points of the movement up to and including 1994. This update has benefited from the views and writings of G. Palmer.

2. The detailed reports on the infractions of the Marketing Code by infant formula companies are mostly in "fugitive literature"—letters, newspaper advertisements, and brief reports in low budget newsletters in many languages. The violations are most accurately reflected in the "SOCs," red and blue folders published by IBFAN since 1988, documenting the State of the Code, by country and by company. The advocacy groups in individual countries are the best sources for these records, particularly ACTION for Corporate Responsibility in the United States, INFACT Canada, IBFAN in Penang, Malaysia, GIFA in

Geneva, Switzerland, and the Baby Milk Action Group in Britain. Their files are treasure troves for studying a social movement, but are not easily made to conform to academic standards of citation.

3. "The Innocenti Declaration was produced and adopted by participants at the WHO/UNICEF policy-makers' meeting on 'Breastfeeding in the 1990s: A Global Initiative,' co-sponsored by the United States Agency for International Development (A.I.D.) and the Swedish International Development Authority (SIDA), held at the Spedale degli Innocenti, Florence, Italy, on 30 July–1 August 1990. The Declaration reflects the content of the original background document for the meeting and the views expressed in group and plenary sessions" (Innocenti Declaration, 1991:273).

REFERENCES

Allain, A.
1991 IBFAN: On the cutting edge. *Development Dialogue* offprint, April:1–36, Uppsala, Sweden.

Apple, R.
1980 To be used only under the direction of a physician: Commercial infant feeding and medical practice, 1870–1940. *Bulletin of the History of Medicine* 54:402–417.

Baby Friendly Hospital Initiative
1994 Progress Report. See Note 3.

Catholic Institute for International Relations
1993 *Baby Milk: Destruction of a World Resource*. London: Russell Press.

Chetley, A.
1986 *The Politics of Baby Food*. London: Frances Pinter.

Cunningham, A. S., D. B. Jelliffe, and E. F. P. Jelliffe
1991 Breast-feeding and health in the 1980s: A global epidemiologic review. *Journal of Pediatrics* 118(5):659–666.

Fildes, V.
1986 *Breasts, Bottles and Babies*. Edinburgh: Edinburgh University Press.

Gerlach, L. P.
1980 The flea and the elephant: Infant formula controversy. *Transaction* 17(6):51–57.

Givens, D., and R. Tucker
1994 Sociocultural anthropology: The next 25 years. *Anthropology Newsletter* 35(4):1.

Harries-Jones, P.
1985 From cultural translator to advocate: Changing circles of interpretation. In *Advocacy and Anthropology*, edited by R. Paine, pp. 224–248. St. John's, Newfoundland: Institute of Social and Economic Research.

IBFAN
1991 Breaking the rules. Penang. See Note 3.

INFACT, Canada
1982 See Note 3.

Innocenti Declaration
1991 Innocenti Declaration: On the protection, promotion and support of breastfeeding. *Ecology of Food and Nutrition* 26:271–273.
Margolis, L. H.
1991 The ethics of accepting gifts from pharmaceutical companies. *Pediatrics* 88(6):1233–1237.
Minchin, M.
1985 *Breastfeeding Matters*. Sydney, Australia: George Allen and Unwin.
Muller, M.
1974 *The Baby Killer*. London: War on Want.
Palmer, G.
1993 *The Politics of Breastfeeding*. London: Pandora Press. Post, J.
1985 Assessing the Nestlé boycott: Corporate accountability and human rights. *California Management Review* 27(2):113–131.
Radford, A.
1992 *The Ecological Impact of Bottle Feeding*. WABA Activity Sheet #1. Penang, Malaysia.
Sussman, G. D.
1982 *Selling Mothers' Milk: The Wet-Nursing Business in France, 1715–1914*. Urbana, IL: University of Illinois Press.
UNICEF News Release
1994 See Note 3.
United States Congress
1978 *Marketing and Promotion of Infant Formula in the Developing Nations*. Washington, DC: U. S. Government Printing Office.
Van Esterik, P.
1986 Confronting advocacy confronting anthropology. In *Advocacy and Anthropology*, edited by R. Paine, pp. 59–77. St. John's, Newfoundland: Institute for Social and Economic Research.
1989 *Beyond the Breast-Bottle Controversy*. New Brunswick, NJ: Rutgers University Press.
1992 *Women, Work and Breastfeeding*. Cornell International Nutrition Monograph No. 23. Ithaca, New York.
1994 Breastfeeding in feminism. *International Journal of Gynecology and Obstetrics* (Supplement) 47:41–54.
1993 A fresh look at the risks of artificial infant feeding. *Journal of Human Lactation* 9(2):97–107.
Williams, C.
1986 Milk and murder. In *Primary Health Care Pioneer: The Selected Works of Dr. Cicely Williams*, edited by N. Baumslag, pp. 66–70. Geneva, Switzerland: World Federation of Public Health Associations.
World Alliance for Breastfeeding Action
1994 *Protect Breastfeeding: Making the Code Work*. World Alliance for Breastfeeding Action, Action Folder. Available through La Leche League International.
World Commission on Environment and Development
1987 *Our Common Future*. New York: Oxford Press.

7

Beauty and the Breast: The Cultural Context of Breastfeeding in the United States

Katherine A. Dettwyler

"The giving of birth and nurturing of my baby empowered me as a woman in ways that I can't quite explain. All I know is that when I would sit up at night, nursing him, when all the house was quiet, I had an uncommon sense of being engaged in the single most important activity there is in life." (Anonymous respondent, Women's Committee of the American Studies Association, 1988)

"I could never be a woman 'cause I'd just stay home and play with my breasts all day." (Telemacher, 1991)

"So what is it about this small gland of postnatal nourishment that puts a great nation in a dither? Perhaps the problem has to do with generations of men who didn't get enough nipple when it really counted." (O'Brien, 1995)

INTRODUCTION

Today, few people would argue that formula/bottle-feeding is superior, or even equivalent, to breastfeeding. The nutritional, immunological, and emotional benefits of breastfeeding are well documented, and a number of breastfeeding promotion programs have been established. However, breastfeeding continues to decline in most regions of the world, both in terms of percentages ever breastfeeding and duration of breastfeeding. Even in the United States, the trend of the 1970s and 1980s toward increased breastfeeding (mostly among well-educated, middle- and upper-class women) peaked in 1984 at 59.7% breastfeeding in the hospital and 8.0% breastfeeding at 12 months. Hospital and 12-month figures declined from 1985 to 1990, when they were 51.5 and 6.2%, respectively. There are, however, reasons for optimism. In 1991 and 1992, breastfeeding rates in the hospital rose again, particularly among women enrolled in the Women, Infants, and Children Program (WIC) (Ross Labs Mothers' Survey, 1993). A high percentage of WIC participants are African American, Hispanic, and Asian, and of low socioeconomic status. These increases among WIC participants followed the 1991 release of $8 million in funds authorized by Congress in 1990 for the promotion of breastfeeding by the WIC program. Also, in 1991, the U.S. Department of Health and Human Services defined a lengthy list of objectives for improving the health of people in the United States, known as the *Healthy People 2000 Report*. One of these objectives is to "increase to at least 75% the proportion of mothers who breastfeed their babies in the early post-partum period and to at least 50% the proportion who continue breastfeeding until their babies are five to six months old" (U.S. Public Health Service, 1991).

The decision of whether to bottle- or breastfeed is often presented in the literature as being primarily based on nutritional and economic issues. Breastfeeding promotion programs often focus on education, teaching about the nutritional and immunological superiority of breast milk over formula or powdered milk, especially in third world contexts. They may also discuss the contraceptive value of breastfeeding, or its relative economic benefits, since it is far cheaper to provide extra food to the nursing mother than to provide formula and extra medical care for her child. The focus of breastfeeding promotion campaigns is almost always the mothers, based on the assumption that women are free to make decisions about how to feed their children based upon personal knowledge and preference. Breastfeeding is promoted as the "simple and natural" infant feeding choice, which every woman would choose if only she were convinced of its nutritional and immunological superiority over bottle-feeding with formula, and would succeed if only she were given adequate encouragement and support.

In reality, breastfeeding is both a "simple and natural" process that flows from our human biological status as mammals, and a heavily *culturized* behavior that can be so modified by cultural perceptions away from a "natural process" as to be almost unrecognizable.[1] Recent cross-cultural studies have shown that breastfeeding behaviors and, indeed, the decision of whether or not to breastfeed initially, are always embedded within a wider cultural context. In addition to nutritional, immunological, contraceptive, and economic considerations, there are, in all cultures, a number of factors and beliefs not directly related to breastfeeding, that nevertheless affect women's decisions about how to feed their children. Every cultural group holds beliefs about the primary function of women's breasts, and the proper separation of private and public domains: How are breasts defined? Are they defined as practical, useful parts of the body, similar to arms and legs? Are they viewed as functioning primarily for the purpose of feeding children? Or are breasts defined as sexual organs, functioning primarily to attract and keep male attention? How is breastfeeding defined? Is it defined as "something all women do, wherever they happen to be with their children"? Or is it viewed as an activity that should be kept private, an activity that is not acceptable in public contexts?

In some cultures, the primary function of the human breast as the physiological link between mother and child after birth has been overshadowed, or even denied, by the force of cultural beliefs assigning a sexual role to female mammary glands. In Western cultures in particular, the image of the female breast as an erotic sexual organ has become pervasive, to the extent that some people would even deny that the breast has any function in child rearing. The biological and psychological consequences for women and children living in these cultures are staggering. If we are to achieve the goals outlined in the *Healthy People 2000 Report*, breastfeeding promotion programs will need to address the wider cultural context of breastfeeding. In this chapter, I will focus on these issues, particularly as they affect women's decisions about breastfeeding in the United States.

ALL GOD'S MAMMALS GOT BREASTS

I begin with a fundamental question: What are breasts for? Or, put another way, why do human females have breasts? Breasts are known technically as mammary glands. They give their name to the class Mammalia, the zoological class to which humans belong. Mammals are characterized by having a constant internal body temperature, hair or fur, a four-chambered heart, giving birth to live young instead of laying eggs, and nourishing their young for some time after birth through secretions of the mammary glands. Mammals, or "animals with mammary glands," first appear in the fossil record more than 65 million years ago. Humans belong to the taxonomic order Primates, which also includes prosimians such as lemurs and lorises, New World and Old World monkeys, and the Lesser and Great Apes. Compared to members of the other orders, primates have longer periods of gestation and infant dependency, and longer life spans. Our closest primate relatives, chimpanzees and gorillas, nurse their offspring for 5 to 6 years (Goodall, 1986; Harvey and Clutton-Brock, 1985; Nishida, 1979; Stewart, 1988).

Humans, like all primates, belong to Ben Shaul's Group II category: mammals who remain in continuous contact with their offspring, such that the offspring can nurse "on demand," whenever they want (Ben Shaul, 1962). Human milk is relatively low in fat and protein and relatively high in carbohydrates, especially lactose, and it reflects our primate heritage, with infants that are born relatively undeveloped, nurse frequently, grow slowly, and do not need a high milk fat content for warmth (compared to pinnipeds, for example).

Why do women (and all female mammals) have breasts?[2] The breasts continue the nutritional and immunological functions of the placenta after the child is born. In addition, the process of breastfeeding involves the child in multisensory interactions with the mother. Prior to the last two generations in Western/industrialized countries (and still today in most of the world), breastfeeding was (and remains) absolutely critical for child survival itself. Even in Western/industrialized countries, breastfeeding is necessary for optimal child health and growth, from both nutritional and immunological perspectives. In addition, the tactile, olfactory, auditory, visual, and gustatory interactions between mother and child that take place during the breastfeeding process are required for proper physical, cognitive, and emotional development of the child. The Harlows' studies of infant rhesus monkeys who were offered two "mothers"—a wire model who gave milk and a cloth-covered model who did not—showed conclusively that the nutritional value of mother's milk was only one component of the mother–child relationship, from the perspective of the infant, who spent most of its time on the cloth mother (Harlow, 1958; Harlow and Harlow, 1969). In addition, carefully controlled studies of humans have consistently shown that breastfed children score better on standardized tests of mental development than formula-fed children, with children breastfed the longest showing the greatest achievements (Bauer, Ewald, Hoffman and Dubanoski, 1991; Lucas, Morley, Cole, Lister and Leeson-Payne, 1992; Morley, Cole, Powell and Lucas, 1988; Morrow-Tlucak, Houde and Ernhart, 1988; Rodgers, 1978; Rogan and Gladen, 1993; Taylor and Wadsworth, 1984; Temboury, Otero, Polanco and Arribas, 1994).

From the evolutionary perspective of the mother, breastfeeding her offspring maximizes the mother's reproductive success through three mechanisms. First, breastfeeding for several years maximizes the health and fitness of each of her children, promoting survival, proper growth, better short- and long-term health, and better cognitive development.

Second, breastfeeding precipitates the release of two hormones in the mother, oxytocin and prolactin. These hormones affect maternal feelings and behavior, leading to more appropriate child-promoting behaviors on the part of the mother, and strong feelings of acceptance and nurturance in the child (Argiolas and Gessa, 1991; Newton, 1978; Panksepp, 1992). Third, breastfeeding provides a natural child-spacing mechanism through the suppression of ovulation while the child is young and nursing intensively (see Ellison, Chapter 11, for a thorough review of the links between breastfeeding and human fertility), again promoting the survival and optimal development of the currently youngest offspring, and maximizing the mother's reproductive success over the course of her lifetime.

From the biological perspective, it is clear that human females have breasts for the primary purpose of nurturing their children. From the cultural perspective, however, breasts themselves, as well as the process of breastfeeding, can come to have other meanings. As the following examples from Mali, Sierra Leone, and Nepal show, beliefs about the links between breastfeeding and kinship, the need for economic liaisons with men, and the necessity of combining breastfeeding with work, are among the wide variety of factors that affect breastfeeding in non-Western contexts.

THE WIDER CULTURAL CONTEXT OF BREASTFEEDING: THREE NON-WESTERN EXAMPLES

I have studied breastfeeding in Mali (West Africa) firsthand, and I have read the extensive literature on breastfeeding in other cultures as well. In Mali, as in most cultures around the world, breasts hold no sexual connotations for either men or women. Sexual behavior does not involve the breasts, which are perceived as existing for the sole purpose of feeding children. When I told my friends and informants in Mali about American attitudes toward women's breasts, especially sexual foreplay involving "mouth to breast contact" by adult men, they were either bemused or horrified, or both. In any case, they regarded it as unnatural, perverted behavior, and found it difficult to believe that men would become sexually aroused by women's breasts, or that women would find such activities pleasurable.

In Mali, where breasts have retained their primary biological function, women at home may wear no clothing above the waist, and in public contexts are able to breastfeed freely without anyone even noticing. In Mali, women breastfeed in the markets, on long treks to gather firewood, on public transportation, and even at work in offices. In Mali, wherever one sees women, one sees breastfeeding women. The Bambara word for breast milk, *shin ji* (literally "breast water"), is used to refer not only to breast milk itself, but also to one's closest kin, those who not only share common parentage, but who share the more significant bond of having been nurtured at the breasts of the same woman.

In Mali, beliefs concerning kinship and biological relatedness are very influential. Malian women place a high value on the "kinship" bond that develops between a mother and her child as she breastfeeds. Nursing from the same woman likewise creates bonds of kinship between otherwise unrelated individuals. To not breastfeed would mean giving up the tenuous connection a mother has to her children in a strongly patrilineal society, and render the child unrelated to the mother. Thus, a decision not to breastfeed carries a significant social cost, as well as costs in terms of the health of both mother and child (Dettwyler, 1988). Many other societies share similar beliefs about the nature of breastfeeding and kinship (cf. Counts and Counts, 1983).

Caroline Bledsoe's work on the meaning of "tinned milk" among the Mende of Sierra Leone (West Africa) provides an entirely different perspective on breastfeeding versus bottle-feeding (Bledsoe, 1987). Among the Mende, women choose to use tinned milk to feed their children for reasons related to their economic dependence on men, and the traditional Mende postpartum sex taboo. In Mende culture, people believe that semen can contaminate the breast milk and make the child sick. This belief is widespread in West Africa, including Mali, and the "disease" caused by too early resumption of sexual activity has symptoms Western health workers would classify as "malnutrition" (Dettwyler, 1990).

Among the Mende, the semen of a man other than the child's father is thought to be especially harmful. Mende women, to prevent accusations of causing a child's illness from breast milk contaminated by semen, wean the child at a very young age and give tinned milk instead. Early weaning reduces the chance that malnutrition will be attributed to the mother's resumption of sexual activity with her husband or, particularly, with a boyfriend. In addition, male provisioning of tinned milk is interpreted as a public sign that a man acknowledges paternity, and serves to strengthen ties between father and child, and between mother and father (Bledsoe, 1987).

Some women wean their children onto tinned milk early because they recognize the contraceptive effect of breastfeeding, and want to decrease child spacing, and thus increase their fertility. For economic security, most women must ally themselves with a man; they do this partly through sexual relations. Thus, they give their child tinned milk so that they will be free to establish or continue a sexual and economic bond with their husband or other adult male. When Mende women talk about the decision to breastfeed, or when to wean, their discussions are couched almost entirely in phrases referring to the resumption of sexual intercourse (see Treckel, 1989 for fascinating parallels between the Mende beliefs and the beliefs of men and women in colonial North America). Nutritional, immunological, and economic factors directly related to the cost of tinned milk were not particularly relevant for Mende women (Bledsoe, 1987).

The work of Catherine Panter-Brick in Nepal illustrates another recent trend in breastfeeding studies. Following in the tradition of Konner and Worthman's studies of the !Kung (1980) and Vitzthum's studies of Quechua nursing patterns (1986, 1988, 1989, 1994), Panter-Brick (1991) has conducted careful, longitudinal, observational studies of breastfeeding behavior among women belonging to two different castes in rural Nepal. Using a time-allocation method, she quantified nursing frequency and duration for infants and toddlers among Tamang agro-pastoralists, who travel extensively up and down mountains to cultivate their crops and herd their animals, and among Kami women, the wives of blacksmiths, who spend most of their time working in and around their homes.

Tamang children travel with their mothers, and are nursed whenever their demands coincide with their mothers' ability to stop work temporarily. Mothers and children are often away from the home where supplementary foods might be available, thus Tamang mothers rely more heavily on breast milk, and wean their children at a much later age (up to 35 months) compared to Kami mothers (up to 25 months).

Kami women, staying at home, would seem to be in a better position to nurse at leisure, but they also find it easier to provide supplementary foods at home, and wean their children earlier than Tamang women do. However, Kami women also nurse their children for comfort (as opposed to hunger) more often than Tamang women, who, because of work constraints, nursed their children primarily when it seemed to serve a nutritional purpose, or to put the children to sleep so they would not disturb their work patterns (Panter-Brick, 1991; Catherine Panter-Brick, personal communication, 1994).

This type of quantified study of breastfeeding behavior is very time-consuming and difficult to interpret in terms of its nutritional and fertility-related implications. One problem is that it is often impossible to distinguish among (1) a child nursing vigorously and receiving substantial quantities of breast milk, (2) a child nursing for comfort, or pleasure, or while asleep, who is not extracting significant quantities of milk, and (3) a child who is suckling from a woman who is not, in fact, lactating.

The nutritional consequences for the child, and the fertility consequences for the mother, of different combinations of frequency, duration, and intensity of breastfeeding sessions may be impossible to determine. However, Panter-Brick's careful work clearly shows that "breastfeeding" is not *one* behavior, even in one population (1991), and does not serve only one (nutritional) purpose. Her work also reminds us not to make assumptions about the relationship between the type and quantity of women's work and the frequency or duration of breastfeeding episodes, or the consequences for weaning age, or about socioeconomic status and feeding patterns (Panter-Brick, 1992).

THE WIDER CULTURAL CONTEXT OF BREASTFEEDING: THE UNITED STATES

Like Mali, Sierra Leone, and Nepal, breastfeeding in the United States is embedded in a wider cultural context, one that is very different, but no less powerful in shaping breastfeeding behaviors. In the United States, the wider cultural context of breastfeeding is shaped by four fundamental assumptions that underlie beliefs about breasts: (1) the primary purpose of women's breasts is for sex (i.e., for adult men), not for feeding children, (2) breastfeeding serves only a nutritional function, (3) breastfeeding should be limited to very young infants, and (4) breastfeeding, like sex, is appropriate only when done in private.

Assumption 1: Breasts are Primarily for Sex

In the United States, many people, including many women, define women's breasts primarily as sex objects, as a focus of eroticism. Western culture is obsessed with the sexual nature of women's breasts and their role in attracting and keeping male attention, as well as their role in providing sexual pleasure for men and women (see Jelliffe and Jelliffe, 1979; Latham, 1975; and Van Esterik, 1989 for other discussions of these and closely related topics). This is reflected in many different arenas of American culture, both by the "normal" circumstances under which breasts are exposed in the United States, by the phenomenon of breast augmentation surgery (female mammary mutilation), by the association of breasts with sexual pleasure, and by the reactions of people when they do see women using their breasts to feed their children.

"Normal" Circumstances of Breast Exposure in the United States. Under "normal" circumstances in the United States, women's breasts are cov-

ered up by clothing. Among "respectable" women, partial exposure of the tops and sides of the breasts is acceptable in public only in the evening, and only in explicit, sexually alluring circumstances. For example, a woman may wear a low-cut evening gown to a fancy party, with substantial cleavage exposed, and be admired by onlookers, especially if her breasts are large. The same dress worn to church, or to teach elementary school, would be considered inappropriate. Similarly, a scanty bikini top may be all right for the beach, but not for the office. Even the most daring evening or beach wear must, however, completely cover the nipple and areola of the breasts.

In the context of pornography, women do expose their breasts, including the nipple and areola. The massive pornography industry in the United States includes magazines, books, videotapes, films, topless dancers, sex-shows, lingerie-night at the Hilton lounge, and so on. In all of these venues, much of the allure is focused on women's breasts, particularly, once again, on large breasts. Large breasts are portrayed in the media as sexy, beautiful, and essential for attracting the attention of men.

If you do not have large breasts, you are urged to acquire them through exercises, padded bras, inflatable bikini tops, or breast augmentation surgery. Teen magazines advise their young readers how to achieve the appearance of large breasts through various avenues, assuming that the girls already understand the value and desirability of large breasts (*Teen Magazine*, 1993).

In advertising, scantily clad women, almost always with large breasts, are used to sell everything from lingerie to cigarettes to beer. In 1992, the news program "20/20" aired a segment involving interviews with high-fashion models who claimed that they could not get as much work, and were not hired for the better-paying lingerie and swimsuit modeling jobs, unless they had large breasts. This is particularly difficult for most models to achieve because they are also required to have almost no body fat. Thin bodies can be achieved through dieting, but that also reduces the size of a woman's breasts. Thus, models often resort to breast augmentation surgery with silicone or saline implants to be successful at their careers. The image of the ultrathin woman with large breasts has come to stand for beauty, sexiness, and success as a woman. In at least one instance, an article in *Time* Magazine even referred to women's breasts as "human genitalia" (Quinn, 1992).

Breast Augmentation Surgery (Female Mammary Mutilation). The use of surgery to make one's breasts larger, and therefore to make one more attractive, is not limited to high-fashion models. Students in my anthropology classes at Texas A&M report that it is customary for upper-class parents in the Dallas–Fort Worth area to give their daughters breast implant surgery as high school graduation gifts. It is explicitly recognized by both parents and daughters that the young women will get more dates and be more popular in college if they have larger breasts. As one student put it: "Among the wealthier families, the boys get hot cars for graduation, and the girls get big breasts."

In 1992, it was estimated that between 1.6 and 2.0 million U.S. women already had breast implants, and the demand keeps growing, at the rate of 150,000 each year. Eighty percent of these breast implant operations are purely for enhancing the size of perfectly normal breasts. The other 20% are for reconstructive surgery following removal of a breast due to cancer, and are typically *not* classified as "cosmetic," even though the implant does not contribute in any way to the woman's physical health. In the early 1990s, the safety of silicone breast implants, manufactured by Dow-Corning Corporation and other breast implant manufacturers, was questioned, following media reports of complications including scar formation, hardening of the implant, migration of the implant, silicone leakage, and autoimmune disease. The focus in the media was on whether the breast implant manufacturers conducted thorough safety trials, and why they ignored the results of their own preliminary studies showing that the implants were prone to failure (Byrne, 1992; Chisholm, 1992).

The original disclosure of these findings resulted in a 90-day moratorium on implant surgery, and discussion then focused on whether implants should be banned altogether, and whether women who were not having problems with their implants should have them removed. Throughout these discussions, very little was said about *why* so many women felt the need to surgically alter their bodies to meet an unrealistic cultural ideal. For example, *Mirabella* magazine published an extensive article in August 1991, complete with photographs, on the dangers of implant surgery, without ever raising the underlying issue of *why* women might want this surgery (Drawbridge, 1991).[3] A notable exception was an article in *McCall's* magazine titled "Why Women Want Man-Made Breasts" (Mithers, 1992), which briefly discussed the cultural pressure on women in the United States to have large breasts.

The American Society of Plastic and Reconstructive Surgeons (the group of surgeons, almost exclusively male, who make money from breast augmentation surgery) told the Food and Drug Administration that "There is a substantial and enlarging body of medical information and opinion to the effect that these deformities (small breasts) are really a disease" (Ehrenreich, 1992). Women with perfectly normal, functioning breasts were told that they had micromastia (literally "small breasts" in Latin), a disease for which the only cure was breast augmentation surgery (Ehrenreich, 1992). In another statement, the Society claimed that "If left uncorrected these deformities [small breasts] can cause a total lack of well-being" (Cited in Mithers, 1992).

In the United States, both in the public eye, and in the eyes of the medical establishment, not only are breasts most commonly viewed as sexual organs, but small breasts are viewed as a disease, and providing all women with large breasts is considered a public health issue. Adding their voices to the breast implant controversy were a number of women who demanded that their "right to choose to have implants" be restored. Some women cited "mental health" issues in defense of their right to have surgery to make their breasts larger, claiming that their body image and self-esteem would be permanently damaged if they were not able to have large breasts.

How can we understand this Western cultural perspective of women's breasts as sex objects, a perspective that has led to more than two million women voluntarily mutilating their bodies in pursuit of a male-defined sexually attractive ideal? A comparison to an analogous complex of beliefs and behavior in a very different cultural context may help us think about these issues from a broader perspective.

Are Mammary Glands Intrinsically Erotic in Humans? First, despite what the typical Western male thinks, including U.S. anthropologist Owen Lovejoy (1981) and British physician Peter Anderson (1983)—see further discussion below—there is no evidence that the human female breast is *intrinsically* erotic. Men and women in Western, industrialized countries are taught by their culture to think of breasts this way, from a very early age, but it is only a cultural belief of limited distribution, shared by relatively few cultures around the globe.

A perfect analogy to the way Western culture eroticizes breasts is the now-defunct practice of foot-binding in China, which persisted from some time prior to A.D. 960 until well into the twentieth century (Anagnost, 1989; Levy, 1992). Young girls in upper-class families in China had their feet bound so that, as adults, they would have tiny, severely deformed feet. The binding process, usually performed by their mothers, took place when the girls were between 6 and 8 years of age. Tight bandages bound the four lateral toes underneath the foot. "While subject to sores and putrescence which caused them further suffering, their feet were forced into a succession of progressively smaller shoes until they achieved the desired three inches in length, a process that took about two years" (Anagnost, 1989:331).

Tiny feet were usually a sign of high status, a symbol of wealth, as they marked a family who could afford to forego the agricultural labor of its women. They were also viewed as "an effective way of ensuring the virtue of women by circumscribing their movement . . . a sign of feminine virtue and respectability. . . . The smallness of one's feet therefore became an acutely conscious measure of feminine presentability, and this is important to remember when trying to understand how foot binding could have been *a form of oppression that women enacted against themselves*" (Anagnost, 1989:330, emphasis added). Among the lower classes, women were "merely hobbled" (Anagnost, 1989:331), and were still expected to work in the fields.

Tiny feet, known as "Golden Lotuses," were also highly valued, even worshipped by men, as the ultimate in erotic stimulants (Levy, 1992). The practice of foot-binding took a perfectly healthy, functional organ, the foot, and mutilated it through the cruelest torture into something useful only for male sexual pleasure. Women without bound feet were ridiculed and shamed for their big feet (Gordon and Hinton, 1984). Women with bound feet could not walk properly and could not stand for long hours on their feet; some were in constant pain for much of their lives. Men also claimed that it was easy to keep a woman with bound feet "in line" as all a husband had to do during an argument with his wife was stomp on her foot, and she would submit to his wishes (Gordon and Hinton, 1984).

Most Americans view Chinese foot-binding as the barbaric practice of backward people. Yet breast augmentation surgery, or female mammary mutilation, as it is more properly called, is *essentially the same thing* (Table 7.1). A perfectly healthy, functional organ, the breast, is mutilated through surgery into something useful only for male sexual pleasure. Rarely is the lactational function of the breast preserved, or even considered, in breast augmentation surgery. Women with small breasts are

Table 7.1. Comparison of Breast Augmentation Surgery (Female Mammary Mutilation) and Chinese Foot-Binding

Feature	*China*	*United States*
Body part	Feet	Breasts
Normal biological function	Locomotion	Lactation
Culturally defined function	Sexual stimulant	Sexual stimulant
Cultural modification	Foot-binding	Breast augmentation surgery
Effects on normal function	Often completely impaired	Often completely impaired
Primary promoters	Usually women, for their daughters	Usually women, for themselves
Effects on health	Scarring, infections, pain	Scarring, infections, pain, perhaps autoimmune disease

made to feel inadequate, unattractive, even abnormal. The largeness of one's breasts therefore becomes "an acutely conscious measure of feminine presentability." A body part that is not intrinsically sexually stimulating to the male of the species is culturally defined as being so, but only in certain (deformed/abnormally large and pert) configurations. Women go to great lengths to achieve this ideal, even to the point of permanent mutilation and long-term damage to their health.[4]

The Western preoccupation with breasts as sexual organs spills over into anthropological theory as well, where it is reflected in many (usually male) anthropologists' recreations of early hominid behavioral evolution. The prime example is the model proposed by Owen Lovejoy, based in part on elaborate speculation by zoologist Desmond Morris in his popular book *The Naked Ape* (Morris, 1967). Lovejoy (1981) suggests that prominent breasts among female Australopithecines helped attract males in the first place, and then helped cement the pair-bond relationship necessary for further physical and cultural evolution toward modern humanity (Lovejoy, 1981). This model is still often presented in introductory anthropology textbooks (for example, Nelson and Jurmain, 1991:264). The aspect of the model dealing with the "erotic value of prominent breasts in early hominid females" is seldom questioned.

How valid is this perspective? The mammary glands play no role in sexual behavior in any species other than humans. Among humans, the cross-cultural evidence does not support the notion that male attraction to female breasts is a widespread, universal phenomenon across all populations of the human species. People in most cultures do not regard female breasts as sexually stimulating, manipulation of the breasts is *not* a common aspect of sexual behavior in most cultures, and women in most human populations do not have particularly prominent breasts. Why, then, do anthropologists such as Lovejoy construct elaborate scenarios of hominid evolution to explain the Western *cultural* phenomenon of defining breasts as erotic?

In 1983, British physician Peter Anderson wrote an article titled "The Reproductive Role of the Human Breast," published in *Current Anthropology*. Early in the introduction he cites Lovejoy's 1981 article. Later, in a section titled "The Erotic Role of the Human Breast," he cites Ford and Beach (1952)[5] as his reference for the claim that "*In many cultures* the size and shape of the woman's breasts are important criteria of sexual attractiveness" (Anderson, 1983:26, emphasis added). Anderson's article is often cited when people want to claim that attraction to human female breasts is a biological propensity of human males. What did Ford and Beach actually say on this subject?

In their cross-cultural survey of patterns of sexual behavior in 190 cultures around the globe, Ford and Beach had this to report about the role of female breasts in sexual attraction: "*In a few cultures* the size and shape of the woman's breasts are important criteria of sexual attractiveness" (Ford and Beach, 1951:87, emphasis added). In their Table 5 (p. 88), they cite 13 cultures, out of the 190 surveyed, where men viewed women's breasts as sexually attractive. In nine of these cultures men preferred large breasts, in two cultures men preferred long, pendulous breasts, and in another two cultures men preferred "upright, hemispherical breasts." Clearly, "a few cultures" was transmuted to "many cultures" by Anderson because the reality undermined the purpose of his argument, which was to explain male attraction to female breasts in a pan-human, evolutionary manner.

Similarly, the cross-cultural evidence does not support the notion that women's breasts play an important role in sexual behavior in humans. Once again, Anderson's article is often cited in this context, and Anderson cites Ford and Beach (1952) to back up his statement that "*in most cultures* stimulation of the woman's breasts is a common precursor to intercourse" (Anderson, 1983:26, emphasis added). Ford and Beach's cross-cultural survey actually said: "Manual or oral stimulation of the woman's breasts by the man frequently precedes or accompanies intercourse *in the United States*. . . . Stimulation of the woman's breasts by her partner is a common precursor or accompaniment of intercourse *in some societies* other than our own" (Ford and Beach, 1951:46, emphasis added). In a footnote, the authors again list 13 societies, out of 190, in which women's breasts are stimulated before or during sexual intercourse. Of these 13 societies, only three are also listed among the 13 where breasts are considered sexually attractive. Once again, Anderson has transmuted "some societies" to "most cultures," yet his miscitation is often cited and repeated.[6]

Finally, the anatomical reality is that most women do not have particularly "prominent" breasts unless they are in certain biological categories (overweight, pubescent, pregnant, or lactating), or use cultural adjustments (push-up bras, inflatable bikini tops, or breast implants). In Mali, people referring to the age of a young woman will make reference to whether her breasts have "fallen" yet or not, recognizing that only young, nulliparous girls have prominent breasts. Someone whose breasts have "fallen" is merely an older woman, however, not someone to be reviled, and a woman's sexual attractiveness depends on her face and thighs, not on the size or shape of her breasts.

"Why do human females, alone among the primates, have 'prominent' breasts?" When the question is posed, we need to look first to whether, or to what extent, this is even true. Second, we should begin from the assumption that since breasts serve the biological function of child survival, then prominent breasts, to the extent that they exist in humans, probably serve some adaptive role in child survival. Perhaps the breasts are a convenient and handy place to store excess fat when available, fat that can be easily and quickly mobilized into the breast milk during times of nutritional stress. Along the same lines, it is most probable that the nipples contain erectile tissue to facilitate the child's latching-on to nurse, and that the contrasting color and texture of breast versus areola function as visual and tactile "bull's eyes" to help the child find the nipple, not as "epigamic features" to attract male attention, as some have claimed (Montagna and MacPherson, 1974, for example).

Are mammary glands *intrinsically* erotic in humans? The ethnographic evidence clearly says "no." As Anderson himself points out, "We seem to be the only mammal in which the mammary gland has this erotic function" (1983:26). Even among humans, according to Ford and Beach's survey (1951), only 13 out of 190 cultures report that men view women's breasts as being related to sexual attractiveness, and only 13 out of 190 cultures report male manipulation of female breasts as a precursor or accompaniment of sexual intercourse. Given that the ethnographic evidence suggests that in only a small percentage of human societies is the mammary gland viewed as erotic or sexual, we are led to the conclusion that such behavior has a purely cultural basis, with a limited distribution. Obviously, humans can *learn* to view breasts as sexually attractive. We can learn to prefer long, pendulous breasts, or upright, hemispherical breasts. We can learn to prefer large breasts. All of these views can be culturally imposed, just as some Chinese men learned to view tiny, deformed feet as sexually attractive. Once we understand that these behaviors have a *cultural* basis, we can stop searching for creative, evolutionary, adaptive, explanations of why they exist.

Because these views are culturally imposed, we can stop searching for adult male-based explanations of why it would be adaptive for women to have prominent breasts, to have erectile tissue in their nipples, and for the areola to be a different color and texture than the rest of the breast. Because these views are culturally imposed, we can choose not to accept the idea that large breasts are desirable, and worth the high cost to women's and children's health. Because these views are culturally imposed, we can consciously choose the alternative route of using cultural beliefs to reinforce, rather than deny, the biological function of women's breasts as body parts designed for nurturing children.

Is Breastfeeding Sexually Stimulating? In almost every discussion of breastfeeding published in a Western context, the issue is raised of whether the activity of breastfeeding itself is sexually pleasurable or stimulating to the mother. Given our cultural context of viewing breasts as erotic, this is not surprising. What is surprising is that so few people, scientists and medical professionals included, have recognized the culture-bound nature of the question.

For example, Hytten claims: "Many women enjoy breast-feeding. They derive considerable sensual, even erotic pleasure from the suckling and a sense of pride and satisfaction when the baby is obviously thriving. Such a picture is held up by enthusiasts for breastfeeding as the norm, yet for the majority of women breast-feeding offers no such pleasures" (Hytten, 1991:131). Hytten then goes on to claim that many women experience discomfort and pain while breastfeeding, and that breastfeeding also exhausts them, leaving one with the overall impression that breastfeeding is *not* pleasurable for the mother.

In addition, some opponents of "prolonged" breastfeeding have argued that the mother is continuing to breastfeed an older child to satisfy her own sexual needs, because she finds breastfeeding sexually satisfying (see Chapter 2, this volume, for a fuller discussion of this perspective).

We can approach this question by breaking it into several component parts. First, are the breasts particularly sensitive? Second, is it the case that breastfeeding is always, or even usually, pleasurable for the mother? Third, are all physically pleasurable feelings necessarily *sexual* feelings?

Are the Breasts Particularly Sensitive? It is often assumed that breasts are particularly sensitive and are richly endowed with sensory nerves, but this does not seem to be the case. Montagna and MacPherson conducted anatomical and histological analyses of human breast tissues, and found no evidence that the breasts are particularly sensitive. They write:

> There is a widespread notion that breasts, nipples, and areolae in particular, are erogenous areas, highly sensitive to tactile stimulation. Thus they are assumed to be rich in cutaneous sensory nerves. Physiologic data, however, contradict this assumption. Morphologic preparations show only a few recognizable nerve end organs at the tip of the nipple around the galactophores of the glands of Montgomery. In most of the other areas of the breast except around the vellus haris there are relatively few superficial nerves of any kind. (1974:10)

These authors also cite other research showing that the nipples, areolae, and peripheral breast areas are relatively insensitive to warmth, cold, pain, and pressure (Montagna and MacPherson, 1974:15). According to Montagna and MacPherson, the tips of the nipples themselves are the most sensitive part of the breast. During breastfeeding, the nipples are being compressed between the base of the infant's tongue and his/her palate.

That human females can *learn* to associate oral and manual manipulation of their breasts during foreplay with sexual arousal and pleasure is well-known. They can also learn to associate many other activities with sexual arousal and pleasure ("dirty" language, earlobe nibbling, pornographic films, sexual fantasies, or bondage, for example). This does not automatically mean that the breasts are particularly sensitive, or that the sensations a mother experiences from breastfeeding her child should be interpreted as *sexual* pleasure.

Is Breastfeeding Always, or Even Usually, Pleasurable for the Mother? Certainly breastfeeding can be pleasurable for women. The intense, intimate bond that exists between a mother and her nursing child can be a source of great pleasure to the mother. To be cuddled up with one's child, knowing that your body is capable of sustaining life and health in this new person you have created, can be an immense source of pride and satisfaction for the mother, as Hytten noted above. Many women enjoy breastfeeding their children, and well they should. It is the one thing, other than giving birth itself, which women can do that men cannot. It can be a great boost to self-esteem, and many women report feeling linked to all other women, especially to their own mothers and grandmothers, as they sit and nurse their children. An acquaintance of the author expresses it this way: "I enjoy breastfeeding my two-year-old because I love what it does for him. It relaxes him, it calms him down, it makes him happy. He knows without any doubt that his mommy loves him" (Anonymous, personal communication).

The explanation of these feelings of empowerment and well-being is partly cultural and partly physiological. During breastfeeding sessions, two hormones are released by the mother's pituitary gland. Oxytocin is released in response to the physical stimulation of the child's suckling of the breast. In many women, just the sight, sound, or even thought of their child can trigger oxytocin release and milk let-down. Oxytocin has been described as "the hormone of love," by Niles Newton, who devoted her life to the study of the role of oxytocin in breastfeeding and maternal behavior (Newton and Newton, 1948; Romano, 1990). Oxytocin stimulates a mother's let-down or milk-ejection reflex. It also stimulates contraction of the uterus, which is essential to expulsion of the placenta and prevention of hemorrhaging immediately postpartum. In addition, oxytocin triggers nurturing behavior and affectionate feelings toward others. Both men and women release oxytocin in conjunction with eating, and with orgasm (Newton, 1978).

It is clear from animal and human studies that high circulating levels of oxytocin contribute to general feelings of well-being in breastfeeding mothers (Insel and Shapiro, 1992; McCarthy, Kow and Pfaff, 1992). What is not clear is that either the surge of oxytocin itself, or its immediate consequences, is recognized as physically pleasurable by the mother. The milk let-down reflex, when the milk-producing cells high on her chest release milk into the milk ducts of her breasts, is usually described by women as a "warm, tingling sensation." For some women, it can be painful or unpleasant. The effect of oxytocin on the uterus is most clearly felt immediately postpartum. These strong uterine contractions can be as painful as intense labor. In any case, the immediate or longer-term effects of oxytocin released by breastfeeding cannot automatically be interpreted as feelings of *sexual* pleasure in the breastfeeding woman.

A second hormone, prolactin, is released by the mother's pituitary in response to the removal of milk from the breast by the child. Prolactin acts as the mediator between the child's demand for milk and the mother's supply. The more milk the child removes, the more prolactin is released, and the more milk the mother produces. Breast milk production is a demand-driven system. In addition, prolactin acts—either directly or through some intermediary—to suppress ovulation in the woman (see Chapter 11, this volume). Like oxytocin, prolactin acts to relax the mother and induce feelings of well-being and calm. Thus, there are both psychological and physiological factors that contribute to breastfeeding being pleasurable for women, but these are all vague, overall feelings of well-being, not specifically physical pleasure from the act itself.

Sometimes the physical sensation of the child nursing is pleasurable because it evokes all these "warm fuzzies." Sometimes it is pleasurable in the same way as many different forms of physical contact are pleasurable: like taking off your shoes, like a hug from a friend, like someone holding your hand, like scratching an itch. All of these descriptions have been offered by breastfeeding women as they try to describe "what it feels like."

Some authors have argued that breastfeeding *must* be pleasurable for the mother, or the species would not have survived. For example, Riordan and Rapp (1980:109) claim: "The objective of this article is to explore the hypothesis that one of these [feminine reproductive functions], breastfeeding/lactation, is a sexually pleasurable process for the mother in addition to providing nourishment for her infant. Included in this hypothesis is the assumption that the very survival of *Homo sapiens* has been dependent on these sensual reinforcements of breastfeeding. If it were not so, man would have joined the dinosaurs in extinction long ago." (1980:109). La Leche League International's statement on "Breastfeeding and Female Sexuality" includes a similar statement: "The human race would not have survived if breastfeeding was not enjoyable for mothers" (La Leche League International, 1992). In a similar vein, Newton and Newton write: "The survival of the human race, long before the concept of "duty" evolved, depended upon the satisfactions gained from the two voluntary acts of reproduction—coitus and breastfeeding. These had to be sufficiently pleasurable to ensure their frequent occurrence" (1967:1180).

All of these statements reveal a fundamental misunderstanding of the mechanisms of evolution by natural selection. Natural selection operates on populations to increase the frequency of alleles (variant forms of genes) that increase reproductive success. To the extent that breastfeeding behavior in humans has a genetic basis, natural selection will act to increase the frequency of any alleles that contribute to breastfeeding success. Throughout the prehistory and history of the species, and continuing today, women who breastfed their children had greater relative reproductive success than women who did not. That is, breastfeeding provided a health advantage to the child, and a reproductive advantage to the breastfeeding mother, so that she ended up with more children surviving to adulthood—the measure of reproductive success—than women who did not breastfeed. Whether breastfeeding was pleasurable to the mother or not is a moot point. As long as breastfeeding conferred a reproductive advantage, the behavior would have been selected for, whether or not it was pleasurable to the woman.[7] One cannot argue from an evolutionary perspective that breastfeeding must have been "sensual" or conveyed "sexual pleasure" to the breastfeeding mother in order for the species to survive.

At the same time, many women report that they are afraid to attempt breastfeeding, because they have heard that it is painful. Others say that they fully intended to breastfeed, but gave it up in defeat after a few days, because their nipples hurt. It is the case that the physical sensation of the child nursing can be painful due to sore nipples. Every lay publication on breastfeeding has a section on how to prevent and treat sore nipples. Sore nipples are usually the result of improper positioning of the infant on the breast, which can be easily corrected if the mother is referred to someone capable of diagnosing and correcting the problem. Sore nipples can also be caused by "nipple confusion" in infants who have been given pacifiers and bottles. When a child accustomed to a pacifier or bottle nipple is put to the breast, he may suck only on the end of the nipple, rather than taking the entire nipple and much of the areola into his mouth. This can result in sore nipples in the mother and poor growth in the child, who is not able to remove breast milk from the breast efficiently. Nipple confusion of this kind is easily avoided by not using pacifiers or bottles.

In addition, sometimes nipples get sore simply because the child is nursing very often or has been nursing in a particular way (turning his head to look at something without releasing the nipple, for example). Sometimes sore nipples are a symptom of a fungal infection known as thrush (*Candida*). Sore nipples may be the result of anxiety on the mother's part, which interferes with the milk let-down reflex, requiring the infant to suck harder and harder to extract milk. Contrary to popular belief, the child's teeth are *not* usually a source of pain for the mother. The child's lower teeth are covered by his or her tongue during active suckling, and the upper teeth are placed high on the areola. If the child does bite the mother, as children sometimes do, it hurts, whether or not the child has teeth—a young infant can clamp down with toothless gums and cause just as much pain as an older child who bites. Thus, breastfeeding a child can be painful for the mother, but these sources of pain are easily correctable *if* the mother gets appropriate advice from a knowledgeable and supportive source.

Sometimes the physical sensation of the child nursing is annoying. The mother is tired, she needs to be doing something else, the baby has been nursing all day because of a growth spurt, or a new tooth, or an illness, and she just wishes she could be somewhere else, doing something else; or she is awakened during the night by the child waking up, once again, and latching on.

Sometimes the physical sensation of the child nursing is simply neutral. It does not feel like much of anything, one way or the other. Especially after a mother has nursed several children, and is well into her second or third year of nursing a child, the physical sensations may be negligible, as the nipple becomes desensitized due to prolonged contact. This is probably the most common experience of most women for most of their breastfeeding careers. "You can tell the baby is nursing, but that's it," as one woman told me. Some authors, committed to the idea that breastfeeding is sexually pleasurable to women, have even explained away the reports of many women that breastfeeding is *not* sexually pleasurable by suggesting that these mothers are in denial, or feel too guilty or embarrassed to admit to having sexual feelings while breastfeeding (Riordan and Rapp, 1980). A simpler explanation is that these women are telling the truth.

Thus, it appears that the physical sensations evoked by a child breastfeeding range from physically pleasurable to painful, annoying, or neutral. For most women, most of the time, the physical act of breastfeeding is either pleasurable or neutral.

We can go on to ask, if a mother *does* experience physically pleasurable sensations during breastfeeding, are these feelings necessarily *sexual* feelings?

Are All Physically Pleasurable Feelings Necessarily Sexual Feelings? Is there anything *intrinsically* erotic or sexually stimulating about pleasurable feelings arising from manual and oral stimulation of the nipples and areola, or do people in some cultures *learn* to respond in a sexual way to such behavior? To put it another way, if your only experience of breast stimulation has been in a sexual context, then when you experience those feelings during breastfeeding, will you tend to interpret those feelings as *sexually* pleasurable?

An analogy may help us think about this issue in an objective manner. Is there anything *intrinsically* erotic or sexually stimulating about a back rub? Among some couples, back rubs can be a prelude to sexual intercourse, and the feelings evoked by a back rub under such circumstances—the privacy of a bedroom, a desirable partner, strong emotional involvement, perhaps even candle light, scented oils, a little wine, a little Louis Armstrong—can certainly be interpreted as erotic and sexually stimulating. Conversely, *the very same physical motions, the very same physical feelings,* equally as physically pleasurable, administered by a trainer in a gym after a workout, or by a physical therapist subsequent to an injury, normally do not evoke erotic feelings, nor are they usually interpreted as sexually stimulating. To claim that breastfeeding a child, or getting a back rub from a professional masseuse/masseur, is *intrinsically* erotic is to confuse content with context. Similarly, if a woman construes the physical sensations of a child breastfeeding as sexually stimulating, it is most likely because she has internalized her culture's beliefs that breasts are primarily for sexual pleasure, and because all of her prior experience with "mouth-to-nipple" contact was in a sexual context.

Riordan and Rapp state that in "many paintings of nursing dyads that abound in collections of great art, we may note a mood of introspection and a faint, bemused expression of pleasure on the mother's face" (1980:109). They argue that these expressions represent *sexual* pleasure, but they provide absolutely no justification for their interpretation. It does a great disservice to women everywhere to interpret the feelings of pleasure they enjoy from nursing and nurturing their children at the breast as sexual feelings.

The physical sensations of an infant or child nursing at the breast can be pleasant, of course. They can also be painful, or annoying, or totally neutral, depending on the context, the mother's mood, and the child's position at the breast (see above). By the same token, the sensations of a back rub can be physically pleasant, or painful, or annoying, or neutral, depending on the context, one's mood and the skill of the masseuse. The breasts are not particularly sensitive body parts; and while breastfeeding can be physically pleasant, it isn't always. When it is pleasurable, these feelings should not automatically be interpreted as *sexual* feelings.

As has been shown above, the overwhelming notion that female breasts are sexual organs is reflected in pornography, advertising, evening wear, the demand for breast implants, and anthropological theories of early hominid evolution.

It is also reflected clearly in common public attitudes toward women who choose to go against the cultural norm, who choose to follow instead the biological norm, and use their breasts for feeding their children. At the same time that breasts, especially large breasts, are worshipped as evidence of female sexual attractiveness, the role of breasts in nourishing and nurturing children is often misunderstood.

Reactions of People to Women Breastfeeding Their Children. In the Western cultural context, many people are not comfortable seeing a woman breastfeeding. They are embarrassed; they do not know where to look, or what to say or do. Many public accommodations have rules against breastfeeding, and women are asked to leave or to cease breastfeeding. In restaurants, women have been told that they are "offending" their fellow diners by breastfeeding their children, and must cease or leave the restaurant. In her nationally syndicated advice column, Ann Landers tells mothers to nurse their children only in private, and to use the rest rooms if they must nurse their children while out in public. Another alternative she offers is for mothers to pump their milk at home and give it to their children in bottles, so as not to offend anyone.

All researchers who study breastfeeding in the United States can cite numerous instances of women being arrested, fired from their jobs, or harassed, simply because they were breastfeeding outside their homes (Jelliffe and Jelliffe, 1979:302). In the late 1980s, news personality Debra Norville was dismissed from her job as co-host of the Today show, in part because she posed for *People Weekly* with "one of her breasts exposed" (she was breastfeeding her newborn). The situation had not improved much by the early 1990s, as the following examples reveal: A woman breastfeeding in a grocery store was told by a store employee, "Don't you know that's what bottles are for?" A ten-year-old boy observed a classmate's mother nursing her infant, and remarked, "that's disgusting." He then turned around and made a joke about *Playboy* centerfolds to the other boys in the class, who snickered. The mother of a toddler was asked by the director of her son's day-care center not to breastfeed him in the classroom, in front of the other children. The director said she was afraid the children "would get the wrong idea." A university English professor was reprimanded by her department head for breastfeeding her 1-month-old infant during a writing workshop she was conducting for graduate students.

Given the typical cultural context in the United States concerning the primary purpose of breasts, is it any wonder that using your breasts to feed a child seems odd, strange, perhaps even bizarre? Is it any wonder that doctors are so quick to recommend artificial infant-feeding products, and are so reluctant to help women work through breastfeeding problems? Is it any wonder that so many women are reluctant to even consider breastfeeding? In addition to this cultural context, another assumption underlies much of the research and rhetoric surrounding the relative merits of breast milk and infant formula—the belief that breastfeeding serves only a nutritional purpose.

Assumptions 2 And 3: Breastfeeding Serves Only a Nutritional Function and Is Only for Young Infants

Even for people who do get beyond the idea that breasts are only for sexual purposes, another assumption clouds their thinking about breastfeeding: the notion that the process of breastfeeding itself serves only one purpose, a nutritional purpose, the transfer of breast milk from mother to infant.[8] This assumption has far-reaching implications for the cultural context of breastfeeding in the United States.

If your culture teaches you that the only function of breastfeeding is nutritional, and if it also teaches you that artificial feeding products are nutritionally equivalent to breast milk, then there would be no particular reason to choose one method over the other. If breastfeeding serves only nutritional purposes, then children should not want to nurse unless they are hungry, and mothers should not feel obligated to allow children to suckle if they have recently been fed.

If you accept the nutritional superiority of breast milk over artificial infant-feeding products, but still believe that breastfeeding serves only a nutritional purpose, then there is not much point in breastfeeding beyond the age of 12 months, when most children can drink from a cup, and begin to eat solid foods, and you may conclude that the sooner the child is weaned from the breast, the better.

Where does this belief come from, that breastfeeding serves primarily (or exclusively) a nutritional function? A powerful force to be considered in any discussion of breastfeeding in the Western, industrialized world is the infant formula industry. Prior to the vociferous "Infant Formula Controversy" of the 1970s and 1980s, manufacturers of artificial feeding products promoted their wares as being "scientific formulated," and superior to breast milk. Women were encouraged to doubt their own abilities to feed their children, and "insufficient" or "weak" milk were common diagnoses in mothers having problems breastfeeding their infants. Since the controversy, infant formula manufacturers have bent over backward to acknowledge the superiority of breast milk in print and television advertising, and on the labels of their products. The formula companies vie with one another to claim that their product most closely mimics mother's milk, and ask "If it doesn't come from you, shouldn't it come from Gerber?" Recent advertisements compare the various nutritional components of one particular infant formula with those found in human milk, to demonstrate that this formula is most like mother's milk.

The infant formula industry even produces informational pamphlets, aimed at pregnant women, that extol the virtues of breastfeeding, "until you switch to bottles." However, a close examination of the images of breastfeeding women in advertisements for artificial feeding products and articles about infant-feeding choices in "baby" or "new parent" magazines is highly revealing. In the infant formula promotion literature, breastfeeding is often described and portrayed as a "quasi-sexual" behavior, an intimate, private experience between mother and child. Beautiful perhaps, laudatory even, but still, like sex, an activity best done while wearing a modest white negligee and in the privacy of one's own bedroom, and, of course, only with a very young infant. And breastfeeding is portrayed as having exclusively nutritional purposes.

The images of women breastfeeding their children that are used in infant formula advertising almost invariably show Caucasian women. They are shown breastfeeding newborns or young infants (as opposed to older infants, toddlers, or older children), they are pictured wearing modest, frilly, usually white, nightgowns or negligees, and the setting is usually a rocking chair in a middle- or upper-class baby's room. The not-so-subtle message is that nursing a child is not something one does while dressed in street clothes, not something one does while working, not something one does outside of the bedroom, let alone out in public or at work, and definitely not something one does with a child old enough to walk and talk.

For many women, the perception is perpetuated that breastfeeding is restrictive, confining, and limits one's activities outside the home. Likewise, the message is clear: breastfeeding is only for young infants, and the natural course of events is to wean the infant off the breast and onto a bottle of infant formula.[9]

In a recent pamphlet published by Ross Labs (1989), there is only one photo of a woman nursing who is not dressed in a negligee, sitting in the bedroom. This woman is dressed in regular clothing, and is shown sitting in her kitchen nursing her infant. In the background, her husband is cooking dinner. This may be meant to promote the image of the liberated, sensitive man, who is willing to help out his wife. But to many women, the message it sends is that "if you want to breastfeed, you'll need someone to help with your regular chores." Help with the housework, whether from a spouse or from relatives, friends or paid workers, certainly makes it easier on the mother to tend to the baby, including breastfeeding, but in the West, such help remains a luxury that many women will not have. For a man, it may imply that he will have to do more work around the house if his wife breastfeeds, which many men are not willing to do. Other pictures in this brochure show men interacting with their children primarily by giving the baby a bottle, rather than some other mode of interaction such as diaper changing, bathing, dressing, or playing. For men who want to be involved, the message is that if your wife breastfeeds, you will not be able to help feed the baby, you might have to change diapers instead.

Along similar lines, several studies have been published recently focusing on how to support the husband of the breastfeeding woman, who may feel "left out" of the relationship between mother and child, or even jealous of the child's access to his wife's breasts (Jordan, 1986; Jordan and Wall, 1990, 1993; Walker, 1991). In the guise of promoting breastfeeding, these studies offer recommendations on how to help men cope with their feelings of envy and jealousy. For example, one author notes, "The changes [of pregnancy and lactation] may be especially problematic if the breasts have been a source of great sexual pleasure for the man. . . . During lactation, the presence of milk may serve as a constant reminder to the father that the breasts "belong" to the infant" (Jordan, 1986:95). Jordan's solutions include weekly nights out for the couple without the infant, and trips out alone for the mother, leaving the father to give the infant breast milk in a bottle, so that the father "does not feel totally deprived of the closeness engendered by the feeding experience" (Jordan, 1986:96). None of the suggestions for helping the couple deal with the father's feelings addresses the simpler, more basic, and permanent solution of changing what we teach our sons about the purpose of female breasts.

The fundamental idea that the infant formula companies want doctors and their patients to believe is that breastfeeding serves only a nutritional function, and that their product so closely mimics breast milk as to be interchangeable, or even superior. The infant formula companies have a vested interest in promoting the "commodification" of breast milk. They also want to promote the idea that breastfeeding is restrictive and confining to women, and that women should be worried about the quantity or quality of their breast milk.

Nutritionists also promote the idea that breastfeeding serves only nutritional purposes. For example, in 1994, Samuel Fomon, a highly respected expert on child nutrition, made the following statements: "One of the goals of nutritional management of the infant is to promote eating in moderation. Therefore, as soon as the mother feels confident about her ability to breast feed her infant, usually by 10 days after delivery, she should begin to encourage the infant to terminate the feeding at the earliest indication of the infant's willingness to do so" (Fomon, 1994:1). Such statements reflect a purely nutritional approach to breastfeeding, as well as a woeful lack of knowledge of the literature on breastfeeding and growth published during the last decade. The DARLING study of Dewey and colleagues (Dewey, Heinig, Nommsen, Peerson and Lonnerdal, 1992; Heinig, Nommsen, Peerson, Lonnerdal and Dewey, 1993) showed conclusively that it is *bottle-fed* infants who consume excess amounts of formula, and who have problems with obesity. Breastfed infants in the DARLING study were significantly leaner for the same length and head circumference than the bottle-fed infants, and consumed far fewer calories and fat. The work of Woolridge and colleagues (Drewett and Woolridge, 1979, 1981; Woolridge, 1992 and Chapter 8, this volume; Woolridge, Ingram and Baum, 1990) has shown that breastfed children are quite capable of controlling their own intake, without arbitrary rules imposed from outside. The literature on the physiological mechanisms of breast milk content and appetite control in human children (Woolridge, 1992) shows that breastfed children do not have to be "taught" to eat in moderation—they have built-in mechanisms to monitor and control the intake of nutrients, when allowed to nurse on demand. Likewise, Fomon's advice is not supported by the anthropological and animal science literature on feeding frequency and duration (Ben Shaul, 1962; Trevathan, 1987; Wood, Lai, Johnson, Campbell and Maslar, 1985), which suggests that frequent feedings are appropriate for the human species. Comparative primate data indicate that several short nursing bouts per hour, around the clock, constitute the "natural" rhythm for higher primate breastfeeding frequency (Stewart, 1988), and a number of human populations still breastfeed in this manner (Konner and Worthman, 1980; Wood et al., 1985). There is no evidence that terminating a breastfeeding session "as soon as possible" is advisable from either the perspective of the child, in terms of growth and health, or the mother, in terms of maintaining milk supply and lactational amenorrhea. Most significantly, Fomon ignores the nonnutritional functions of breastfeeding—physical, social, psychological, and emotional development of the child, immunological protection, and of course the birth-spacing mechanisms of child suckling.

A final example comes from the work of Louis Lefebvre (1985), who proposed that frequent parent–offspring food sharing among certain nonhuman primates functions to promote early weaning. This hypothesis assumes that the primary, if not the only, function of breastfeeding is nutritional. Early weaning would be adaptive from the mother's perspective, as she could then invest in a subsequent offspring. Lefebvre tested this hypothesis using data from 52 primate species, and concluded that the hypothesis could not be supported. He concluded that parent–offspring food sharing serves some other purpose in nonhuman primates. Significantly for my argument here, he did *not* conclude that breastfeeding might serve nonnutritional purposes.

Assumption 4: Breastfeeding Should Be Done Only in Private

The image of breastfeeding as a quasi-sexual behavior that should be kept private has profound implications for whether women who work outside their homes can successfully breastfeed their children.

Women's work outside the home is often viewed as a barrier to successful breastfeeding, and, in industrialized countries, solutions range from longer maternity leave to having employers provide breast pumps and private places to pump, or even on-site child-care facilities, where children can be nursed during breaks or at lunch. Underlying these approaches is the assumption that breastfeeding is essentially incompatible with simultaneous work activity. But breastfeeding is not *intrinsically* incompatible with work outside the home. Rather, it is often *culturally defined* as incompatible in the United States.

An honest answer to the question, "Is breastfeeding compatible with women's work outside the home?" is a resounding "It depends." It depends on whether the work can be interrupted. It depends on whether the work can be done while sitting in one place, and whether it requires both hands or arms free. It depends on whether the work is physically dangerous. It depends on beliefs about the dangers to children outside the home—these may be "real" or "supernatural" dangers to children taken outside the home before a certain age, ranging from fear of exposure to germs to fear of supernatural spirits.

Likewise, if breastfeeding is defined as a "private" activity, and work involves "public" or "professional" contexts, then breastfeeding *becomes* incompatible with women's work by cultural definition. In the United States, all activities connected with child rearing are devalued. In addition, professional workplace culture in the United States demands an almost complete separation of private and professional lives. Only in the last decade have on-site child-care and leave to take care of sick children been accepted as legitimate demands by workers.

Whether breastfeeding is compatible with women's work also depends on who controls her work—does the woman have to answer to someone else for the amount and quality of her work, or does she set her own pace and goals? And it depends on the nature, the temperament, of a particular baby, who may or may not be amenable to adapting to his or her mother's needs and his or her culture's ideas about how children should be fed. It also depends on the nature, the temperament, of a particular mother, who may be able to accomplish her work while breastfeeding her child simultaneously, or who may be able to interrupt her work often to nurse her child without losing her momentum.

Breastfeeding is not "one thing" for all women or for all children. Medical personnel, and even some La Leche League leaders, may promote the idea that infants should be nursed on a schedule, and that 4- or 3- or 2-hour schedules are reasonable. Some children are happy to nurse for 20 minutes or so, only every 3 to 4 hours, which some women still find too often, or too daunting. Other children want to nurse vigorously for only a few minutes, but more often, maybe even every hour. And then there are children who like to nurse either continuously, or at least every 45 minutes to an hour, and nurse less vigorously, but for longer stretches. Some children have more need to suck than others, which probably reflects an underlying need for some or all of the nutritional, immunological, social, and emotional benefits of breastfeeding. Some children can be mollified with a rubber pacifier or their fingers or thumbs, while other children insist on "mom." Some mothers allow the child to meet all of his or her sucking needs at the breast, some teach and promote self-comforting behaviors, while still others punish the child for thumb-sucking or finger chewing. Some infants are content to lie around watching the world or playing with toys while awake, while others want to be held and have continuous interaction with another person. Many parents in the United States prefer a placid, nondemanding baby, while in other cultural contexts a baby with a quiet temperament stands a poorer chance of surviving than one who cries and demands attention more often (de Vries, 1987). Despite reams of advice on how to "achieve" the kind of child you prefer, or your culture says is best, most women find that they must adapt, in part, to the child they got.

In the United States, it is often assumed by medical personnel, employers, and women themselves, that women must give up breastfeeding when they return to work after a typical 6-week maternity leave. They are told their milk will "dry up" unless they pump their milk several times a day. Pumping milk at work is only possible for women with the available time to pump, a private place to pump, and a refrigerator to store their milk. Many women do not have these luxuries. Another, less advertised, solution, is for women to maintain their milk supply for months or even years after returning to work full-time by nursing their children as often as possible when they are together. This technique works well, particularly if the child is able to nurse on demand throughout the night. This simple solution, of course, runs up against another deeply held, but scientifically unsupported, American cultural belief—that children should sleep by themselves, in a separate room, and that they should sleep through the night as soon as possible (see Chapter 10, this volume, for a discussion of one of the biological side-effects of this cultural pattern).

One solution to the problem of sustaining breastfeeding in conjunction with maternal employment outside the home is to allow the woman to have her child with her at work. As discussed above, this would not be feasible in all circumstances, but certainly would work in many contexts if child rearing were more highly valued by the culture, if breastfeeding were defined as a legitimate, important aspect of child rearing, and if breasts could be culturally redefined as body parts elegantly designed for feeding children, not as sex objects.

THE CULTURE OF MISINFORMATION

Where do these cultural assumptions about breasts come from, and how are they perpetuated? In the United States, a "Culture of Misinformation" surrounds breastfeeding. Not only are breasts defined as primarily sexual objects, and breastfeeding defined as a private activity with nutritional value only, but *accurate* information about breastfeeding is very difficult to come by. When making infant feeding decisions, women and men bring to the process a wide array of misinformation gleaned from parents, in-laws, siblings, friends, neighbors, talk shows, magazines read in doctors' offices, newspaper advice columns, television specials, etc. Unfortunately, much of this misinformation is either factually incorrect, incomplete, or a matter of personal opinion presented as "scientific" doctrine (see Jelliffe and Jelliffe, 1986, for a more thorough discussion of the misinformation about, and bias against, breastfeeding evident in scholarly publications).

Medical personnel, the people we most trust to provide us with objective, accurate information, constitute one of the primary sources of incorrect information concerning breastfeeding. Part of the problem is that issues of breastfeeding in the United States are usually considered the expert domain of the pediatrician, despite the fact that medical students receive little or no training in nutrition generally, and most receive no training at all in the normal physiological process of breastfeeding, or in how to handle problems that patients may present (Freed, 1993; Stanfield, 1984). Even if pediatricians were to be specifically trained in breastfeeding, most infant feeding decisions are made during pregnancy, before the pediatrician is involved, and are shaped by values learned in early childhood. Obstetricians and gynecologists may ask pregnant women whether they are "planning to breastfeed or bottle-feed" and duly note it on their chart, but most do not discuss the health risks to the child (and to the mother) of choosing infant formula. The impression is given that the two products (breast milk and infant formula) and the two processes (breastfeeding and bottle-feeding) are equivalent, and the woman is entirely free to make her own decision based on personal preferences.

Even doctors who extol the "advantages of breastfeeding" to their pregnant patients say that they do not discuss the "risks of using artificial infant feeding products" because they do not want to make women feel guilty if they choose not to breastfeed. But when doctors do this, they are forgetting the doctrine of "informed choice." At least in Texas, before your child gets an immunization, you must read several pages of tiny print outlining all the possible risks, and then sign permission. But before you decide to use infant formula, no one even mentions that there may be adverse consequences. How, then, can women and their partners make informed choices?[10]

Some doctors are merely unwilling to discuss the pros and cons of alternative infant feeding choices with patients, what we might call a "sin of omission." Others actually provide misinformation about breastfeeding, what we might call a "sin of commission." I can cite numerous examples drawn from among my own acquaintances over the course of several years (1991–1993) in a town of approximately 100,000 people: An obstetrician told a woman expecting twins that she could expect to spend a minimum of 10 hours a day nursing her children. When the twins were born in early 1994, she was told by her pediatrician that she could not breastfeed them in the hospital because, if she did, he would not know how much or what they were getting to eat (Anonymous, personal communication). Another doctor at a major teaching hospital told the mother of a premature infant that breast milk was the *cause* of her infant's necrotizing enterocolitis, and the baby needed to be entirely on formula (Anonymous, personal communication). In fact, it has been well documented through careful scientific research that breast milk *protects* newborns against necrotizing enterocolitis (Lucas and Cole, 1990). Another doctor told a breastfeeding woman that spices in her food were the cause of her infant's intestinal bleeding (Anonymous, personal communication), without mentioning that infant allergic reactions from dairy products in the mother's diet are the *primary* cause of blood in the stools in breastfed infants (Host, Husby and Osterballe, 1988; Jakobsson and Lindberg, 1978; Juto and Holm, 1992; Lifschitz,

Hawkins, Guerra and Byrd, 1988). She was advised to wean the infant onto a cows' milk-based infant formula. Naturally, the problem worsened, and the child was switched to soy-based formula, and finally to corn-based formula. One pediatrician told a nursing mother that there was no point in nursing after 3 months because the baby's immune system had taken over by that time (Anonymous, personal communication), despite evidence that passive immunity from mother to infant through the breast milk lasts for about 6 months, and active immunity for as long as 6 years (Doren Fredrickson, personal communication).

Finally, despite the attempts of the Baby-Friendly Hospital Initiative, many hospitals persist in practices that are well-known to interfere with the establishment of lactation, including separating mother and infant during the critical first hours following birth, giving bottles of plain or glucose water, and routinely using pacifiers in the nursery, often despite repeated attempts by mothers to have their infants with them to nurse. The American Formula Manufacturers Association and the American Hospital Association are currently lobbying the U.S. government to disallow the Baby-Friendly Hospital Initiative in the United States.

Less obvious than lobbyists' attempts to disallow the Baby-Friendly Hospital Initiative, and extremely difficult to document, is the role that infant formula company advertising dollars play in editorial decisions of the entire genre of popular magazines aimed at the expectant and new mother market. Accurate nutritional and medical information about breast milk and breastfeeding, compared to the use of artificial infant feeding products, is seldom provided in these magazines.[11]

Because of this "Culture of Misinformation" surrounding breastfeeding, many women approach the decision and/or the first attempt at breastfeeding with minds full of contradictory, incorrect, or incomplete information. Breastfeeding in the United States can truly be described as a "lost cultural art." It is a learned behavior, full of cultural meaning, yet most women in the United States grow up without the experience of learning about breastfeeding through observing relatives, friends, or neighbors breastfeed. This is due, in part, to the fact that their mothers used bottles, and in part to small family size and close spacing of children, which means that many women have no younger siblings, or if they do, they were not old enough to remember even if their younger siblings were breastfed. It is also due to our tendency to keep breastfeeding a private activity, to be so discrete that even when breastfeeding in public, no one can tell. Thus, breastfeeding is not readily observable. Yet, we expect women to be able to master this complex behavior without any education, support, or encouragement, or in the face of active discouragement—no wonder so many are not successful, or never even try. Combine this with the near constant bombardment of messages equating breasts with adult sexuality, and the stage is set for misunderstanding about the role of breasts in human reproduction.

In the fall of 1993, one of the undergraduate students in my "Women and Culture" course was totally flabbergasted to discover that the biological function of women's breasts was for feeding children. With obvious shock and disgust evident in her voice she asked, "You mean women's breasts are like a cow's udder?" That a young woman could reach college without ever having even heard of women using their breasts to feed their children is a sad commentary on American culture.

DISCUSSION, CONCLUSIONS, AND IMPLICATIONS

In conclusion, many different cultural beliefs, on a variety of subjects only peripherally related to breastfeeding per se, affect women's choices and women's success in breastfeeding their children. In the United States, the promotion of breastfeeding based on education about the nutritional and immunological superiority of breast milk can only go so far toward increasing the number of children who breastfeed in this country. To make serious progress we will need to change the underlying cultural context of breastfeeding in the United States: the assumption that women's breasts are sexual objects valued only in the context of sexual pleasure, rather than for feeding children, the assumption that breastfeeding serves only a nutritional function, the assumption that breastfeeding is appropriate only for young infants, and the assumption that breastfeeding is appropriate only in private. Finally, we can do much to combat the "Culture of Misinformation," by providing, to all parties concerned, accurate, current information about the biological costs to women and children of choosing not to breastfeed.

Cause for Optimism?

Unlike Kennell and Klaus (1983), I do believe that an understanding of the evolutionary background of the human species carries clear implications for cultural change in the United States. Nevertheless, I would be pessimistic about the potential for cultural change in the United States concerning attitudes toward breastfeeding were it not for the major changes I have witnessed in my own lifetime with respect to tobacco smoking. Like artificial infant feeding, the risks of tobacco smoking were difficult to pin down epidemiologically, and were not accepted by the medical establishment for many years. Like artificial infant feeding, an extremely powerful financial lobby worked very hard to counter the medical and public acceptance of the growing scientific literature on the health risks of tobacco smoking (see Fredrickson, 1993 for the genesis of this idea that there are striking similarities between the two issues). Despite these difficulties, public attitudes toward tobacco smoking have changed radically in the past 20 years. The number of people who smoke has dropped sharply during this time; many restaurants, including McDonald's, department stores, hospitals, public buildings, and workplaces have voluntarily banned smoking. Smoking is no longer allowed on most airplanes. Because of studies documenting the detrimental effects of second-hand smoke on nonsmoking bystanders, especially children, President Clinton is currently considering legislation that would outlaw smoking in all public buildings, and the Food and Drug Administration is considering whether or not to classify nicotine as a drug.[12] Because I have lived through this radical shift in public opinion, beliefs, and behaviors concerning smoking, I can imagine the same thing happening with bottle-feeding.

In the early 1990s, one can find evidence that we have reason to be optimistic that public attitudes toward breastfeeding are changing in the direction of more direct support. Two well-publicized cases in 1994 involved breastfeeding mothers being ejected from public buildings and even threatened with arrest for breastfeeding in public. They made the national news because the mothers did not slink home, embarrassed. The first case involved a New York shopping mall, where a woman breastfeeding her 3-month-old son was asked to leave by a security guard because she was "exposing herself" (AP wire story, 1994). The next day, more than 40 women gathered at the mall and staged a "nurse-in" to protest against the mall's attitude toward public breastfeeding. Similarly, in Texas, a woman was asked by a security guard to leave Houston's Museum of Natural Science because she was nursing her 6-month-old infant. The next day, more than 150 women and children gathered across the street from the museum and staged a "nurse-in" to protest against the museum's application to nursing infants of their policy prohibiting "eating" in the exhibits. The museum's response was that nursing mothers should go to the restroom to nurse their children. The fact that more and more women are standing up for their right to breastfeed their children in public, and finding widespread support from other people, is a cause for optimism. In addition, thousands of instances of women nursing their children in public without being harassed go unreported, and, therefore, unnoticed.

There are other reasons for optimism as well. Laws in most states have vague indecent exposure statutes that often define any exposure of the nipple and areola in public as "indecent exposure." Although breastfeeding in public is not against the law in any state, hypothetically, the indecent exposure laws could be used to characterize breastfeeding as indecent exposure. Beginning as long ago as the 1980s, in a quiet effort to clarify the issues, a number of states and local jurisdictions have been amending their indecent exposure statutes to explicitly exclude breastfeeding. As of 1995, New York, Florida, North Carolina, Nevada, Texas, Michigan, and Virginia were among the few states to specifically protect women who breastfeed in public (Elizabeth Baldwin, personal communication, 1995). Technically, all women have a constitutional right to breastfeed, and there are no laws anywhere in the United States that prohibit breastfeeding or limit the length of time a mother can nurse her child. The New York state law passed in 1994 defines any attempt to prevent a woman from breastfeeding a child, in any location where the woman has a right to be, as a violation of her civil rights, and includes stiff penalties for violation of the law (Elizabeth Baldwin, personal communication, 1994). In New Jersey and Pennsylvania legislation is being written to protect women's rights to breastfeed their children in public.

More and more official bodies are recognizing that breastfeeding is not just a "lifestyle choice" for women, but a health choice for both mothers and children. In Florida, state law requires medical professionals to go beyond providing information and education about breastfeeding and to "actively encourage" mothers to breastfeed. In Dade County, Florida, local ordinances provide incentive programs that allow hospitals to advertise themselves as "Baby-Friendly" if they meet the guidelines of the "Baby-Friendly Hospital Initiative" at the 80% level of compliance. Hopefully this will encourage other hospitals to take responsibility for this issue, rather than waiting for it to be mandated.

In the past several years, over two dozen large corporations have provided pumping breaks, breast pumps, private pumping rooms, and breast milk storage facilities for mothers who are breastfeeding their children. The World Alliance for Breastfeeding Action's (WABA) theme for 1993 was the promotion of a "Mother-Friendly Workplace." In the mid-1990s, the trend is for more and more companies to support the working mother, a change that has come about because society is recognizing that breastfeeding is a positive health choice for both mothers and children. Once again, Florida is leading the way with legislation pending to designate the entire state as a supporter of WABA's "Mother-Friendly Workplace" initiative. Because of these shifts in public, corporate, and legislative attitudes and policies, I am optimistic for the future of the cultural context of breastfeeding in the United States.

In the not too distant future, I can imagine a day when a young couple enters a restaurant with an infant or young child, and notes the sign on the front door: "This is a Breastfeeding Friendly Establishment." I can imagine a day when all 50 states have legislation guaranteeing a mother's right to breastfeed her child in public. I can imagine a day when infant formula is available by doctors' prescription only. I can imagine a day when all cans of infant formula carry a series of rotating warning labels from the Surgeon General that clearly state: "Use of infant formula may be hazardous to your infant's health. Infant formula is known to be a contributing factor in many cases of infant illness and death, including cancer and Sudden Infant Death Syndrome. The use of infant formula is known to reduce children's IQ as much as lead poisoning does, and hinders the development of strong affective bonds between mother and child." I can imagine a day when parents would have to sign a release when they buy infant formula, relieving the formula company of responsibility for causing higher rates of infant morbidity and mortality.[13] I can imagine a day when heavy taxes are levied on the sale of every can of infant formula, both to discourage its use and to help offset the enormous medical costs incurred by those who use it. I can imagine a day when insurance companies charge higher life-long premiums for health care coverage of bottle-fed children. I can imagine a day when all pregnant women are fully informed of the costs of bottle-feeding, in terms of both their own health, and their children's health. I can imagine a day when doctors no longer worry about "making mothers feel guilty for choosing not to breastfeed," any more than they worry today about "making mothers feel guilty for choosing not to use an infant car seat." I can imagine a day when women who work outside the home can take their children to work with them; a day when every employer has on-site child care, and women can have their children with them as they work, or can go to a nearby location to breastfeed their children as often as they like. I can imagine a day when women in the United States can choose to take a year or more of maternity/nursing leave, with a guarantee that their job will be waiting for them when they return. On good days, I can even imagine that this maternity/nursing leave will be paid leave, as it is already in most European countries! I can imagine a day when children are so used to seeing women nursing their children in public, including at work, that they just assume that is the way things have always been. I can imagine a day when movies, television shows, and children's books portray mothers, including nonhuman animal mothers, nursing their children as a matter of course, instead of giving them bottles.[14] I can imagine a day when anthropology students will learn about "the great breast implant debacle of the late twentieth century" as yet another example, along with Chinese foot-binding and female genital mutilation, of cultural beliefs gone astray to the detriment of women and children. I can imagine a day when children grow up appreciating women's breasts for the wondrous, amazing, life-sustaining organs that they are. I can imagine a day when all the world's children, including those in the United States, start out breastfeeding, and are allowed to breastfeed for as long as they need.

What can we do to make these imaginations become reality? Among the first steps might be the following:

We can speak out against the prevailing cultural view that breasts are "naturally" sex objects, and that "breast–mouth" contact is, by definition, sexually charged. It is inappropriate to take the very Western cultural idea that breasts are sexual organs and turn it into a "Law of Nature," applicable to all people, at all times. It is inappropriate to let the very Western cultural idea that breasts are for men overshadow their primary biological function for feeding children, just as it was inappropriate for people in Chinese society to let the cultural idea that deformed feet were sexually stimulating overshadow their primary biological function for walking. Women and children are harmed by Western beliefs about breasts, both directly and indirectly, both physically and emotionally.

I am not suggesting that it is wrong or immoral or perverted to experience sexual pleasure from manual or oral manipulation of the breasts as part of sexual behavior. I am insisting, however, that we recognize this as *learned behavior*, learned in a particular cultural context. I am not suggesting that men and women in any culture should give up this aspect of their sexuality; I am suggesting that they should recognize this role of the breasts as a very distant, secondary *lagniappe*. Can't we "have our cake and eat it, too?" one may ask. Perhaps, I would respond, but with caution. Perhaps, but only to the extent that using our breasts for these purposes does not lead to the excesses represented by female mammary mutilation, widespread dissatisfaction among women with the way their bodies look, men who judge a woman's value on the size of her breasts, and widespread misunderstanding of the primary function of women's breasts, which leads to breastfeeding being defined as sexual behavior. The costs of these cultural beliefs, in terms of women's physical health and self-esteem, and children's health, are, it seems to me, too high a price to pay.

Women deserve to have their bodies accepted as they are, and not feel compelled to submit to the knife in pursuit of the perfect body. The size of a woman's breasts is not related to her ability to produce breast milk. We can teach our daughters that whatever the size of their breasts, they will be able to sustain and nurture their children through their breast milk. If we can teach our children that breasts are for feeding children, then the phenomenon of female mammary mutilation and the issue of breast implant safety will simply fade away, as the desire and demand for artificially inflated breasts disappears.

We can educate ourselves, and others, about all the different roles that breastfeeding plays in normal, healthy child development. Breastfeeding is more than just the transfer of nutrients from mother to child. Not only nutritionally, but immunologically, physically, cognitively, and emotionally, breast milk is vastly superior to artificial infant feeding products, and breastfeeding is much more than just a way to feed a child, much more than just a "lifestyle choice." Women need to know about the advantages of breast milk and breastfeeding; they need to know that breast milk protects children against a variety of illnesses and parasites as long as they are ingesting it, and that an early diet of breast milk sets the stage for life-long health advantages through a strengthened immune system. Women also need to know about the very real "risks" of bottle-feeding, including higher morbidity and mortality during childhood, higher rates of cancer and diabetes in adulthood, and poorer cognitive development. Women need to know that infant formula is not "almost as good" as breast milk. They need to have realistic expectations about how often and for how long human children need to nurse, so that they will nurse often enough to produce enough milk, of sufficiently high fat content, to satisfy their child's needs. They need to know that breast milk continues to be an important source of clean, cheap, and convenient nutrition for their children as long as they are producing milk, and that breast milk can be a critical source of nutrients for a sick child. They need to know that breastfeeding releases a flood of hormones that promotes maternal behavior and that will help them cope with the many demands of child rearing. Women need to know that breastfeeding quiets a noisy or fussy child, relaxes an anxious child, comforts a sick, injured, or frightened child, and conveys unequivocally that the child is safe and loved. They need to know that a child who has the "safe haven" of his or her mother's arms is a secure, independent child, one who has the self-confidence to reach out and explore the world. Finally, women need to know that meeting their children's needs through breastfeeding, as long as children express those needs, is both normal and appropriate.

Everyone, from doctors and lactation consultants down to the youngest school children, needs to know that breastfeeding is not only for newborn infants. All of the evidence from our closest living relatives in the animal kingdom, the nonhuman primates, suggests a natural weaning age between 2.5 and 7 years of age. Cross-cultural evidence from around the world suggests that 2 to 4 years of breastfeeding is typical of modern humans.[15] The question "Is that child *still* nursing?" needs to be stricken from our conversations. Parents and health professionals need to recognize that the benefits of breastfeeding (nutritional, immunological, cognitive, emotional) continue as long as breastfeeding itself does, and that there never comes a point when you can replace breast milk with infant formula, cows' milk or any other food, or breastfeeding with a pacifier or teddy bear, without some costs to the child.

We can work to counter the artificial separation of private and public domains, the cultural perception that our private lives have no relevance for our professional lives, and that our roles as "mothers" render us "unprofessional." Women can make a statement by breastfeeding their children wherever they happen to be, whatever they happen to be doing, to show others that breastfeeding is important and can be accomplished by normal women living in the real world. Women can continue to lobby for realistic maternity/nursing leave, and employment opportunities that allow them to care for their children at the same time. All women, whether breastfeeding or not, whether mothers or not, as well as all men, need to understand the importance, for all members of society, of nurturant child rearing practices.

This is not a male versus female issue; most of the outspoken critics of breastfeeding in public, and breastfeeding older children, are women, just as women are the ones clamoring for their right to have their breast size increased through surgery. Likewise, some researchers have suggested that breastfeeding advocacy represents a call for women to return to their "traditional," circumscribed roles as housewives and mothers. In this chapter, I explicitly reject this interpretation. Women should not have to choose between nurturing their children in the best possible way and pursuing other interests outside the home. Just as an earlier generation of women thought that they had to choose between having a family and having a career, today's generation of working mothers often think they must choose between breastfeeding their children and having a career, but it does not have to be that way. It is up to us to change the cultural context of breastfeeding, and of work, in the United States, so that breastfeeding is compatible with the modern workplace. Rather than concluding that an advocacy of breastfeeding means a return to the days of "a woman's place is in the home," one can argue that an advocacy of breastfeeding means a change in a culture's valuation of child rearing as an activity, and a change in the valuation of the important contributions that only women can make to the social reproduction of a society.[16]

We can teach fathers other ways to nurture and care for their children besides giving them a bottle. We can show them that their cultural beliefs about the sexual nature of women's breasts are cultural beliefs, not biological givens. Men need to know that however much sexual pleasure they may derive from women's breasts, breasts were designed, first and foremost, to feed children. Every father can be taught that the long-term health of his spouse and children should overshadow his culturally taught sexual desires for access to his wife's breasts.

We can teach our sons that they should not judge a woman's character or sexual attractiveness on the basis of her breast size. We can teach our daughters to value their bodies, to have confidence in their bodies, and to not be ashamed of using their bodies as they were designed. We can make sure that children have many opportunities to see women breastfeeding, in many different contexts. We can answer our children's questions about breasts and breastfeeding in a forthright, practical, straightforward manner.

Finally, we can continue to combat the "culture of misinformation" that surrounds breastfeeding among medical professionals and the lay public. Medical students and other health professionals need general nutrition education, as well as specific classroom and clinic education in breastfeeding (Freed, 1993; Stanfield, 1984). If doctors do not know how to effectively treat a particular problem, they can refer their patients to the experts—La Leche League International, lactation consultants, or other local women who have experience breastfeeding—rather than just recommending weaning. Women need to have their problems with breastfeeding met with serious concern and treatment, from knowledgeable, experienced people. Women's and new parents' magazines can make available objective, accurate information about breastfeeding, not bow to the power of the infant formula industry.

I realize that what I am calling for constitutes nothing less than a cultural revolution. Just as women have held rallies and marches to "Take Back the Night," we can "Take Back Our Breasts." We can restore our breasts to their rightful place as the most important point of contact between mother and child after birth. We can do as much as possible to facilitate breastfeeding for all women, and to make sure that women have all the information they need to make informed choices about infant feeding. No child should have to settle for bottle-feeding because his mother thought it was "just as good." No child should have to settle for bottle-feeding because his mother thought she "didn't have enough milk." No child should have to settle for bottle-feeding because his mother thought breastfeeding would be painful, or could be done only in private. No child should have to settle for bottle-feeding because his mother was not allowed enough maternity leave, and/or could not find child care near her workplace. No child should have to settle for bottle-feeding because her father wants her mother's breasts all to himself.

The path to a "Breastfeeding Friendly" society is open before us. We have only to take the first steps.

ACKNOWLEDGMENTS

I wish to thank my children's grandmothers, Mary Elizabeth Hunter Small and Jeanne Betty Hughes Bulger, for breastfeeding their own children in the 1950s, when it was not the cultural norm in the United States, and for their generous and wholehearted support as I breastfed three of their grandchildren. I also wish to thank Martha Toomey, who first introduced me to breastfeeding and to La Leche League, and served as one of my most important role models for mothering. I owe a huge debt of gratitude to Cathy Liles, Professional Liaison for La Leche League of Texas, and a dear friend, who provided essential information, references, and feedback about the ideas that are expressed in this paper. Finally, I wish to thank Elizabeth Baldwin, Virginia Vitzthum, Betty Crase, Rowena Tucker, Sarah Hrdy, Patricia Stuart-Macadam, Roy Stuart, Doug Jones, the members of LactNet, and others whose responses to various incarnations of this paper improved this, the final product. I did not always follow their advice, however, and any errors or deficiencies remain my own responsibility. Special acknowledgment is due to my husband, Steven P. Dettwyler, who has a hard time accepting that breasts may not naturally be erotic, but who is, at least, willing to consider the notion.

NOTES

1. In some cases, inaccurate culture beliefs about how to breastfeed can even render breastfeeding unsuccessful. For example, if women are told to nurse for 5 minutes on each side, every 4 hours, and to give the baby a pacifier in between if she or he cries, then they soon find that they have a dwindling milk supply, sore nipples, and a baby with an improper suck, slow weight gain, and at risk for dehydration, brain damage, and death.

2. Research into the evolutionary origin of the mammary gland suggests that mammary glands evolved before viviparity, and the original purpose of early proto-lacteal secretions was to kill microbes in the nest and on the surface of eggs. Ingestion of the secretions by the young, once they had hatched, helped establish optimal intestinal flora in the young. Only later did the nutritional and immunological functions of lactation evolve, including the evolution of α-lactalbumin from lysozyme, allowing the synthesis of lactose (Blackburn, Hayssen and Murphy, 1989; Blackburn, 1993).

3. The Mirabella article is accompanied by an explicit photograph of a plastic surgeon inserting a silicone-filled implant into a breast. A box on one page notes "For women thinking about implants, bigger isn't the most important issue. They want younger-looking breasts" (1991:108). On p. 106 are "before and after" photographs labeled "*Above left*: Before implant surgery to lift drooping breasts and, *right*, six months later." Yet to anyone familiar with breastfeeding and lactation, it is clear from the photographs that the implants have changed the breasts' appearance to mimic *lactating* breasts.

4. My source of inspiration for this analogy was William A. Haviland's comparison of Chinese foot-binding to North American corset wearing (Haviland 1994:501).

5. In this chapter, I have cited Ford and Beach (1951), *Patterns of Sexual Behavior* published in New York by Harper & Row, Publishers. Anderson cites Ford and Beach (1952), *Patterns of Sexual Behaviour*, published in London by Eyre and Spottiswoode. Caro (see below) cites Ford and Beach (1952), *Patterns of Sexual Behaviour*, published in London by Metheun. The Metheun edition was actually published in 1965, as a reprint of the 1951 Harper & Row edition. As far as I can determine, despite the discrepancy of dates of publication and spelling of the word "Behavior" in the title, these are all the same publication.

6. T.M. Caro, in his 1987 article "Human breasts: Unsupported hypotheses reviewed," continues the miscitation of Ford and Beach (1952) without reference to Anderson (1983). He writes: "Men often become sexually aroused when they view women's breasts (Schmidt & Siqusch, 1970) and when they touch them (Masters & Johnson, 1966), and this latter activity is *a common precursor to sexual intercourse in a large number of societies* (Ford & Beach, 1952)" (Caro, 1987:272–273, emphasis added). Either Caro is really citing Anderson misciting Ford and Beach, or else he has also, like Anderson, miscited Ford and Beach's published work to suit his own purposes.

7. It is *possible* that women varied genetically with respect to their enjoyment of breastfeeding, and that those who found breastfeeding pleasurable would have been more likely to practice it, and so would have had greater reproductive success than women who found it unpleasant and were therefore less likely to practice it. This would have resulted in a higher frequency of the alleles that coded for breastfeeding enjoyment in subsequent generations. However, this scenario is not inevitable. It is also *possible* that women uniformly found breastfeeding to be unpleasant, yet varied genetically with respect to their persistence in the face of discomfort. Those who persisted even when it was painful would still have enjoyed a reproductive advantage. This would have resulted in a higher frequency of the alleles that coded for persistence in breastfeeding in the face of discomfort. This scenario is just as likely as the first one.

8. To argue that breastfeeding has only one legitimate function, a nutritional one, is analogous to insisting that sexual intercourse has only one legitimate function, a procreative one. If the only legitimate function of sex is procreative, then why have sex unless the woman is ovulating and both partners wish her to become pregnant? In fact, it would be a lot less hassle if the woman used a semen donor and artificial insemination. Just as sex serves many functions besides the transfer of semen from male to female, so breastfeeding serves many functions besides the transfer of nutrients from mother to infant. See Weichert (1975) for a similar discussion.

9. The images found in a La Leche League International brochure titled "Can Breastfeeding Become the Cultural Norm?" (Gotsch, 1989) serve as a contrast to those presented in the infant formula literature. La Leche League International is the network of breastfeeding women who provide information and support to other women who want to breastfeed their children, often against

great pressure from their family and friends not to breastfeed. In the brochure, women are shown in a park, in a mall, and dressed at home, nursing their children. The women are dressed in regular clothes, and are out in the world. For many years La Leche League's only advice to working mothers wanting to breastfeed was "try to stay at home." Over the last decade, La Leche League has begun to provide support and information to working mothers, and has taken a more active position in encouraging mothers to continue breastfeeding when they go back to work.

10. Marsha Walker writes: "Few parents are aware that hazards exist with artificial feeding. Health care professionals dodge the issue of the differences between formula and breast milk by not informing parents of the hazards of artificial feeding. The excuse is that this information might make bottle-feeding mothers feel guilty. This paternalistic view seeks to protect women from knowing the possible consequences of making "poor" choices for themselves and their infant, and robs parents of the right to informed decision-making. Withholding information generates more anger than guilt in parents when they find out that there really is a difference" (Walker, 1993:103).

11. See Dettwyler (Chapter 2, this volume), for a critique of the misinformation provided in one particular popular magazine article purportedly promoting breastfeeding.

12. Joel Achenbach, in his newspaper column "Why Things Are," writes of smoking: "Maybe cigarette smoking will turn out to be a strictly 20th century fashion, like jousting in the 11th century, or dying of plague in the 14th. Our guess is that within a quarter of a century smoking will be considered a bizarre and antiquated behavior" (The *Bryan/College Station Eagle*, July 31, 1994).

13. Van Esterik (1994b) makes a similar suggestion for mothers in the hospital.

14. In the children's book *Little Rabbit's Baby Brother*, by Fran Manushkin (1986), Mother Rabbit lays in a supply of bottles and formula in preparation of the new baby's arrival. Of course, the baby rabbit also wears "Happy Hare Diapers." The implication is that when rabbits act like humans, they feed their offspring with infant formula using a bottle. Van Esterik cites other popular media examples promoting bottle-feeding (1994b).

15. See Chapter 2 as well as the chapters by Fildes (Chapter 4) and Stuart-Macadam (Chapters 1 and 3), this volume, for documentation and further discussion.

16. Van Esterik (1994a:4) makes a similar point: "Some feminists have criticized breastfeeding advocates, arguing that they want to tie women down, and keep them at home to feed babies and change dirty diapers. This is not the case. Women's groups needs to make sure that their efforts on behalf of breastfeeding are not used by traditionalists and conservative policymakers against women's interests." Van Esterik has written most eloquently on breastfeeding and feminism and breastfeeding and women's work (see Van Esterik 1989, 1992, 1994a, b, c, 1995, and Chapter 6, this volume. She is currently examining why breasts and breastfeeding are most notable by their absence in current feminist literature, as well as the links between breastfeeding and women's empowerment.

REFERENCES

Anagnost, A.
1989 Transformations of gender in modern China. In *Gender and Anthropology: Critical Reviews for Research and Teaching*, edited by S. Morgen, pp. 313–342. Washington, DC: American Anthropological Association.

Anderson, P.
1983 The reproductive role of the human breast. *Current Anthropology* 24(1):25–45.

AP Wire Story
1994 Breast-feeding moms gather for nurse-in at N. Y. mall. *The Bryan/College Station Eagle*, March 7, p. A2.

Argiolas, A., and G. L. Gessa
1991 Central functions of oxytocin. *Neuroscience and Biobehavioral Reviews* 15:217–231.

Bauer, G., S. Ewald, J. Hoffman, and R. Dubanoski
1991 Breastfeeding and cognitive development of three-year-old children. *Psychological Report* 68:1218.

Ben Shaul, D. M.
1962 The composition of the milk of wild animals. *Zoological Yearbook* 4:333–342.

Blackburn, D. G.
1993 Lactation: Historical patterns and potential for manipulation. *Journal of Dairy Science* 76:3195-3212.

Blackburn, D. G., V. Hayssen, and C. J. Murphy
1989 The origins of lactation and the evolution of milk: A review with new hypotheses. *Mammal Review* 19 (1):1-26.

Bledsoe, C. H.
1987 Side-stepping the postpartum sex taboo: Mende cultural perceptions of tinned milk in Sierra Leone. In *The Cultural Roots of African Fertility Regimes*, Proceedings of the Ife Conference, Nigeria, February 25–March 1, 1987, edited by J. Akin Ebigbola and Etienne van de Walle, pp. 101–124. Ile-Ife, Nigeria: Department of Demography and Social Statistics, Obafemi Awolowo University.

Byrne, J. A.
1992 The best laid ethics program. *Business Week*, March 9, 67–69.

Caro, T. M.
1987 Human breasts: Unsupported hypotheses reviewed. *Human Evolution* 2(3):271–282.

Chisholm, P.
1992 Anatomy of a nightmare. *Maclean's* 105:42–43.

Counts, D. A., and D. R. Counts
1983 Father's water equals mother's milk: The conception of parentage in Kaliai, West New Britain. In *Ideologies of Conception in Papua New Guinea*, edited by D. Jorgensen. *Mankind* 14(1):46–56.

Dettwyler, Katherine A.
1988 More than nutrition: Breastfeeding in urban Mali. *Medical Anthropology Quarterly*, 2(2):172–183.

1990 Traditional perceptions of malnutrition in Mali. Paper presented at the meeting of the American Anthropological Association, New Orleans, Louisiana, November 1990.

de Vries, M. W.

1987 Cry babies, culture, and catastrophe: Infant temperament among the Masai. In *Child Survival: Anthropological Perspectives on the Treatment and Maltreatment of Children*, edited by N. Scheper-Hughes, pp. 165–185. Boston: D. Reidel.

Dewey, K. G., M. J. Heinig, L. A. Nommsen, J. M. Peerson, and B. Lonnerdal

1992 Growth of breast-fed and formula-fed infants from 0 to 18 months: The DARLING study. *Pediatrics* 89(6):1035–1041.

Drawbridge, J.

1991 Implants: Dangerous curves. *Mirabella* August:104–108.

Drewett, R. F., and M. W. Woolridge

1979 Sucking patterns of human babies on the breast. *Early Human Development* 3:315–320.

1981 Milk taken by human babies from the first and second breast. *Physiology and Behavior* 26:327–329.

Ehrenreich, B.

1992 Stamping out a dread scourge. *Time* 139(7):88.

Fomon, S. J.

1994 Recommendations for nutrition management of normal infants. Paper presented at the 21st Annual Texas Human Nutrition Conference, Texas A&M University, February 18th, 1994.

Ford, C. S., and F. A. Beach

1951 *Patterns of Sexual Behavior*. New York: Harper & Row.

Fredrickson, D. D.

1993 Breastfeeding research priorities, opportunities, and study criteria: What we learn from the smoking trail. *Journal of Human Lactation* 9(3):147–150.

Freed, G. L.

1993 Breastfeeding: Time to teach what we preach. *Journal of the American Medical Association* 269(2):243–245.

Goodall, J.

1986 *The Chimpanzees of Gombe: Patterns of Behavior*. Cambridge, MA: The Belknap Press of Harvard University Press.

Gordon, R., and C. Hinton

1984 *Small Happiness* (film). Philadelphia, PA: Long Bow Group.

Gotsch, G.

1989 "Can Breastfeeding Become the Cultural Norm?" La Leche League International, No. 61. Franklin Park, Illinois.

Harlow, H. F.

1958 The nature of love. *American Psychologist* 13:673–685.

Harlow, H. F., and M. K. Harlow

1969 Effects of various mother-infant relationships on rhesus monkey behavior. In *Determinants of Infant Behavior*, Vol. 4, edited by B. M. Foss, pp. 15–36. London: Methuen.

Harvey, P. H., and T. H. Clutton-Brock
1985 Life history variation in primates. *Evolution* 39(3):559–581.
Haviland, W. A.
1994 *Anthropology*, 7th ed. Ft. Worth: Harcourt Brace College.
Heinig, M. J., L. A. Nommsen, J. M. Peerson, B. Lonnerdal, and K. G. Dewey
1993 Energy and protein intakes of breast-fed and formula-fed infants during the first year of life and their association with growth velocity: The DARLING study. *American Journal of Clinical Nutrition* 58:152–161.
Host, A., S. Husby, and O. Osterballe
1988 A prospective study of cow's milk allergy in exclusively breast-fed infants. *Acta Paediatrica Scandinavica* 77:663–670.
Hytten, F.
1991 Science and lactation. In *Infant and Child Nutrition Worldwide: Issues and Perspectives*, edited by Frank Falkner, pp. 117–140. Boca Raton, FL: CRC Press.
Insel, T. R., and L. E. Shapiro
1992 Oxytocin receptors and maternal behavior. In *Oxytocin in Maternal, Sexual, and Social Behaviors*, Annals of the New York Academy of Sciences, Vol. 652, edited by C. A. Pedersen, J. D. Caldwell, G. F. Jirikowski, and T. R. Insel, pp. 122–141. New York: The New York Academy of Sciences.
Jakobsson, I., and T. Lindberg
1978 Cow's milk as a cause of infantile colic in breast fed infants. *Lancet* 2:437–439.
Jelliffe, D. B., and E. F. P. Jelliffe
1979 *Human Milk in the Modern World*. Oxford: Oxford University Press.
1986 The uniqueness of human milk up-dated: Ranges of evidence and emphases in interpretation. *Advances in International Maternal and Child Health* 6:129–147.
Jordan, P. L.
1986 Breastfeeding as a risk factor for fathers. *Journal of Obstetric, Gynecologic, and Neonatal Nursing* 15(2):94–97.
Jordan, P. L., and V. R. Wall
1990 Breastfeeding and fathers: Illuminating the darker side. *Birth* 17:210–213.
1993 Supporting the father when the infant is breastfed. *Journal of Human Lactation* 9(1):31–34.
Juto, P., and S. Holm
1992 Gliadin-specific and cow's milk protein-specific IgA in human milk. *Journal of Pediatric Gastroenterology and Nutrition* 15:159–162.
Kennell, J. H., and M. H. Klaus
1983 Early events: Later effects on the infant. In *Frontiers of Infant Psychiatry*, Vol. 1, edited by J. D. Call, E. Galenson, and R. L. Tyson, pp. 7–16. New York: Basic Books.
Konner, M., and C. Worthman
1980 Nursing frequency, gonadal function, and birth spacing among !Kung hunter-gatherers. *Science* 207:788–791.
La Leche League International
1992 Breastfeeding and female sexuality. Franklin Park, IL: La Leche League International.

Latham, M. C.
1975 Introduction. In *The Promotion of Bottle Feeding by Multinational Corporations: How Advertising and the Health Professions have Contributed*, edited by T. Greiner, pp. i–iv. Ithaca, NY: Cornell International Nutrition Monograph Series, No. 2.
Lefebvre, L.
1985 Parent-offspring food sharing: A statistical test of the early weaning hypothesis. *Journal of Human Evolution* 14:255–261.
Levy, H. S.
1992 *The Lotus Lovers: The Complete History of the Curious Erotic Custom of Footbinding in China*. New York: Prometheus Books. Reprinted from the 1966 edition, which was titled *Chinese Footbinding: The History of a Curious Erotic Custom*, published in New York by Walton Rawls.
Lifschitz, C. H., H. K. Hawkins, C. Guerra, and N. Byrd
1988 Anaphylactic shock due to cow's milk protein hypersensitivity in a breastfed infant. *Journal of Pediatric Gastroenterology and Nutrition* 7:141–144.
Lovejoy, C. O.
1981 The origin of man. *Science* 211:341–350.
Lucas, A., and T. J. Cole
1990 Breast milk and neonatal necrotizing enterocolitis. *Lancet* 336:1519–1523.
Lucas, A., R. Morley, T. J. Cole, G. Lister, and C. Leeson-Payne
1992 Breast milk and subsequent intelligence quotient in children born preterm. *Lancet* 339:261–264.
Manushkin, F.
1986 *Little Rabbit's Baby Brother*. New York: Crown.
Masters, W. H., and V. E. Johnson
1966 *Human Sexual Response*. London: J. & E. Churchill.
McCarthy, M. M., L. -M. Kow, and D. W. Pfaff
1992 Speculations concerning the physiological significance of central oxytocin in maternal behavior. In *Oxytocin in Maternal, Sexual, and Social Behaviors*, Annals of the New York Academy of Sciences, Vol. 652, edited by C.A. Pedersen, J. D. Caldwell, G. F. Jirikowski, and T. R. Insel, pp. 70–82. New York: The New York Academy of Sciences.
Mithers, C. L.
1992 Why women want man-made breasts. *McCall's* 119:83,84,86,88,90,91,141.
Montagna, W., and E. E. MacPherson
1974 Some neglected aspects of the anatomy of human breasts. *Journal of Investigative Dermatology* 63:10–16.
Morley, R., T. J. Cole, R. Powell, and A. Lucas
1988 Mother's choice to provide breast milk and developmental outcome. *Archives of Disease in Childhood* 63:1382–1385.
Morris, D.
1967 *The Naked Ape*. New York: McGraw-Hill.
Morrow-Tlucak, M., R. H. Houde, and C. B. Ernhart
1988 Breastfeeding and cognitive development in the first two years of life. *Social Science and Medicine* 26:635–639.

Nelson, H., and R. Jurmain
1991 *Introduction to Physical Anthropology*, 5th ed. St. Paul, MN: West Publishing Company.
Newton, M., and N. Newton
1948 The let-down reflex in human lactation. *Journal of Pediatrics* 33:693–704.
Newton, N.
1978 The role of the oxytocin reflexes in three interpersonal reproductive acts: Coitus, birth and breastfeeding. In *Clinical Psychoneuroendocrinology in Reproduction*. Proceedings of the Serono Symposia, Vol. 22, edited by L. Carenza, P. Pancheri, and L. Zichella, pp. 411–418. New York: Academic Press.
Newton, N., and M. Newton
1967 Psychologic aspects of lactation. *New England Journal of Medicine* 277(22):1179–1188.
Nishida, T.
1979 The social structure of chimpanzees of the Mahale Mountains. In *The Great Apes*, edited by D. A. Hamburg and E. R. McCown, pp. 73–121. Menlo Park, CA: Benjamin/Cummings.
O'Brien, G.
1995 Nipple phobia. *Playboy*, January 1995:42–43.
Panksepp, J.
1992 Oxytocin effects on emotional processes: Separation distress, social bonding, and relationships to psychiatric disorders. In *Oxytocin in Maternal, Sexual, and Social Behaviors*, Annals of the New York Academy of Sciences, Vol. 652, edited by C. A. Pedersen, J. D. Caldwell, G. F. Jirikowski, and T. R. Insel, pp. 122–141. New York: The New York Academy of Sciences.
Panter-Brick, C.
1991 Lactation, birth spacing and maternal work-loads among two castes in rural Nepal. *Journal of Biosocial Science*, 23:137–154.
1992 Women's work and child nutrition: The food intake of 0–4 year old children in rural Nepal. *Ecology of Food and Nutrition* 29:11–24.
Quinn, M.
1992 Rock to the rescue. *Time* 139(22):89.
Riordan, J. M., and E. T. Rapp
1980 Pleasure and purpose: The sensuousness of breastfeeding. *Journal of Obstetric, Gynecologic, and Neonatal Nursing* 9:109–112.
Rodgers, B.
1978 Feeding in infancy and later ability and attainments: A longitudinal study. *Developmental Medicine and Child Neurology* 20:421–426.
Rogan, W. J., and B. C. Gladen
1993 Breastfeeding and cognitive development. *Early Human Development* 31:181–193.
Romano, R.
1990 Oxytocin—The hormone of love. *New Beginnings* May–June:78–79.
Ross Labs
1989 Breastfeeding: Feeding your baby "the natural way." Columbus, OH: Ross Laboratories.

Ross Labs Mothers' Survey
1993 Breastfeeding: Trends in incidence and duration. Columbus, OH: Ross Laboratories.
Stanfield, J. P.
1984 Training of doctors in maternal and child health (MCH) in medical schools. *Advances in International Maternal and Child Health* 4:96–109.
Stewart, K. J.
1988 Suckling and lactational anoestrus in wild gorillas (*Gorilla gorilla*). *Journal of Reproductive Fertility* 83:627–634.
Taylor, B., and J. Wadsworth
1984 Breastfeeding and child development at five years of age. *Developmental Medicine and Child Neurology* 26:73–80.
Teen Magazine
1993 Your body. *Teen Magazine*, October 1993, p. 25.
Telemacher, H.
1991 "L. A. Story." Commercial release film. Steven Martin played the part of Harris Telemacher.
Temboury, M. C., A. Otero, I. Polanco, and E. Arribas
1994 Influence of breast-feeding on the infant's intellectual development. *Journal of Pediatric Gastroenterology and Nutrition* 18:32–36.
Treckel, P.
1989 Breastfeeding and maternal sexuality in colonial America. *Journal of Interdisciplinary History* XX:I (Summer 1989):25–51.
Trevathan, W.
1987 *Human Birth: An Evolutionary Perspective*. Hawthorne, NY: Aldine de Gruyter.
United States Public Health Service
1991 *Healthy People 2000 Report*. Department of Health and Human Services, Publication No. (PHS) 91-50212. Washington, DC: Superintendent of Documents, U.S. Government Printing Office.
Van Esterik, P.
1989 *Beyond the Breast-Bottle Controversy*. New Brunswick, New Jersey: Rutgers University Press.
1992 *Women, Work, and Breastfeeding*. Cornell International Nutrition Monograph No. 23. Ithaca, New York.
1994a *Breastfeeding: A Feminist Issue*. WABA Activity Sheet #4. Penang, Malaysia.
1994b Lessons from our lives: Breastfeeding in a personal context. *Journal of Human Lactation* 10(2):71–74.
1994c Breastfeeding and feminism. *International Journal of Gynaecology and Obstetrics Supplement* 47:541–554.
1995 Thank you breasts: Breastfeeding as a global feminist issue. In *Ethnographic Feminisms*, edited by S. Cole and L. Phillips. pp. 75–91. Ottawa, Canada: Carleton University Press.
Vitzthum, V.
1986 Breastfeeding patterns in a rural highland Peruvian community. Abstract. *American Journal of Physical Anthropology* 69(2):275.

1988 Variation in infant feeding practices in an Andean community. In *Multidisciplinary Studies in Andean Anthropology,* edited by V. J. Vitzthum. *Michigan Discussions in Anthropology* 8:137–156.

1989 Nursing behavior and its relation to the duration of post-partum amenorrhea in an Andean community. *Journal of Biosocial Science* 21:145–160.

1994 The comparative study of breastfeeding structure and its relation to human reproductive ecology. *Yearbook of Physical Anthropology* 37:307–349.

Walker, M.

1991 Letter concerning "Breastfeeding and fathers: Illuminating the darker side." *Birth* 18(3):175.

1993 A fresh look at the risks of artificial infant feeding. *Journal of Human Lactation* 9(2):97–107.

Weichert, C.

1975 Breast-feeding: First thoughts. *Pediatrics* 56(6):987–990.

Women's Committee of the American Studies Association

1988 *Personal Lives and Professional Careers: The Uneasy Balance.* College Park, MD: American Studies Association.

Wood, J. W., D. Lai, P. L. Johnson, K. L. Campbell, and I. A. Maslar

1985 Lactation and birth spacing in highland New Guinea. *Journal of Biosocial Science, Supplement* 9:159–173.

Woolridge, M. W.

1992 Returning control of feeding to the infant. Paper presented at the La Leche League of Texas Area Conference, Houston, Texas, July 24–26, 1992.

Woolridge, M. W., J. C. Ingram, and J. D. Baum

1990 Do changes in pattern of breast usage alter the baby's nutrient intake? *Lancet* 336:395–397.

8

Baby-Controlled Breastfeeding: Biocultural Implications

Michael W. Woolridge

"the infant should be fed every two hours in the day, and once at night. At about the sixth week the interval between the day feedings should be increased to two and a half hours, . . . until the infant is about twelve weeks old, when it need only be fed, in the day, every three hours."

Ralph Vincent (1913:41)

"Clock-like regularity of feeding, with intervals of four hours (or at least three hours) from the beginning of one feeding to the beginning of the next. There must be no night feeding."

Sir F. Truby King (1913–1940)[1]

"Public opinion has changed very rapidly on this subject—not many years ago the mother was asked to feed two-hourly, night and day. What wonder that breast-feeding went out of fashion! Then the three-hourly interval was recognised as best, while now the four-hourly has been approved."

Mabel Liddiard (1923–1954)[1]

INTRODUCTION

For several decades, as the above quotes demonstrate, the medical profession sought to regulate the breastfeeding process for women, imposing arbitrary rules with little physiological basis. Norms were defined and efforts made to constrain all nursing couples to adhere to these norms, as if they promised a fail-safe solution to breastfeeding management. Even when notes of reason were first sounded (as in the quote below) they were not readily heeded; perhaps autocratic management held its own attractions, or perhaps prescriptive practices were too entrenched.

> The disadvantage of a rigid schedule for feeding is that the time of feeding or the intervals between feedings may not correspond with the infant's natural "hunger rhythm". This results in prolonged crying; and the infant develops various types of feeding difficulties. (Nelson, 1933–1945:92)

One possible explanation still holds true today: people are intrinsically uncomfortable with flexible patterns of management that require them to find their own solutions, rather than rely on simple "rules-of-thumb."

I suspect that many such restrictive practices were designed to compress breastfeeding into the minimum time necessary, so that the mother invested the least amount of time in what was perhaps viewed as an "asocial" activity (though "antisocial" may be more accurate), leaving her free to engage in more socially acceptable activities the rest of the time (undertaking all the other infant and family related duties that had fallen to her). This rather skeptical view assumes that breastfeeding patterns in a Western industrialized setting have been culturally imposed and do not in any way reflect biological patterns: how true is this?

I believe that we now appreciate better the substantial time investment that may be necessary to sustain the process of breastfeeding, although the actual time is still underestimated. Increasingly, society at large must learn to appreciate the commitment the mother is making on behalf of her infant's current and future health and should not place other demands and pressures on her at this time. This is commonly afforded to women in rural traditional communities where cultural taboos proscribe her from undertaking household chores for up to 6 weeks, a period that accords with the time taken to establish lactation and achieve a "steady-state" for volume output (Drewett, Amatayakul, Wongsawasdii, Mangklabruks, Ruckpaopunt, Ruangyuttikarn, Baum, Imong, Jackson and Woolridge, 1993; Neville, Keller, Seacat, Lutes, Neifert, Casey, Allen and Archer, 1988).

It is also to be hoped that in recent years there has been a growing realization that the infant is a sentient individual with sensitivities, feelings, and rights, like an adult. Just as one would not expect adults to conform to the same fixed patterns of ingestion, why expect infants to be constrained in this way? I readily acknowledge that the desire to suck can be triggered by many different factors, and to satisfy different goals—the relief of some state (hunger, distress), as a self-calming behavior—but on this occasion I wish to restrict my discussions to the primary target of securing dietary needs. If we are unable to acknowledge the need for flexibility in relation to satisfying this primary requirement we are certainly facing an uphill struggle in relation to the other needs of the infant.

There are two particular hypotheses I wish to explore in this chapter; the first is "Effective triggering of appetite control by the intake of milk fat is the key factor in determining whether the breastfed infant satiates and remains settled after a feed."

INTERPRETING THE INFANT'S FEEDING CUES CORRECTLY

To my knowledge, the term "demand-feeding," widely accepted and understood by professionals and the public alike, has never been formally defined—although it came into popular use in the mid-1950s (Illingworth and Stone, 1952). It is often implied, by its detractors, as being synonymous with "chaotic feeding," when in practice it should simply mean that an individual nursing couple is encouraged to settle on the pattern or routine that suits them best, rather than having some arbitrary, external, or culturally prescribed definition of what constitutes an acceptable feeding regimen imposed upon them.[2] Rather too often, culture has imposed a pattern on the nursing couple, rather than allowing them to "titrate" the routine that suits their individual needs. The practical dilemma when implementing this strategy is that the infant becomes the principal, if not sole determinant of when the mother initiates a breastfeed, and the infant's behavior, in particular crying, is the most potent and specific cue in regulating the process.

Throughout this century [designated as "The Century of the Child" (Beekman, 1977)] there is a distinct chance that we have commonly misinterpreted crying and unsettled behavior of the infant in association with breastfeeding. We have taken it either to indicate undernutrition—"not enough milk"—or to reflect nonnutritional needs—the desire for comfort, reassurance, and the relief of distress. We are forced into this interpretation when undersupply is patently not true, as shown, for example, by copious urine production.

Both of these are indisputably correct *in a proportion of cases*, the latter perhaps more commonly than the former, but there is an alternative intermediate explanation that has never been acknowledged. There are many reasons why a baby may engage in contact-seeking and self-calming behavior, crying until contact and reassurance is secured from his or her mother, and showing a desire to suck, which is commonly interpreted as hunger. Hunger remains the primary message, however, and to date we have failed to appreciate the implications of appetite control and of the cues that signal satiety. Only when we have interpreted this message correctly can we progress to understand the others. At present I feel we are faced with a confusing array of explanations for the unsettled breastfed infant, and yet experience from clinical practice suggests that tackling the simplest explanation first resolves a surprisingly high number of problems. So I am simply aspiring to apply the principle of Occam's razor: to dispense with the most straightforward explanation first, before proceeding to more complex theories.

ADAPTIVE MECHANISMS FOR SELF-REGULATING INTAKE

It has long been established that adults on free-running, *ad libitum* food regimes exhibit a relatively stable body weight (Le Magnen, 1983). If perturbed from this by enforced over- or underconsumption, individuals depart from their ideal weight, but when the forced situation is relaxed they return to their previous stable weight (Harris and Martin, 1984). We may presume that many cultural factors cause adults to depart from their ideal weight: views about when to eat (adult consumption in the West seems rarely to be triggered by hunger), and how much to eat (the ready availability of food, as well as wide variety, may help to encourage nonessential overconsumption). We may presume that babies do not possess cultural beliefs about how they should feed and should simply demand what is needed to meet their nutritional requirements.

It would seem that the infant has twin dietary objectives: to satisfy day-to-day metabolic needs (and potentially thirst) and to meet growth needs. I will assume at this stage that the human newborn on an exclusive liquid diet (breast milk is recognized to have a low solids content) is likely to satisfy requirements for water intake in the process of meeting nutrient requirements. We may ask whether the newborn has independent and mature motivational states for both hunger and thirst, but there would appear to be no simple answer (Friedman, 1975). Contrary to the situation in hospital, however, after discharge into the community, there is often greater concern for the newborn of becoming critically dehydrated, due to inadequate intake, than of suffering fatal hypoglycemia. It may be that thirst is wholly subservient to the hunger state in the early newborn period while the infant is exclusively breastfed (Drewett, 1993).

The precise nutrient requirements of the individual infant cannot be predicted on a day-to-day basis, let alone in the long term. One might expect that nature has invested in infants the ability to regulate their own intake and certainly there is a growing body of evidence that they do in fact possess an appetite-control mechanism (Fomon, Filmer, Thomas, Anderson and Nelson, 1975; Tyson, Burchfield, Sentance, Mize, Uauy and Eastburn, 1992; Woolridge, Ingram and Baum, 1990) by which they regulate their intake of calories, or possibly fat. Based on this we have argued, as have others, that patterns of breastfeeding management that allow infants to self-regulate their intake are much more preferable to uniformly applied rules that attempt to regiment the individual variability out of infants (Woolridge and Baum, 1992). This necessitates schemes of baby-controlled feeding—"demand" or "baby-led" feeding.

But why should this be so critical to a baby's well-being? If babies are able to self-regulate their intake the underlying mechanisms should be adaptive, in which case infants should be capable of adapting their feeding to accommodate a variety of imposed feeding regimens. This has in fact been demonstrated: when alternative rigid patterns of breast usage were imposed experimentally, infants were able to modify their feeding to achieve a stable fat intake despite significant shifts in the volume of milk available and the fat concentration of that milk (Woolridge, Ingram and Baum, 1990). This study, however, was of normal babies of normal mothers who were experiencing trouble-free breastfeeding. If we were to place these mothers on a Gaussian or "normal" distribution, we should probably place them among the 68% lying $\pm$ 1 SD either side of the middle of the distribution of physiological normality. But if a particular mother were to lie much closer to one or the other end of the normal range ($> \pm$ 2 SD) then the imposition of rigid patterns (inappropriate to that mother's physiology) might prevent her baby from securing his or her desired intake.

Experience from clinical practice suggests that we encounter this situation repeatedly with cases of intrinsic under- or oversupply. It is essential to remove artificial constraints on feed frequency and duration, and to advise on the pattern of breast usage that most suits that individual mother's physiology. However, such changes are often effective only when offered as an adjunct to advice on ways to improve practical aspects of her technique.

My clinical experience is based on over 1500 referrals to a breastfeeding clinical support service that I operated in Bristol, U.K., over a 7-year period. Referrals were made by hospital and community health care staff of women with seemingly intractable breastfeeding problems. In our clinic in Bristol, changes in the mother's breastfeeding technique have been largely instrumental in effecting improvements, and they are usually essential, because without these changes in technique, changes in feed patterning are likely to be ineffectual.

Returning to the main theme of this chapter, for many years the baby's volume of milk intake was often considered the only variable open to manipulation, specifically by increasing feed frequency. For some while, in contrast, we have based our clinical practice upon the principle that milk *quality* is also open to manipulation, most conspicuously by effecting *improvements in technique,* but also by changing *the pattern of breast usage.*

FAT AND/OR CALORIES AS THE KEY TRIGGER OF SATIETY

Culturally, we seem wedded to the belief that the breastfed baby who is crying and unsettled after feeds is "not getting enough milk," the sole emphasis being on inadequate volume intake. If we accept that babies possess an appetite control mechanism and that the trigger for satiety is either fat or calories, then the baby who remains unsettled after feeds, *may,* more specifically, be failing to achieve his or her targets for fat (or calorie) intake. A shortfall in fat can occur despite adequate volume intake. This is a common outcome when long-term mismanagement creates an imbalance in milk *quality,* the predominant cause of which is prolonged ineffective breast emptying.

One possible reason for this misconception is that, scientifically, we have tended to focus on population-based studies and the causes of differential growth within a population, rather than on clinical studies and ways to improve the weight gain of poorly growing breastfed infants.

To counter the belief engendered by this approach I offer the following summary statements:

> On a *population basis* differences in *volume intake* are the principal determinant of infant growth. **Inter-individual differences in volume intake are associated with inter-individual variation in infant size.** Differences in achieved weight gain are predominantly due to differences in volume intake between infants. (Jackson, Imong, Silprasert, Wongsawasdii, Chiowanich, Ruckphaopunt, Williams, Woolridge, Drewett, Amatayakul et al., 1988c)

In contrast:

> On an *individual basis* changes in *milk quality* are the principal determinant of differences in achieved weight gain. **Intra-individual differences in breast milk quality are associated with intra-individual changes in weight gain.** Improving the quality of mouth to breast apposition (i.e., fixing, positioning) and modifying the nursing pattern to optimize breast milk quality are the vital areas of clinical management.

A settled infant is likely to have fulfilled his or her immediate dietary targets, and the appetite-control mechanism will have been effectively triggered. I still feel that we have yet to appreciate the "currency" of this appetite control—this is likely to be *calories*, but may, more particularly, be *fat*. I suspect that in the public perception *volume intake* is regarded as the critical factor, so invariably it is assumed that any woman whose baby remains unsettled after feeding has inadequate milk volume to satisfy her baby's needs. Much more specifically there may be a small but critical shortfall in her baby's fat or caloric intake with the result that satiety is not reached. I feel this point needs to be stated quite emphatically, as it has not been made distinctly enough in the past.

In this context, a critical difference between breastfeeding and bottle-feeding is that a bottle of formula is of uniform caloric density, so that nutrient intake bears a linear relationship to volume intake. In contrast, breast milk increases in caloric density during the feed as the volume available diminishes, so that calorie intake shows a curvilinear relationship to volume intake, with the later stages of the feed making a disproportionate contribution to the baby's intake of calories. Concomitantly, restriction of milk volume removal from the breast results in disproportionate caloric restriction. Though there are likely to be many explanations, including those operating at an emotional level, this is a potential physiological explanation for why unsettled behavior is perceived more commonly for the breastfed than for the bottle-fed infant (Barr, Kramer, Pless, Boisjoly and Leduc, 1989).

To prevent any potential calorie restriction two critical facets of breastfeeding must be correctly managed: the quality of mouth to breast apposition throughout the feed,[3] and the absence of time restrictions on feeding. Although both are critical to effective volume removal from the breast, in the absence of correct positioning the length of the feed will make a relatively small contribution. In simple terms, a poorly "fixed" baby may secure an adequate volume of milk, but is likely to encounter a shortfall in fat intake and so will remain unsettled after feeding through ineffective triggering of appetite control. An outcome such as this invariably reflects an imbalance between the effectiveness of milk removal by the infant and the sensitivity of the mother's secretory capacity; over time, a progressively greater imbalance in intake can arise, which may lead ultimately to acquired undersupply. At any stage during this process the mother may perceive herself as having insufficient milk to satisfy her baby, when in point of fact there may be no limitation on the volume of milk available to her infant.

While I readily acknowledge that a whole range of social factors (cultural views about crying babies), psychological factors (locus of control, self-esteem), and emotional factors (current susceptibility) will influence this (Gussler and Briesemeister, 1980; Hillervik-Lindquist, 1991), I do not feel we can afford to ignore the most direct physical cause of genuine symptoms of undernutrition—caloric restriction—nor blame the mother for interpreting these symptoms by a culturally prescribed set of criteria. We would do better to recognize that our own understanding of the situation may at worst be incomplete and at best be insufficiently specific to address the most direct cause first. While there is, as yet, scant empirical evidence to support this conjecture, clinical experience indicates that sound physiologically based management of breastfeeding, based on this principle, holds the key to resolving problems of apparent insufficiency with a disconcertingly high frequency.

Certainly, when a baby is suffering from discomfort and distress unrelated to any parameter of hunger, crying is their singular most effective mode for communicating these needs. Once contact has been reestablished, sucking is the commonest route by which comfort, reassurance, and gratification are achieved. Sucking, being a highly pleasurable activity for the baby, is one of the most effective soothing, comforting, and self-calming behaviors in which the baby can indulge. The mother will invariably interpret her infant's desire to suck as hunger, and if she is unable to satisfy this by further prolonged feeding, not uncommonly she will believe that she has insufficient milk. I hope to demonstrate that prolonged feeding is not the primary means for achieving effective milk removal, but is in fact secondary to improving the quality of mouth to breast apposition.

We have previously argued that either excessive breast milk intake due to overfeeding, or an imbalance in intake resulting from ineffective breast emptying, can itself be the origin of gastrointestinal pain and discomfort, causing the baby to appear to want constant feeding (Woolridge and Fisher, 1988). But in this case, as in all other aspects of clinical management, our primary aim should be to ensure that the infant's principal dietary needs are met. Only when reassured that these needs have been appropriately and effectively met should we proceed to address alternative, nonhunger causes of the baby's distress.

If our aim is to ensure adequate fat intake what are the proximate determinants of the fat content of breast milk?

POINT ESTIMATES OF BREAST MILK FAT CONCENTRATION

A descriptive study of the changes in breast milk fat concentration among women in northern Thailand confirms the above principles by identifying the determinants of breast milk fat concentration in individual women. We were concerned with determining the optimal sampling

Table 8.1. Predictors of Fat Concentration

a. *Prefeed*
 Significant predictors
 1. Interfeed interval ($p < 0.001$)—inversely related (the longer the interval the lower the prefeed fat)
 2. Postfeed fat at previous feed ($p < 0.001$)
 3. Day/night ($p < 0.001$)—positively related to sleep (i.e., *higher* at night)
 Not significant predictors
 1. Volume intake at previous feed

b. *Postfeed*
 Significant predictors
 1. Prefeed fat concentration at current feed ($p < 0.001$)
 2. Volume intake at current feed ($p < 0.001$)
 3. Day/night ($p < 0.001$)—negatively related to sleep (i.e., *lower* at night)
 4. Duration of current feed ($p = 0.03$)

technique for collecting representative data on milk quality (Jackson, Imong, Silprasert, Preunglumpoo, Leelapat, Yootaboot, Amatayakul and Baum, 1988a). In practice, fat concentration is one of the principal determinants of caloric concentration (Hernell, 1990), fat contributing 54% of the total energy content of milk (Oftedal, 1984), so as fat is the most variable constituent in breast milk it causes the greatest variation in calorie intake. Prentice, Prentice and Whitehead (1981) established for women in The Gambia that the feed closest to 1300 hours (1:00 PM) was the most typical for milk fat concentration throughout the 24 hours. While valuable for population-based studies, this is not appropriate for individual studies, as there may well be interindividual variation in this parameter. Our study (Jackson, Imong, Silprasert, Ruckphaopunt, Wool-ridge, Baum and Amatayakul, 1988b) identified those variables of breastfeeds that were most closely associated with milk fat concentration in individual women (Table 8.1a, all correlations are positive unless otherwise stated).

Prefeed fat[4] is inversely related to the length of the interfeed interval,[5] which means that *feed frequency influences milk fat concentration*. Thus feed frequency, one of the key parameters of feed patterning, shows a direct relationship to milk fat concentration and so would appear capable of exerting a direct influence on milk quality.

It is apparent that feed duration is capable of influencing postfeed fat concentration, over and above that accounted for by the volume removed, although its influence is small relative to interfeed interval and volume removed (Table 8.1b). This suggests that improving the effectiveness of milk removal is the more important clinical target and that extending feed duration indefinitely will not compensate for ineffective milk removal resulting from poor physical attachment.

Table 8.2. Predictors of Mean Feed Fat Concentration

Significant predictors	
1.	Time since last feed ($p < 0.001$)—inversely related
2.	Fat concentration at end of previous feed ($p < 0.0001$)
3.	Volume intake at previous feed ($p < 0.0001$)
4.	Volume intake at current feed ($p = 0.03$)
Not significant predictors	
1.	Feed duration
2.	Day/night—opposing effects cancel out

Overall, the fat concentration of milk taken at feeds would appear to be maximized *both* by increasing feed frequency *and* milk volume removal (which itself is a combination of unrestricted feed duration and optimal positioning), yet in Western hospitals it has been common in the past to impose restrictions on both feed frequency and feed duration to the likely detriment of the baby's fat intake. Such restrictions may well have resulted in iatrogenic problems of breastfeeding, which would include fat restriction (resulting in unsettled behavior), symptoms of breast milk insufficiency, and underfeeding. Furthermore, a reduced fat intake would also compromise the intake of fat-soluble vitamins; currently there is concern over the intake of the fat-soluble vitamin K (see Cunningham, Chapter 9, this volume) and yet many "normative" data on the incidence of hemorrhagic disease of the newborn were collected at a time when it was routine to impose strict regimens on the breastfed infant (Woolridge and Baum, 1992).

The effect of sleep on fat levels is intriguing. It is probable that if a mother lies supine (face up) for a relatively long period, fat may tend to settle out in a position more proximal to the nipple ("creaming" effect).[6] If the mother routinely switches her side-lying position, the effect may be similar. This would have the effect of elevating the prefeed fats, with a concomitant reduction in the postfeed fats, although the mean feed fat, derived by averaging the prefeed and postfeed values, should be similar day and night as shown in the analysis below (Table 8.2).

MEAN FAT CONCENTRATION OF MILK TAKEN BY BABY

The predictors of fat concentration in the prefeed and postfeed breast milk samples are important, as these are point markers that generate the mean feed fat concentration. However, if over the course of the day these were to vary inversely with respect to each other (as with the influence of sleep), then the mean fat concentration of the milk might remain stable. So, ultimately, we must consider the factors that predict the mean feed milk fat concentration, as it is these that tell us whether milk quality is open to manipulation by changes in feeding practice.

The factor that shows the highest association is the time elapsed since the previous feed and this shows an inverse relationship to mean feed fat concentration—the greater the interval the lower the average fat content. Thus, the more frequent the feeds, the higher the fat content. This is intriguing, because at one time it was very common for women who felt their supply was inadequate to be advised to increase the frequency of feeding on the sole assumption that it boosted milk volume; rather more explicitly it is likely to have increased fat concentration, in the short term, in addition to increasing supply in the longer term.

Several studies have shown that interfeed interval predicts volume intake (Butte, Garza, Smith and Nichols, 1984; Pao, Himes and Roche, 1980)—the shorter the interval the lower the intake at a feed—so volume intake may not be increased in the immediate term by increasing the feed frequency except in a small subgroup of women who are offering clinically too few feeds, whereas more frequent feeding may well improve milk quality. In contrast, maximizing the fat concentration of breast milk is likely to mean that satiety is more reliably triggered, resulting in a more settled baby. As might be inferred from the above, milk volume and milk fat concentration will often be inversely related within an individual.

There is marked diurnal variation in milk fat concentration: the Thai data show that the mean feed fat concentration is above average from 4 PM to midnight and markedly below average between 4 and 8 AM; this is likely to coincide with volume availability. Postfeed fat concentration shows the closest diurnal pattern to this, suggesting that breast emptying may be the predominant influence on fat content, more so than feed frequency.

One might expect the frequent feeding demanded by infants in the late afternoon and early evening (a typical time of day for infants to show unsettled behavior) to be associated with above average milk fat concentration and hence *more* settled behavior.[7] The fact that it is not commonly so makes us question whether volume intake is the more critical variable at this time, because of its ability to affect gross calorie intake, or whether unsettled behavior is actually unrelated to any shortfall in intake. Evidence exists that the timing and duration of crying, unsettled or fussy behavior show both a diurnal peak (6–9 PM) and a developmental peak (2–12 weeks), which is the same irrespective of feeding method (St. James-Roberts, 1989). This evidence suggests that unsettled behavior late in the day, commonly reported for infants in a Western industrialized setting, can be independent of intake.

Data from eight studies on the diurnal pattern in milk fat concentration are reviewed by Jackson et al. (1988b, Fig. 4) and they show surprisingly little consistency. Some of the differences can be explained on the basis that different milk sampling strategies were employed. As fat is the most variable constituent in breast milk, changing with the efficiency of breast emptying, the method used to obtain breast milk samples is critical and no one method can be described as representing the "gold standard" (Garza, Woolridge, Butte, Ferris and Casey, 1985). There are also marked differences in breastfeeding management between the studies, although the five studies from women subject to scheduled feeding in an industrialized setting show some uniformity in pattern. Disconcertingly, in the two studies that are most directly comparable in terms of both sampling technique and nursing pattern—The Gambia and Thailand—the diurnal patterns are 180° out of phase, an observation that is difficult to explain. Suffice it to say that no clear biological pattern has emerged of changes in breast milk fat concentration over the course of the day and night.

An issue that remains to be resolved is whether milk quality, in terms of fat, can be specifically manipulated in the long term by changing feed frequency and the pattern of breast usage. The experimental study of Woolridge, Ingram and Baum (1990) would suggest that it can, as the mean feed fat concentration *was* affected significantly by changing the pattern of breast usage, although it was variable across individual women.

It remains unclear, and needs to be tested empirically, which variable is capable of affecting quality the most—feed frequency, volume removed, or feed duration? In the experimental study (Woolridge et al., 1990) a derived measure—the Index of Emptying (%)—showed more significant variation as a function of the experimental conditions than did any measured variable. This derived measure reflects how consistently extreme fat values are reached at each feed, indicating the uniformity with which stored milk is extracted over the day. A high IE% would reflect reliable milk delivery at each feed, while a low IE% would indicate that milk delivery was inconsistent. So, the answer to the question posed above may well be that whichever factor(s) is(are) capable of affecting breast *emptying* the most will also have the greatest effect on milk quality. I suspect this would be different for different women. While certain women do feed too infrequently, others are already feeding very frequently, making it inappropriate for them to attempt to increase this. Some exhibit what may be viewed as premature breast switching, while others persist with the same side for what may appear an inappropriate length of time. Ultimately, consistency of milk extraction will reflect an interaction between the amount of milk available ("milk supply"), the infant's motivation to feed and tendency to remove milk ("infant demand"), and the physical approximation of the baby's mouth to the breast ("positioning," "latch-on," or "attachment") affecting the baby's ability to remove milk from the breast. All these assume that the infant is given unrestricted access to the breast so that milk transfer can be maximized, while also permitting time for other nonnutritional needs to be met. The imposition of time restrictions implies that someone external to the infant is a better judge of the infant's needs and feeding efficiency.

Despite the changes introduced by the experimental conditions, in the study above, the infants adapted their feeding to ensure a stable fat intake. Clinical experience would suggest that one often encounters infants who are unable to self-regulate fat intake adequately. This may partly be explained because clinicians are more likely to be dealing with women at extreme ends of the physiological spectrum, whose infants might find it more difficult to achieve their desired intake of fat by having to accommodate extremes of volume intake.

WHAT BECOMES OF MILK FAT THAT IS NOT REMOVED AT A FEED?

One issue that many people find difficult to grasp is how impairment of milk quality comes about, as it seems to imply there is a flaw in the basic mechanism of milk secretion. The clinical hypothesis of Woolridge and Fisher (1988) was prompted by the observation that failure to correct practical aspects of feeding could lead to a progressive decline in milk quality (fat content) to the detriment of the infant. Caloric restriction is the primary cause of impaired growth, with ingestion of predominantly low fat milk causing several other infant symptoms—colic, vomiting, diarrhea, and flatulence—that are often attributed to lactose malabsorption (maldigestion). While commonest among women with an abundant milk supply, prolonged mismanagement ultimately leads to limitation of supply through reduced infant demand. Shortly after publication of the hypothesis, the following quote came to light, which indicated that ours was not a novel observation:

> The first milk drawn off is relatively dilute; the last milk is so rich in fat that it may almost be considered as cream. With feeble suction and insufficient emptying of the breast this last concentrated milk is not obtained, and the food of the sick child becomes relatively dilute. (Cameron, 1913:911)

The concept that impaired breast drainage resulted in the long-term compromise of milk fat content was implicit in the hypothesis. The logical dilemma that this raises is "What happens to the fat that is not removed, will it not remain available to be removed at subsequent feeds?" There is little evidence to challenge the basic assumption that milk is synthesized at a relatively standard and uniform composition, relative, that is, to the variation induced by the process of storage and delivery (principally in fat content, although there are commensurate changes in the aqueous fraction). If the baby fails to secure the high fat milk at a feed, then surely it should remain accessible within the breast to be removed at the subsequent feed. Clinical experience indicates that this does not happen, as one can observe a progressive decline in milk quality that can be reversed by addressing causes of ineffective milk delivery. Two possible explanations might account for why this does not happen—either fat that is not removed is reabsorbed, or it exerts negative feedback on fat synthesis—the latter is the more probable.

Fat in the milk is derived from two sources—from dietary lipids present in the plasma as triglycerides, and by *de novo* synthesis from blood glucose (Williamson, Munday and Jones, 1984). Although there would seem to be an ongoing level of conversion of glucose to lipids within the mammary tissue (lipogenesis), this is likely to be reduced or inhibited by the presence of plasma triglycerides. In essence, therefore, the glandular tissue of the breast must possess an elaborate switching mechanism that mediates between uptake of plasma triglycerides and lipogenesis. The presence of a high concentration of unremoved fat droplets in the proximal alveoli may equate with high plasma lipids and either inhibit or reduce lipogenesis from glucose, or decrease uptake of plasma lipids.

Uptake of plasma triglycerides for incorporation into milk fat droplets is regulated by lipoprotein lipase (LPL) in the mammary tissue. Hamosh, Clary, Chernick and Scow (1970) demonstrated that if milk removal is prevented by duct ligation, the accumulated milk inhibits LPL activity, blocking uptake of triglycerides from the blood. So although unremoved fat on its own has not been shown to inhibit LPL activity and fat uptake by the breast, nonspecific milk accumulation does. Other biochemical pathways within breast tissue will be unaffected, so the levels of other milk constituents will remain unaltered.

Thus, a high concentration of unremoved fat droplets lying within the alveolar space, close to the apical cell border, may exert negative feedback on lipid uptake and/or lipid synthesis, causing a progressive reduction in fat secretion. Additionally, because the milk fat droplets are bounded by plasma membrane (Jensen, 1989), the possibility exists that they could recoalesce with the apical cell membrane and be reabsorbed into the secretory cell. This process is likely to occur naturally during breast involution when unremoved milk will be reabsorbed. While possible, I suspect this is unlikely to happen on the time-scale that is relevant here.

If milk quality is compromised by ineffective milk removal from the breast, this would seem to represent a potentially serious flaw in the lactation process and the existence of infants who exhibit adverse symptoms suggests that this apparent "flaw" can produce a clinical entity. We should remain cautious on this, however, as the problem is most commonly manifested when women curtail their feeding artificially to comply with culturally prescribed rules. It would not be a "flaw" if we were able to identify some adaptive benefit to the infant from differential breast emptying; I will venture below that the infant may in fact harness this to his or her potential benefit. If such a process proved to be another facet of self-regulation by the infant, once again the imposition of rigid cultural practices would militate against the normal process.

There is often speculation over what fundamental nursing pattern we might strive for, and to what biological pattern we might be expected to adhere. The nursing patterns of infants in conditions that are climatically very different from those in Western societies are often cited. Yet, if milk quality is influenced by nursing patterns, differences around the world might reflect the nutrient requirements pertaining in a particular climatic location. So a related question that might be addressed is: "Are there climatic adaptations in nursing pattern, depending upon whether it is fat intake or water throughput that is being maximized?" Is it the case that through evolution, nursing patterns have coadapted with milk quality, or is there an optimal pattern for nursing in humans irrespective of geographic location? Even if there were, would it ever be possible to disentangle natural strategies of nursing from culturally prescribed patterns?

This is an extension of the question posed at the start: Are breastfeeding patterns and practices dictated primarily by biology or by culture? We may conjecture that at different climatic extremes different nutritional priorities are placed upon breastfeeding. So, in tropical or arid conditions one might presume that high evaporative water loss would place the emphasis mainly on maximizing water throughput to prevent dehydration. Such adaptation could be achieved by genetic differences in the nutrient density of milk, or in metabolism. If physiological mechanisms constrain within-species differences in milk quality, adaptation might be achieved by changes in nursing pattern, maximizing extremes of the range of nutrient density in accordance with climatic requirements.

While a substantial degree of adaptation in terms of milk quality is likely to be genetic, reflecting the cumulative effects of natural selection, it would not be surprising for nursing patterns to show coadaptation in accordance with the prevailing climate. Such a process could be analogous to that producing difference in milk composition and nursing pattern between closely related species [seals for example (Bonner, 1984)], or as suggested across different classes of mammals (Ben Shaul, 1962; Oftedal, 1984). Similar variation might be expected across the human species along a geographic or climatic cline, or with ethnic subtype. Few studies have focused on ethnic differences in nursing pattern matched for analysis of milk composition, and there is a clear need for more cross-cultural data.

It must be said that what data do exist neither support nor contradict this conjectural viewpoint. The pattern of frequent short nursing episodes of !Kung people is usually quoted as being the fundamental or intrinsic nursing pattern for humans, but we should not exclude the possibility that this is adapted either to a culturally prescribed lifestyle or to physiological requirements. The high feed frequency (4.1 episodes of feeding/hour) would be predicted to maximize fat intake (data in Table 8.1), although the short feed durations (1.9 minutes/feeding episode) might run counter to this (Konner and Worthman, 1980). High feed frequencies have been reported for several other cultures in addition to the !Kung, including the Gainj of New Guinea [2 episodes/hour (Wood, Lai, Johnson, Campbell and Maslar, 1985)] and the Quechua Indians of Peru [2.4 episodes/hour (Vitzthum, 1989)].

In contrast, substantially less frequent suckling episodes have been shown for women in The Gambia [7.1/12 hours at 3 months (Whitehead, Rowland, Hutton, Prentice, Muller and Paul, 1978)], in Guatemala [10.4/24 hours at 3 months (Delgado, Martorell and Klein, 1982)], in rural Bangladesh [9.5/8 hours at 18 months (Huffman, Chowdhury, Allen and Nahar, 1987)], and in urban Chile [8+/24 hours (Díaz, Rodríquez, Marshall, del Pino, Casado, Miranda, Schiappacasse and Croxatto, 1988)]. Feed frequencies in a northern Thai population (subtropical) range from as few as 7 feeds per day, up to 27 feeds per day (Imong, Jackson, Woolridge, Wongsawasdii, Ruckphaopunt, Amatayakul and Baum, 1988), with a median feed duration of 9.5 minutes [range 5–15 minutes/feed, 40–370 minutes/day (Drewett, Woolridge, Jackson, Imong, Mangklabruks, Wongsawasdii, Chiowanich, Amatayakul and Baum, 1989)]. The diversity of these data suggests that cultures experiencing similar climatic conditions may exhibit substantial differences in nursing behavior. This discussion does not address the intrinsic problems of defining nursing episodes and identifying the ratio of "nutritive" to "nonnutritive" sucking or the functional roles that "nonnutritive" sucking may play in lactational infertility.

Data from temperate and Arctic zones are more sparse. Most data relate to industrialized cultures and so cannot be considered free from cultural influence of the type that dictates rigid feeding practices. Data from Inuit suggest that feed patterns in cold, Arctic regions share some features in common with other areas. The data of Berman, Hanson and Hellman (1972) indicate that Inuit infants are typically nursed for 5 minutes from *each* breast every 2–3 hours; it is not known, however, whether the reliable offering of both breasts is traditional or is a recent cultural acquisition from contact with a Western system of medical care. It is not stated whether infants were routinely nursed inside clothing. The feed duration may be regarded as relatively short [cf. Thailand 10 minutes/feed (Imong, Jackson, Wongsawasdii, Ruckphaophunt, Tansuhaj, Chiowanich, Woolridge, Drewett, Baum and Amatayakul, 1989), India 10–15 minutes/feed (Shatrugna, Raghuramulu and Prema, 1982), Boston 10.5 minutes/feed "Standard," 15 minutes/feed for "La Leche League" (Elias, Teas, Johnston and Bora, 1986)], while the interval between feeds among the Inuit is relatively protracted and would not seem to be conducive to maximizing fat intake.

From these relatively sparse data one might discount the conjectured hypothesis of climatic adaptation in nursing pattern. This would further imply that nursing pattern is dictated more by cultural factors such as lifestyle, ease of access to the breast, and other similar practical issues. This would need to be confirmed by cross-cultural studies of milk composition, but to date these are not readily available. What comments do exist tend to emphasize the uniformity in milk composition between cultures (Crawford, Laurance and Munhambo, 1977).

In fact the data presented above suggest that there are greater differences in nursing behavior between traditional populations within a similar climatic range than have been recorded between cultures at the extremes of the climatic range. Nonetheless, it remains difficult to determine the extent to which urbanization, or Western-style practices have influenced these rural cultures. I would venture that at the present time the comparative approach to the study of nursing patterns, and their relationship to climatic, dietary, and cultural factors, produces no readily discernible pattern. Only when our knowledge base has increased dramatically will we be able to arrive at a more sophisticated insight into the relative biological, climatic, and cultural influences on nursing behavior.

As a simple example of cultural differences in nursing pattern, women in an industrialized setting often strictly alternate the breast that is offered at a feed, or which is offered first, whereas in northern Thailand and in many other traditional rural cultures it is common for only one breast to be offered at each feed. While the relatively short interfeed intervals give the opportunity for the contralateral breast to be offered within a relatively short time-span, women often feed with no clear reference to whether the right or left breast is being offered; in other words it is unusual for a woman to exhibit any awareness of laterality. This may result in a mother offering the same breast for several consecutive feeds (extreme runs of 5–7 were recorded), before spontaneously switching and offering the other breast. One may presume this reflects preferred laterality in infant carrying and handling utensils while caring for the infant. Over a 24-hour period, such a bias often balances out so that both breasts are being visited equally frequently, but even if it was sustained, lactation capacity could accommodate the bias through differential output. For women in Western culture we have identified marked asymmetries in breast milk output even without any obvious bias in breast use. A further clear example of an imposed cultural practice is that noted by Prentice et al. (1981) that it is a Moslem tradition for all breastfeeds to be started with the right breast.

EFFICIENCY OF MILK REMOVAL FROM THE BREAST

Returning to the earlier discussion, the factor with which the magnitude of change in fat concentration from the start to the end of the feed was most explicitly related was the volume of milk removed (Jackson et al., 1988b; Prentice et al., 1981; Woolridge et al., 1990). In this context it is interesting to note that some milk usually remains in the breast once a baby has finished feeding and this is generally taken to signify the baby exercising appetite control (Drewett and Woolridge, 1981). Where complete breast expression is used to evaluate breast milk quality, more milk is commonly removed than the infant would take, but it is not clear whether the residual milk represents a physiological reserve within the breast, or is left voluntarily by the infant.

A somewhat surprising outcome was found for a population of Burmese infants showing relatively poor growth, in whom up to 30% additional milk remained unconsumed in the breast, which could be extracted by breast pump after feeds (Khin-Maung-Naing, Tin-Tin-Oo, Kywe-Thein and Nwe-New-Hlaing, 1980). It is possible that the babies were clinically malnourished, and so were unable to remove the residual milk, or that technical aspects of feeding were suboptimal, resulting in inadequate breast emptying at a clinical level across the population: both of these explanations seem improbable.

Alternatively, more effective breast emptying might have given the infants an unnecessary fat burden that would be inappropriate to the tropical climate in which they lived and so they were self-limiting feeds when their fluid requirements were met. This proposition is more attractive and it raises the possibility that the infant might manipulate the quality of its intake through differential breast emptying, something of which the mother might be completely unaware. If correct, then it would fundamentally question the assumption that complete breast expression to estimate breast milk quality accurately mirrors the infant's intake. *Infants may in fact be adopting differential breast emptying as their principal means of self-regulating their intake in terms of nutrient quality.*

The relevant issue for most people from these discussions is: "What is the most appropriate pattern of breastfeeding and feed management for women in the industrialized West?" Are the patterns we have practiced in the recent past physiologically or biologically appropriate, or are they primarily culturally imposed? I suspect the answer to this last question is an emphatic "They are primarily culturally imposed," and probably the ongoing dilemma that we must face is the potential discordance between a pattern that is biologically optimal (in terms of hormone release, maintenance of adequate milk supply, and of lactational infertility) and that which culture seeks to impose for the convenience of those concerned (often dictated by that which can be imposed on the *bottle-fed* baby). We probably have to recognize and accept this dilemma, and at best hope to achieve a compromise.

This problem can be best illustrated by the issue of night feeds. We know that breastfeeds given during the night are associated with increased prolactin release, and that sustaining night feeds is likely to be the best way to maintain lactational amenorrhoea (Elias et al., 1986; and Ellison, Chapter 11, this volume) and probably an adequate milk supply. However, in our culture there is a popular belief that "going through the night" is an indicator of infant advancement and an expectation that this should be achieved as early as possible, despite it being biologically inappropriate. In a rural area of Thailand (Imong et al., 1988, 1989), nighttime feeds are sustained at the same level throughout the first year of life, despite a daytime reduction in the number of feeds, as a result of which nighttime breast milk intake makes up an increasing proportion of the infant's total 24 hour intake in the latter half of infancy (Imong, Jackson, Wongsawasdii, Ruckphaopunt, Amatayakul, Drewett and Baum, 1987; Imong et al., 1989). Despite the retention of nighttime breastfeeds, there would appear to be no contingent increase in the number of infants with sleep pathologies. In fact, sleep dysfunction is largely absent from rural traditional cultures, suggesting that the high incidence of sleep pathologies in Western society may be culturally induced. It is probably our cultural expectation both of how a "good night's sleep" should comprise an uninterrupted period of continuous sleep, and the fact that we attempt to secure or enforce it at a premature stage, that contribute to the development of such problems.

We can readily identify the issues in this area of breastfeeding, but they apply equally well in all other aspects of breastfeeding management that are culturally circumscribed, including the frequency of feeds, the duration of feeds and pattern of breast usage. *Breastfeeding is for the infant, and should be controlled by the infant,* if the infant is to be permitted to self-regulate his or her intake in accordance with his/her changing needs.

CONCLUSION

The picture that emerges is that, unwittingly, by the imposition of cultural expectations on how often and how long babies should feed, we are potentially restricting the baby's milk intake. While the effect on volume intake is acknowledged, that on fat intake is not often appreciated. The fact that breast milk composition (fat concentration) changes in a nonlinear manner during a feed will mean that the baby's intake is restricted disproportionately in fat/calories if the end of the feed is truncated. As it is this constituent that appears to regulate infant appetite, we should not be surprised if a baby whose feeding is culturally restricted appears unsettled or persistently hungry. Studies of the determinants of breast milk fat show that while permitting the baby unrestricted feeding on the breast does improve the mean feed fat concentration, this is not as effective as increasing the efficiency of milk delivery *by making sure the baby is positioned properly at the breast*. As women rarely receive adequate technical instruction on how to improve effective milk delivery, we should not be surprised by the high incidence with which perceived breast milk insufficiency is reported.

For certain women, the clinical outcome of uncorrected ineffective milk delivery is that milk quality becomes compromised, resulting in a progressively lower fat content, further exacerbating the perceived undersupply. Ultimately, if the baby self-limits its intake from the breast as a way of coping with the imbalance between milk volume and composition, this is likely to result in acquired undersupply. This problem is often more common for women with oversupply, but, irrespective of whether this is intrinsic or acquired, the majority *of problem cases* remain correctable by improving technique and removing cultural restrictions on the frequency and duration of feeds.

Regarding climatic adaptation in nursing pattern, there is a paucity of data, and the few available suggest that there is no variation in milk composition comparable to that seen among other animals, where closely related species adapt to different environmental situations, nor is there predictable variation in nursing pattern as seen between animal species. This would seem to suggest that nursing patterns adopted in modern Western settings are, in fact, largely a cultural aberration. By imposing them, we are simply testing the infant's ability to adapt his or her pattern of feeding to the extremes that culture has sought to impose. The message should therefore be—Stop doing it!

Will we ever accept that the infant is capable of self-regulating his or her own intake and so should be permitted to dictate the pace and pattern of breastfeeding? My fear is that we shall never do so. A disturbing return to the old views recommending prescriptive patterns of breastfeeding has recently surfaced in the paper by Pinilla and Birch (1993) in which they suggest that it is possible to constrain infant feeding to a more culturally acceptable pattern by imposing routine. The infant may certainly be able to adapt to sustain his or her intake, but the general concern this raises is that it deemphasizes the infant's rights and wishes in this area. This makes the infant simply a convenience for adults, rather than recognizing the infant as a free-thinking individual from the beginning. The dual error of undervaluing motherhood and infanthood alike is a worrying attribute to be taking with us into the next century.

NOTES

1. Dates relate to all editions in which the text remained essentially unchanged.

2. "Demand feeding" can have negative connotations—the baby is a demanding tyrant, and controls the mother and the household—this is largely because people interpret it too literally, rather than use it in the scientific sense in which it has gained widespread acceptance and usage. Nonetheless, it remains common in international usage, as in Step 8 of the WHO/UNICEF "Ten Steps to Successful Breastfeeding." There is frequent debate at a local level over alternatives, but very little has made it into the academic press, as a result of which there is no uniformity of agreement. "Cue-based" feeding has obvious attractions, while "baby-led" feeding is my preferred term.

3. This phrase itself relates both to the effectiveness of application of baby's tongue and jaws to the milk sinuses lying behind the nipple *and* to the physical relationship of the glandular tissue to the milk sinuses. These aspects are loosely referred to by the terms "fixing," "positioning," "attachment," and "latching-on," although commonly the point of reference may simply be the superficial approximation of the baby's lips to the skin of the breast, other internal structural relationships and the larger picture of the mother–baby and baby–breast posture often being ignored.

4. "Prefeed fat" is defined as the fat concentration of a milk sample manually expressed, immediately prior to feeding, from the breast to be suckled.

5. "Interfeed interval" is defined as the time elapsed between the *end* of one feed and the *start* of the next.

6. Hytten (1954) proposed and tested a physical model of milk storage and delivery. He immersed a natural sponge in whole milk and left it for some period, then gradually compressed milk from the sponge; the first milk draining off was low in fat, similar to foremilk, and with progressive milk removal the fat concentration rose, finally approximating to hindmilk. The explanation he proposed was that fat droplets, being adherent, became adsorbed onto the internal luminal walls of the sponge, and that sustained milk removal was necessary to dislodge the adherent fat. His physical model of storage and delivery duplicated the changes in fat concentration during milk removal sufficiently closely that it has not been necessary to invoke further models.

Several observations can be explained by this model such as the fact that "drip milk" from the breast not being suckled approximates to foremilk (Lucas, Gibbs and Baum, 1978; Stocks, Davies, Carroll, Broderick and Parker, 1983), and that manual massage of the breast can increase the fat content by dislodging adhered fat globules (Bowles, Stutte and Hensley, 1988).

The only aspect that deserves reconsideration in the light of recent research is that synthesized fat droplets are bounded by a plasma membrane and so may not adhere to the luminal walls of the breasts (themselves plasma membranes) in the same physical manner in which free fat droplets would adhere. For this reason, we should not perhaps discount a "creaming" effect (fat, being of lighter density than water, settles out in a counter direction to that in which gravity acts, i.e., at the top).

By report, A.T. Cowie tested this on a cow by maintaining it on its back between milkings, then milking it while supine, and this supported a "creaming effect" in part, but not fully. The observation made in the Thai data that the sleep period has opposite effects on prefeed and postfeed fats is most easily explainable in these terms.

7. There are probably a multiplicity of social factors that also influence unsettled behavior in the late afternoon and evening. Mothers in England always assume that it is due to their supply dropping off at this time of day, but on many occasions this assumption is not validated by weighing.

REFERENCES

Barr, R. G., M. S. Kramer, I. B. Pless, C. Boisjoly, and D. Leduc

1989 Feeding and temperament as determinants of early infant crying/fussing behavior. *Pediatrics* 84:514–521.

Beekman, D.

1977 *The Mechanical Baby: A Popular History of the Theory and Practice of Child Raising*. New York: Meridian.

Ben Shaul, D. M.

1962 The composition of the milk of wild animals. *Zoological Yearbook* 4:333–342.

Berman, M. L., K. Hanson, and I. L. Hellman
1972 Effect of breast feeding on post-partum menstruation, ovulation and pregnancy in Alaskan Eskimos. *American Journal of Obstetrics and Gynecology* 111:524–534.

Bonner, W. N.
1984 Lactation strategies in pinnipeds: Problems for a marine mammalian group. In *Physiological Strategies in Lactation*, edited by M. Peaker, R. G. Vernon, and C. H. Knight. *Symposia of the Zoological Society of London* 51:253–272.

Bowles, B. C., P. C. Stutte, and J. Hensley
1988 Alternate massage in breastfeeding. *Genesis* 9:5–9.

Butte, N. F., C. Garza, E. O. Smith, and B. L. Nichols
1985 Human milk intake and growth in exclusively breast-fed infants. *Journal of Pediatrics* 104:187–195.

Cameron, H. C.
1913 Causes of the failure of women to nurse their infants at the breast. *Lancet* 2:911–914.

Crawford, M. A., B. M. Laurance, and A. E. Munhambo
1977 Breast feeding and human milk composition. *Lancet* 1:99–100.

Delgado, H. L., R. Martorell, and R. E. Klein
1982 Nutrition, lactation, and birth interval components in rural Guatemala. *American Journal of Clinical Nutrition* 35:1468–1476.

Díaz, S., G. Rodríquez, G. Marshall, G. del Pino, M. E. Casado, P. Miranda, V. Schiappacasse, and H. B. Croxatto
1988 Breastfeeding pattern and the duration of lactational amenorrhoea in urban Chilean women. *Contraception* 38:37–51.

Drewett, R. F.
1993 The infant's regulation of nutritional intake. In *Infant Crying, Feeding, and Sleeping: Development, Problems and Treatments*, edited by I. St. James-Roberts, G. Harris, and D. Messer, pp. 83–98. New York: Harvester Wheatsheaf.

Drewett, R. F., and M. W. Woolridge
1981 Milk taken by human babies from the first and second breast. *Physiology and Behaviour* 26:327–329.

Drewett, R. F., M. W. Woolridge, D. A. Jackson, S. M. Imong, A. Mangklabruks, L. Wongsawasdii, P. Chiowanich, K. Amatayakul, and J. D. Baum
1989 Relationships between nursing patterns, supplementary food intake and breast milk intake in a rural Thai population. *Early Human Development* 20:13–23.

Drewett, R., K. Amatayakul, L. Wongsawasdii, A. Mangklabruks, S. Ruckpaopunt, C. Ruangyuttikarn, D. Baum, S. Imong, D. Jackson, and M. Woolridge
1993 Nursing frequency and the energy intake from breast milk and supplementary food in a rural Thai population: A longitudinal study. *European Journal of Clinical Nutrition* 47:880–891.

Elias, M. J., J. Teas, J. Johnston, and C. Bora
1986 Nursing practices and lactation amenorrhoea. *Journal of Biosocial Science* 18:1–10.

Fomon, S. J., L. J. Filmer, Jr., L. N. Thomas, T. A. Anderson, and S. E. Nelson
1975 Influence of formula concentration on caloric intake and growth of normal infants. *Acta Paediatrica Scandinavica* 64:172–181.
Friedman, M.
1975 Some determinants of milk ingestion in suckling rats. *Journal of Comparative Physiology and Psychology* 89:636–647.
Garza, C., M. W. Woolridge, N. F. Butte, A. Ferris, and C. Casey
1985 Sampling milk for energy content. In *Human Lactation: Milk Components and Methodologies*, edited by R. G. Jensen and M. C. Neville, pp. 115–119. New York: Plenum Press.
Gussler, J. D., and L. H. Briesemeister
1980 The insufficient milk syndrome: A biocultural explanation. *Medical Anthropology* 4:145–174.
Hamosh, M., T. R. Clary, S. S. Chernick, and R. O. Scow
1970 Lipoprotein lipase activity of adipose and mammary tissue and plasma triglyceride in pregnant and lactating rats. *Biochimica et Biophysica Acta* 210:473–482.
Harris, R. B. S., and R. J. Martin
1984 Lipostatic theory of energy balance: Concepts and signals. *Nutrition and Behavior* 1:253–275.
Hernell, O.
1990 The requirement and utilization of dietary fatty acids in the newborn infant. *Acta Paediatrica Scandinavica Supplement* 365:20–27.
Hillervik-Lindquist, C.
1991 Studies on perceived breast milk insufficiency. *Acta Paediatrica Scandinavica Supplement* 376:6–27.
Huffman, S. L., A. Chowdhury, H. Allen, and L. Nahar
1987 Suckling patterns and post-partum amenorrhoea in Bangladesh. *Journal of Biosocial Science* 19:171–179.
Hytten, F. E.
1954 Clinical and chemical studies in human lactation. II. Variation in major constituents during a feeding. *British Medical Journal* i:176–179.
Illingworth, R. S., and D. G. H. Stone
1952 Self-demand feeding in a maternity unit. *Lancet* 1:683–687.
Imong, S. M., D. A. Jackson, L. Wongsawasdii, S. Ruckphaopunt, A. Amatayakul, R. F. Drewett, and J. D. Baum
1987 Importance of night-time breastfeeding in a rural Northern Thai community. Paper presented at the 59th Annual Meeting of the British Paediatric Association, York, England, 1987.
Imong, S. M., D. A. Jackson, M. W. Woolridge, L. Wongsawasdii, S. Ruckphaophunt, K. Amatayakul, and J. D. Baum
1988 Indirect test weighing: A new method for measuring overnight breast milk intakes in the field. *Journal of Pediatric Gastroenterology and Nutrition* 7:699–706.
Imong, S. M., D. A. Jackson, L. Wongsawasdii, S. Ruckphaophunt, A. Tansuhaj, P. Chiowanich, M. W. Woolridge, R. F. Drewett, J. D. Baum, and K. Amatayakul

1989 Predictors of breast milk intake in rural northern Thailand. *Journal of Pediatric Gastroenterology and Nutrition* 8:359–370.

Jackson, D. A., S. M. Imong, A. Silprasert, S. Preunglumpoo, P. Leelapat, Y. Yootabootr, K. Amatayakul, and J. D. Baum

1988a Estimation of 24h breast-milk fat concentration and fat intake in rural northern Thailand. *British Journal of Nutrition* 59:365–371.

Jackson, D. A., S. M. Imong, A. Silprasert, S. Ruckphaopunt, M. W. Woolridge, J. D. Baum, and K. Amatayakul

1988b Circadian variation in fat concentration of breastmilk in a rural Northern Thai population. *British Journal of Nutrition* 59:349–363.

Jackson D. A., S. M. Imong, A. Silprasert, L. Wongsawasdii, P. Chiowanich, S. Ruckphaopunt, A. F. Williams, M. W. Woolridge, R. F. Drewett, K. Amatayakul, et al.

1988c Infant weight in relation to nutritional intake and morbidity in northern Thailand. *European Journal of Clinical Nutrition* 42:725–739.

Jensen, R. G.

1989 Milk fat globule membrane. In *The Lipids of Human Milk*, edited by R. G. Jensen, pp. 153–166. Boca Raton, FL: CRC Press.

Khin-Maung-Naing, Tin-Tin-Oo, Kywe-Thein, and Nwe-New-Hlaing

1980 Study on lactation performance of Burmese mothers. *American Journal of Clinical Nutrition* 33:2665–2668.

King, F. T.

1913–1940 *Feeding and Care of Baby*. London: OUP.

Konner, M., and C. Worthman

1980 Nursing frequency, gonadal function, and birth spacing among !Kung hunter-gatherers. *Science* 207:788–791.

Liddiard, M.

1923–1954 *The Mothercraft Manual*. London: J&A Churchill.

Le Magnen, J.

1983 Body energy balance and food intake: A neuroendocrine regulatory mechanism. *Physiological Reviews* 63:314–386.

Lucas, A., J. A. H. Gibbs, and J. D. Baum

1978 The biology of human drip breast milk. *Early Human Development* 2:351–361.

Nelson, W. E.

1933–1945 *Textbook of Pediatrics*. Philadelphia: W. B. Saunders.

Neville, M. C., R. Keller, J. Seacat, V. Lutes, M. Neifert, C. Casey, J. Allen, and P. Archer

1988 Studies in human lactation: Milk volumes in lactating women during the onset of lactation and full lactation. *American Journal of Clinical Nutrition* 48:1375–1386.

Oftedal, O. T.

1984 Milk composition, milk yield and energy output at peak lactation: A comparative review. In *Physiological Strategies in Lactation*, edited by M. Peaker, R. G. Vernon, and C. H. Knight. *Symposia of the Zoological Society of London* 51:33–85.

Pao, E. M., J. M. Himes, and A. F. Roche

1980 Milk intakes and feeding patterns of breast-fed infants. *Journal of the American Dietetic Association* 77:540–545.
Pinilla, T., and L. L. Birch
1993 Help me make it through the night: Behavioral entrainment of breast-fed infants' sleep patterns. *Pediatrics* 91:436–444.
Prentice, A., A. M. Prentice, and R. G. Whitehead
1981 Breast milk fat concentrations in rural African women. I. Short-term variations within individuals. *British Journal of Nutrition* 45:483–494.
St. James-Roberts, I.
1989 Persistent crying in infancy. *Journal of Child Psychology and Psychiatry* 30:189–195.
Shatrugna, V., N. Raghuramulu, and K. Prema
1982 Serum prolactin levels in undernourished Indian lactating women. *British Journal of Nutrition* 48:193–199.
Stocks, R. J., D. P. Davies, L. P. Carroll, B. Broderick, and M. Parker
1983 A simple method to improve the energy value of bank human milk. *Early Human Development* 8:175–178.
Tyson, J., J. Burchfield, F. Sentance, C. Mize, R. Uauy, and J. Eastburn
1992 Adaptation of feeding to a low fat yield in breast milk. *Pediatrics* 89:215–220.
Vincent, R.
1913 *The Nutrition of the Infant.* London: Bailliere, Tindal, and Cox.
Vitzthum, V. J.
1989 Nursing behavior and its relation to duration of post-partum amenorrhoea in an Andean community. *Journal of Biosocial Science* 21:145–160.
Whitehead, R. G., M. G. Rowland, M. Hutton, A. M. Prentice, E. Muller, and A. Paul
1978 Factors influencing lactation performance in rural Gambian women. *Lancet* 2:178–181.
Williamson, D. H., M. R. Munday, and R. G. Jones
1984 Biochemical basis of dietary influences on the synthesis of the macronutrients of rat milk. *Federation Proceedings* 43:2443–2447.
Wood, J. W., D. Lai, P. L. Johnson, K. L. Campbell, and I. A. Maslar
1985 Lactation and birth spacing in highland New Guinea. *Journal of Biosocial Science Supplement* 9:159–173.
Woolridge, M. W., and C. Fisher
1988 Colic, "overfeeding," and symptoms of lactose malabsorption in the breast-fed baby: A possible artifact of feed management. *Lancet* 2:382–384.
Woolridge M. W., J. C. Ingram, and J. D. Baum
1990 Do changes in pattern of breast usage alter the baby's nutrient intake? *Lancet* 336:395–397.
Woolridge, M. W., and J. D. Baum
1992 Infant appetite-control and the regulation of breast milk supply. *Children's Hospital Quarterly* 3:113–119.

9

Breastfeeding: Adaptive Behavior for Child Health and Longevity

Allan S. Cunningham

INTRODUCTION

Salaried employment, feminism, and AIDS have provoked debate about the importance of breastfeeding and milk for child health and survival in the developed world. Maternal work is seen as a barrier to breastfeeding. Breastfeeding is seen as a barrier to the liberation of women. Finally, since the AIDS virus can be transmitted by human milk, the safety of breastfeeding has been called into question. These and other factors have fostered continued discussion about the relative risks and benefits of breastfeeding and bottle-feeding.

There are no dissenters to the proposition that breastfeeding is vital to the health and survival of infants in poor countries, where large numbers of people lack clean water, sewage disposal, and an adequate fuel supply. There is still an articulate minority that doubts the importance of breastfeeding in industrial nations (Bauchner, Leventhal and Shapiro, 1988). In part, these doubts result from naive skepticism that points to historically low infant mortality rates in the face of a decline in breastfeeding. Furthermore, until recently child health experts assumed that excess mortality among bottle-fed infants resulted exclusively from diarrhea and contaminated formula.

We now know that although the differences between illness and mortality rates are narrower in industrial nations compared with poor countries, there are still real differences between breastfed and bottle-fed infants. We know also that it is not only diarrheal disease that accounts for these differences. Every organ system is affected by the differences between infant formula and human milk. It is time to review the facts.

INFANT MORBIDITY AND MORTALITY

Gastrointestinal Illness

Breastfeeding is crucial to worldwide infant survival. In primitive circumstances, mortal illness from gastrointestinal infections results from microbial contamination of the water supply and feeding utensils. Animal milk and proprietary formulas lack protective immunologic factors, and malnutrition acts synergistically with the microbial burden to weaken the bottle-fed infant. This is particularly likely to occur where purchasing power is inadequate to pay for artificial feedings.

In Latin America alone there are more than 500,000 deaths annually from gastrointestinal infections in preschool children (Macedo, 1988). Most of these deaths occur among infants, for whom the mortality risk of bottle-feeding is at least 10 times higher than the risk for breastfed infants (Victora, Smith, Vaughan, Nobre, Lombardi, Teixeira, Fuchs, Moreira, Gigante and Barros, 1987).

In Europe and North America, efficient sewage disposal and abundant supplies of clean water reduce the infant's exposure to bacterial and other pathogens. As a result, the hazards of bottle-feeding and mortality from gastrointestinal infections are sharply reduced—but they are not negligible. At least 400 infants die annually in the United States from diarrheal disease (Ho, Glass, Pinsky, Young-Okoh, Sappenfield, Buehler, Gunter and Anderson, 1988). We can estimate that 250 to 300 of these deaths are attributable to being bottle-fed or, conversely, to not being breastfed (Schlesselman, 1982).

Respiratory Illness

Prior to World War II, infant mortality from acute respiratory diseases was high among infants who were not breastfed (Cunningham, 1981). The parallel decline in breastfeeding and infant mortality rates after World War II permitted a collective amnesia about this fact in Europe and North America. Even today, there is resistance to the idea that bottle-feeding and the failure to breastfeed can cause respiratory illness in infants, in part because of the simplistic notion that feeding relates only to the gastrointestinal tract. Forgotten is the fact that the mouth is the portal of entry for both the digestive and respiratory systems. Forgotten also is the fact that foods are well-known causes of allergic respiratory diseases. Even now, our knowledge about resistance to infections is incomplete and it is hard to appreciate the complex interrelationships among immunologic defense factors and different organ systems.

Modern information indicates that the relative risk of fatal and nonfatal respiratory infections is two- to fivefold among bottle-fed infants in the Western hemisphere (Cunningham, 1979; Cunningham, Jelliffe and Jelliffe, 1991). In the United States alone, this translates to 500 to 600 additional respiratory-related deaths annually because infants are not breastfed (Schlesselman, 1982).

Otitis Media

The middle ear chamber is directly connected to the upper respiratory tract and is an integral part of the respiratory system. The same pathogens that affect the nose, throat, and lower respiratory passages cause middle ear infections. Although it is rarely fatal, otitis media causes considerable morbidity, inconvenience, and expense. It occurs much more frequently among infants who are not breastfed (Cunningham, 1979; Cunningham et al., 1991). The emergence of bacterial resistance to antibiotics has increased the importance of breastfeeding's prophylactic effect.

Bacteremia and Meningitis

Bacteremia is a bacterial infection in the blood, and meningitis is an infection of the membranes surrounding the brain. These conditions are relatively uncommon, but when they do occur, they are frequently fatal, or can lead to brain damage. Investigations into the effects of breastfeeding and bottle-feeding on these illnesses have been late in coming because of the simplistic thinking mentioned above. In cities in the United States, bottle-feeding imposes on infants a fourfold risk of bacteremia and meningitis (Fallot, Boyd and Oska, 1980).

Prior to the development of a vaccine against *Haemophilus influenzae*, the risk to bottle-fed North American infants of bacteremia and meningitis caused by this pathogen was four- to 16-fold, compared with infants who were breastfed (Cunningham et al., 1991).

In premature infant nurseries where there is a high standard of hygiene and medical care, human milk still has an important role to play in the protection of infants against life-threatening bacteremia and necrotizing enterocolitis. Necrotizing enterocolitis (NEC) is a catastrophic intestinal inflammation and is a major cause of bacteremia and fatality (Lucas and Cole, 1990; Narayanan, Prakash, Murthy and Gujral, 1984).

Mortality

It is estimated that in North America breastfeeding decreases infant mortality by four per 1000 (Rogan, 1989). In the United States, where 4,000,000 babies are born every year, this amounts to 16,000 lives annually. Crib death (cot death, SIDS, sudden infant death syndrome) is a major cause of infant mortality, accounting for 5000 to 6000 infant deaths annually in the United States (Wegman 1991). The relative risk of bottle-feeding is about fivefold, translating to 4000 SIDS deaths every year in the United States from bottle-feeding or lack of breastfeeding (Schlesselman, 1982).

For the epidemiologist, crib death is a complex issue. Maternal cigarette smoking is believed to be a causal factor, and lately it has become evident that infant sleeping position plays a role (Mitchell, Scragg, Stewart, Becroft, Taylor, Ford, Hassall, Barry, Allen and Roberts, 1991). It is also a very touchy subject—emotionally and politically. The unexpected loss of an infant is tragic and does not lend itself to candid explanations of preventable causes. Neither do the politics and economics of medical research, the financial support of which depends primarily on focusing on physiologic mechanisms. These factors have conspired to suppress public knowledge of the link between bottle-feeding, lack of breastfeeding, and infant mortality. To some extent, this is an American peculiarity, and British physicians have been more candid about the relationship (Wood and Walker-Smith, 1981). A few studies have looked at infant mortality from crib deaths (SIDS) and other causes in industrial nations. These are summarized in Table 9.1. The relationships among breastfeeding, co-sleeping, and SIDS are covered more fully in McKenna and Bernshaw (this volume).

IMMUNOLOGY

Immunology is just one part of the edifice of knowledge about breastfeeding's protective physiologic mechanisms. This part of the edifice is complex and, at the same time, incomplete. Nevertheless, it is useful to acquire a sense of mechanism—why the provision of human milk to human infants is adaptive behavior (Cunningham, 1981).

Table 9.1. Mortality Risk of Bottle-Feeding in Industrial Nations

Reference	*Age group*	*Relative risk*	*Attributable risk*	*Comment*
Arnon, Damus, Thompson, Midura and Chin (1982)	0–6 mo	7.0		Sudden death
Carpenter, Gardner, Jepson, Taylor, Salvin, Sunderland, Emery, Pursall and Roe (1983)	1 wk–1 yr		0.8/1000	Unexpected death
Madeley, Hull and Holland (1986)	1 mo–1 yr		5.1/1000	Prevention program
Victora et al. (1987)	1 wk–1 yr	2.5–14.2		Infection deaths
Damus et al. (1988)	0–1 yr	3.7–5.0		Sudden death
Rogan (1989)	0–1 yr		4/1000	Mathematical model
Mitchell et al. (1991)	1 wk–1 yr	2.5		Sudden death
Fredrickson, Sorenson, Biddle and Kotelchuck (1993)	0–1 yr	2.0 for each month not breastfed		Sudden death

The body's main portal of entry for invaders, microbial or allergenic, is the mucous membrane of the aeroalimentary system, otherwise known as the respiratory and gastrointestinal tracts. The secretory immune system is the prime defender against invasion. This is a system of antibody-producing cells that lines the mucous membranes of the gastrointestinal and respiratory tracts. These cells produce secretory immunoglobulin A (S-IgA).

Newborn infants have antibodies circulating in the bloodstream that are acquired transplacentally from their mothers. Their secretory immune system, on the other hand, is not yet functional, and requires additional time and exposure to environmental pathogens for its development. Until the newborn can develop her or his own mucosal defenses, she or he depends, normally, on an external source—the S-IgA contained in mother's milk. This is especially important since transplacental immunity is incomplete and imperfect.

Colostrum and human milk contain abundant quantities of S-IgA directed specifically against viruses, bacteria, and other parasitic organisms in the maternal–infant environment. Furthermore, the mammary gland contains the cells that produce S-IgA. The sources of these cells are the enteromammary and bronchomammary axes. Gastrointestinal and respiratory tract pathogens encountered by the mother stimulate the development of cells that line her mucosal surfaces—cells that produce S-IgA. The S-IgA acts as a barrier to invasion of the blood and organ systems. It is the first line of defense. At the same time, some of the S-IgA-producing cells circulate to the mammary gland, where they reside to produce S-IgA for the infant.

This remarkable adaptation is only one important element of the complex array of defense mechanisms provided by human milk. In addition to conferring passive antibody protection on the infant, mother's milk contains soluble immunoregulatory factors that stimulate active development of the infant's own defenses (Pittard, 1979). Moreover, there are other protective factors such as lactoferrin and oligosaccharides that circulate to other mucosal surfaces such as the urinary tract (Coppa, Gabrielli, Giorgi, Catassi, Montanari, Varaldo and Nichols, 1990; Goldblum, Schanler, Garza and Goldman, 1989; Prentice 1987). This explains the clinical observations linking breastfeeding to protection against urinary tract infections (Mårild, Jodal and Mangelus, 1989; Pisacane, Graziano and Zona, 1990).

There are undoubtedly other protective mechanisms. For example, the benign nature of rotavirus infections in breastfed infants has been related to an interaction with the more benign bacterial flora in the nursling's gastrointestinal tract (Duffy, Riepenhoff-Talty, Byers, La Scolea, Zielezny, Dryja and Ogra, 1986). There is even the suggestion that anti-inflammatory substances in human milk modify exuberant and damaging host responses to the food and microbial antigens to which the breastfed infant is exposed (Goldman, Thorpe, Goldblum and Hanson, 1986).

LONG-TERM HEALTH

Students of animal behavior are familiar with imprinting, the process by which events during certain critical periods of development in early life have a lasting effect on patterns of behavior (e.g., goslings hatched in the absence of their mother will follow the first moving object they see, such as a human being or other animal).

This concept has come lately to the field of human pathophysiology and is known as programming (Lucas, 1990). The concept of physiologic programming provides the link between events during infancy, long-term development, and patterns of health and disease. Infant feeding appears to be an important part of this process.

Disorders of Immune Regulation

Autoimmune diseases, subtle immune deficiencies, systemic vasculitis (inflammation of small blood vessels), and allergies are immunoregulatory disorders that have antecedents in early infant feeding practices.

Inflammatory Bowel Disease. In 1961, the observation that patients with ulcerative colitis (a severe inflammation of the large intestine) benefit from dietary exclusion of dairy products prompted Acheson and Truelove (1961) to ask whether early exposure to cows' milk protein was a relevant factor. Their retrospective study revealed that lack of breastfeeding or its early termination was significantly associated with the eventual development of the disease. A similar association was demonstrated among bottle-feeding, lack of breastfeeding, and the development of Crohn's disease, another intestinal inflammatory disease (Koletzko, Sherman, Corey, Griffiths and Smith, 1989).

These inflammatory bowel diseases are immunologically mediated, and the first steps in their pathogenesis may occur as early as the first 2 weeks of life (Jayanthi, Probert and Mayberry, 1991). It is biologically plausible that deprivation of some factor(s) in human milk, or early exposure to foreign antigens such as cows' milk protein, or both, may initiate this process. It is now well-known that foreign proteins, including those from cows' milk, are absorbed from the gastrointestinal tract, especially in young infants. The same proteins cross the placenta to enter the fetal circulation and also enter the milk of nursing mothers after entering their circulation from the gastrointestinal tract.

Celiac Disease. Celiac disease is another chronic gastrointestinal disorder involving malabsorption from the small intestine that is immunologically mediated. Its development is associated with bottle-feeding and the absence of breastfeeding (Greco, Auricchio, Mayer and Grimaldi, 1988).

Schönlein-Henoch Purpura. Schönlein-Henoch purpura is a systemic immunologic vasculitis seen mainly in toddlers and young school-aged children. Compared with children who were exclusively breastfed 5 months or more as infants, the relative risk of developing the disorder is three- to fourfold for children who were bottle-fed (Pisacane, Buffolano, Grillo and Gaudiosi, 1992a).

Juvenile Diabetes. Juvenile diabetes is an autoimmune disorder in which an individual's natural defenses are turned against its own tissues—in this case the insulin-producing beta cells of the pancreas. The secular increase in juvenile diabetes has been correlated with a preceding decline in breastfeeding. Case-control studies and geographic correlations have confirmed this association, and as many as 25% of cases are ascribed to failure to breastfeed (Mayer, Hamman, Gay, Lezotte, Savitz and Klingensmith, 1988). Furthermore, consumption of cows' milk protein has been correlated with the development of juvenile diabetes (Dahl-Jorgensen, Joner and Hanssen, 1991).

Meticulous immunologic study has shown that a peptide fragment at the surface of pancreatic beta cells is identical to a portion of the bovine serum albumin, one of the proteins contained in cows' milk and proprietary infant formulas. Gastrointestinal absorption of this molecule serves to prime the immunologic machinery in genetically susceptible infants. The immunologic system then directs antibody production and cellular elements against the bovine protein and, *pari passu*, against the infant's own pancreatic beta cells. Over time, the beta cells are destroyed, pancreatic insulin production declines, and clinically evident diabetes develops (Karjalainen, Martin, Knip, Ilonen, Robinson, Savilahti, Akerblom and Dosch, 1992).

Malignant Lymphomas. Malignant lymphomas are cancerous disorders of immune regulation. Geographic correlations have been established between dietary consumption of bovine protein (beef and cows' milk products) and high death rates from lymphomas (Cunningham, 1976) and between low breastfeeding rates and high lymphoma death rates (Cunningham, 1986). Celiac disease is an antecedent to malignant lymphomas (Holmes, Prior, Lane, Pope and Allan, 1989). Davis and colleagues in Denver performed a case-control study that revealed a six- to eightfold risk for the eventual development of lymphomas among children under 15 years of age who were breastfed less than 6 months as infants (Davis, Savitz and Graubard, 1988). In Great Britain, a national cohort study of childhood cancer revealed a twofold risk among children who had not been breastfed during the first week of life (Golding, Paterson and Kinlen, 1990). This comparison included, but was not restricted to, lymphomas.

Breast Cancer. Recently, in a case-control study of women in New York state, Freudenheim, Marshall, Graham, Laughlin, Vena, Bandera, Muti, Swanson and Nemoto (1994) identified artificial infant formula feeding in childhood as a significant risk factor for breast cancer in women in adulthood. In this study, the researchers controlled for age, education, age at menarche, age at first pregnancy, number of months they nursed their own children, number of pregnancies, family history of breast cancer, history of benign breast disease, body mass index, and height. After all of these factors had been taken into account, one factor related to early nutrition was found to be associated with a significant reduction in risk. Having been breastfed as a child reduced breast cancer rates in women over 40 years of age by more than 25% (Freudenheim et al., 1994).

Multiple Sclerosis. A single case-control study (Pisacane, Impagliazzo, Russo, Valiani, Mandarini, Florio and Vivo, 1994) has shown that adults with multiple sclerosis received, on average, 4 months less breastfeeding in infancy than a group of matched controls. The study found a relative risk of two- to threefold when individuals are bottle-fed exclusively or receive breast milk for less than 7 months compared with individuals who are breastfed for 7 months or more. The mechanisms suggested for this association are the differences in chemical composition of the cerebral cortex among individuals fed cows' milk formulas, or the absence of the long-term immunologic protection provided by human milk, or both.

Allergic Disorders. Allergies are common immunologic disorders. They are rarely life-threatening, but they account for considerable morbidity, inconvenience, and expense. In the popular mind, breastfeeding is a panacea against the development of allergies. This is a misconception, and the reality is somewhat more complex.

It is clear that during the period infants are exclusively breastfed, allergic reactions to foods are almost completely avoided. This is an important benefit since allergic reactions to animal milks, proprietary formulas, and other foods can be very serious indeed in young infants. The exemption from allergic reactions is not absolute, even for exclusively breastfed infants, since foreign proteins from the maternal diet do enter breast milk and, even in minute quantities, can cause allergic reactions in infants. Cows' milk protein is the most important example (Høst, Husby and Østerballe, 1988).

Allergic reactions to foods may actually be exaggerated in occasional individuals who are breastfed. This can occur because restricted exposure to certain foreign proteins inhibits the development of immunologic tolerance that would otherwise develop in the presence of large amounts of the same proteins. Without immunologic tolerance, there is exaggerated production of immunoglobulin E, the antibody that accounts for most allergic reactions. For some infants, then, allergic reactions to certain proteins will be avoided only by absolute exclusion, even from the maternal diet (Jarrett and Hall, 1986).

Long-term allergy prophylaxis by breastfeeding has been debated (Kramer, 1988). The most recent information indicates that there is significant prophylactic benefit, but that this is far from universal. Breastfed infants from allergic families are only half as likely to wheeze before their first birthday, even if they are breastfed for only a few weeks (Miskelly, Burr, Vaughan-Williams, Fehily, Butland and Merrett, 1988).

In a group of formula-fed premature infants, the relative risk of eczema, asthma, or food allergies by 18 months was fourfold compared with infants given only human milk during the early weeks of life (Lucas, Brooke, Morley, Cole and Bamford, 1990). This benefit was limited to infants from allergic families. The relative risk of asthma at age 3 years is increased by 50% in children receiving no breastfeeding in infancy, regardless of the family allergy history (Infante-Rivard, 1993).

Finally, in another study, 7-year-old children from allergic families were less likely to have a history of wheezing if they had received some breastfeeding in infancy (59%) compared with children who were never breastfed (74%) (Burr, Limb, Maguire, Amarah, Eldridge, Layzell and Merrett, 1993).

It may be that breastfeeding only delays the onset of allergy for several years, mainly in children from allergic families (Björkstėn, 1983). This is disappointing for anyone seeking a panacea. Still, even this limited benefit is "not to be sneezed at."

The possibility that dietary restriction of certain foods, without complete elimination, may lead to exaggerated allergic reactions in some breastfed babies is bothersome. However, this may be a blessing in disguise if it leads to the avoidance of food proteins (e.g., cows' milk) whose long-term effects may threaten survival (Cunningham, 1976; Dahl-Jorgensen, 1991).

Chronic Respiratory Disease. Lower respiratory infections and wheezing in infants and children are the forerunners of chronic respiratory disease in adults (Barker and Osmond, 1986). In this connection the relevance of breastfeeding as a protective strategy is evident (McConnochie and Roghmann, 1986; Mok and Simpson, 1982).

As mentioned previously, the middle ear chamber is part of the respiratory tract. The prevention of chronic and recurrent otitis media by breastfeeding is also a relevant facet of preventing chronic respiratory disease (Saarinen, 1982; Timmermans and Gerson, 1980).

Coronary Artery Disease. Several strands of evidence suggest that infant feeding is relevant to the prevention of coronary artery disease.

Osborn studied the coronary arteries of young people who had died suddenly and traumatically. He combined the postmortem examinations with medical histories, and found a graded increase in coronary abnormalities according to feeding method in infancy (Table 9.2) (Osborn, 1968).

Kawasaki disease is another type of vasculitis that is a precursor to adult coronary disease and is associated with lack of breastfeeding in infancy (Kato, Inoue, Kawasaki, Fujiwara, Watanabe and Toshima, 1992; Kawasaki, Kosaki, Okawa, Shigematsu and Yanagawa, 1974).

Fall and colleagues have found that one antecedent to ischemic heart disease in adults is exclusive bottle-feeding in infancy (Fall, Barker, Osmond, Winter, Clark and Hales, 1992).

Finally, there is evidence that the method of infant feeding has a long-term effect in programming lipid metabolism, since plasma cholesterol levels are lower in young adults who were breastfed (Marmot, Page, Atkins and Douglas, 1980).

Psychomotor and Neurodevelopment. It was once fashionable to feed high protein formulas to newborn infants to accelerate early growth rates. This fad came to an abrupt halt when it was realized that high protein intakes fostered an increase in blood amino acid levels that could permanently damage the central nervous system (Mamunes, Prince, Thornton, Hunt and Hitchcock, 1976). The same observations prompted a reevaluation of whether the low protein content of human milk was a disadvantage.

Table 9.2. Breastfeeding Prevents Coronary Artery Pathology: Cases Studied by Osborn (1968)

Coronary pathology	*No breastfeeding*	*1 month breastfeeding*	*Over 1 month breastfeeding*
None	7	10	14
Intermediate	10	17	9
Severe	25	9	8

Further rethinking was prompted by the observation that breastfeeding mitigated the intellectual deficits in congenital cretinism (Bode, Vanjonack and Crawford, 1978).

Compared with bottle-feeding and artificial formula, breastfeeding and human milk have always been associated with advanced psychomotor development and intellectual superiority. The differences between breastfed and bottle-fed children generally have been small, but they are consistent (Rodgers, 1978). In middle-class populations, test scores of children on scales of cognitive and motor development increase in proportion to the duration of breastfeeding in infancy (Rogan and Gladen, 1993).

It has been difficult to accept the causal nature of the association in view of the difficulty in controlling for the large number of variables that have an impact on mental development, such as socioeconomic status. Nevertheless, good studies have accounted for such factors, and the breastfeeding advantage remains. Moreover, breastfeeding's advantage was first observed by Hoefer and Hardy in 1929, at a time when bottle-feeding was fashionable among the middle and upper classes and breastfeeding was a lower-class, immigrant phenomenon (Hoefer and Hardy, 1929).

The view that human milk per se confers distinct advantages is reinforced by long-term follow-up of tube-fed premature infants. In one study, by the age of 8 years, those who had received their mother's milk in the first weeks of life had a 10-point IQ advantage over the infants given formula, an effect that was independent of the maternal choice to give milk (Lucas, Morley, Cole, Lister and Leeson-Payne, 1992).

Human milk contains various unique factors that affect neurodevelopment. Docosahexanoic acid (DHA), for example, is a long-chain fatty acid that is unique to human milk and that accumulates in the developing brain and retina and is important for their structural development. DHA and other long-chain polyunsaturated fatty acids enhance the mobility of cell membranes at a time when important dendritic connections are being made (Farquharson, Cockburn, Patrick, Jamieson and Logan, 1992; Uauy, Birch, Birch and Peirano, 1992).

PROBLEMS WITH HUMAN MILK

The cliche that "breast is best" still pertains, but human milk is not always perfect. The AIDS virus can be transmitted in human milk and may be a contraindication to breastfeeding if safe alternative feedings are available (Cutting, 1992; Lederman, 1992).

There are rare deficiencies in human milk. Khoshoo, Kjarsgaard, Krafchick and Zlotkin (1992) have reported a zinc-deficiency syndrome, and strict vegetarians may cause a serious vitamin B_{12} deficiency in exclusively breastfed offspring (Higginbottom, Sweetman and Nyhan, 1978). Vitamin-D deficiency rickets has occurred when babies are exclusively breastfed for long periods with inadequate exposure to sunshine (Edidin, Levitsky, Schey, Dumbovic and Campos, 1980). Finally, breastfed infants are uniquely susceptible to a vitamin-K deficiency syndrome known as hemorrhagic disease of the newborn. This is easily prevented by prophylactic administration of vitamin K (Bancroft and Cohen, 1993).

The presence of maternal dietary allergens in human milk has been noted (Høst et al., 1988). The maternal diet may affect milk in other ways, as in the case of ciguatera toxicity in an infant whose mother ate tainted fish (Blythe and DeSylva, 1990). Of course, drugs taken by the mother can enter the milk. The instances in which breastfeeding is contraindicated are rare, but cocaine use is one of them (Chasnoff, Lewis and Squires, 1987).

PROBLEMS WITH FORMULA PRODUCTION

Even when the manufacture and preparation of formulas are flawless, they cannot match the biological superiority of human milk for human infants. When errors are made in the manufacture or preparation of formulas, additional threats to health are imposed. Table 9.3 lists some of these errors.

When properly manufactured, modern formulas are superior to their antecedents, since they are based on the model of human milk. At the same time, it has to be recognized that the progress made in the devel-

Table 9.3. Errors in the Manufacture and Preparation of Infant Formulas

Error	*Illness*	*Reference*
Carnitine deficiency	Hypoglycemia	Slonim, Borum, Tanaka, Stanley, Kasselberg, Greene and Burr (1981)
Taurine deficiency	Retinopathy	Sturman, Wen, Wisniewski and Neuringe (1983)
Inositol deficiency	Lung, retinal disease	Hallman, Bry, Hoppu, Lappi and Pohjavuori (1992)
DHA deficiency	IQ deficit	Lucas et al. (1992)
Chloride deficiency	Growth, neural deficits	Kaleita, Kinsbourne and Menkes (1991)
Copper excess	Cirrhosis	Tanner, Kantarjian, Bhave and Pandit (1983)
Iron excess	Botulism—SIDS	Arnon et al. (1982)
Iron excess	*Salmonella* infection	Haddock, Cousens and Guzman (1991)
Lead excess	Lead poisoning	Shannon and Graef (1992)
Aluminum excess	Brain deposition	Freundlich, Zilleruelo, Abitbol, Strauss, Faugere and Malluche (1985)
Protein excess	IQ deficit	Mamunes et al. (1976)
Phosphate excess	Tetany	Venkataraman, Tsang, Greer, Noguchi, Laskarzewski and Steichen (1985)
Bacterial contamination	*Salmonella* infection	MMWR (1993)
Bacterial contamination	Enterobacter meningitis	Muytjens et al. (1990)
Underdilution	Hypernatremia, intestinal gangrene	Wilcox, Fiorello and Glick (1993)
Overdilution	Undernutrition	McJunkin, Bithoney and McCornick (1987)

opment of proprietary formulas is a process of learning by mistakes. Each new addition to the nutritional composition of formulas is a tacit recognition of a previous deficiency in proprietary formulas.

CONCLUSION

Figure 9.1 shows that low-protein human milk is the tortoise of mammalian growth and development, intended for a slow-growing, long-

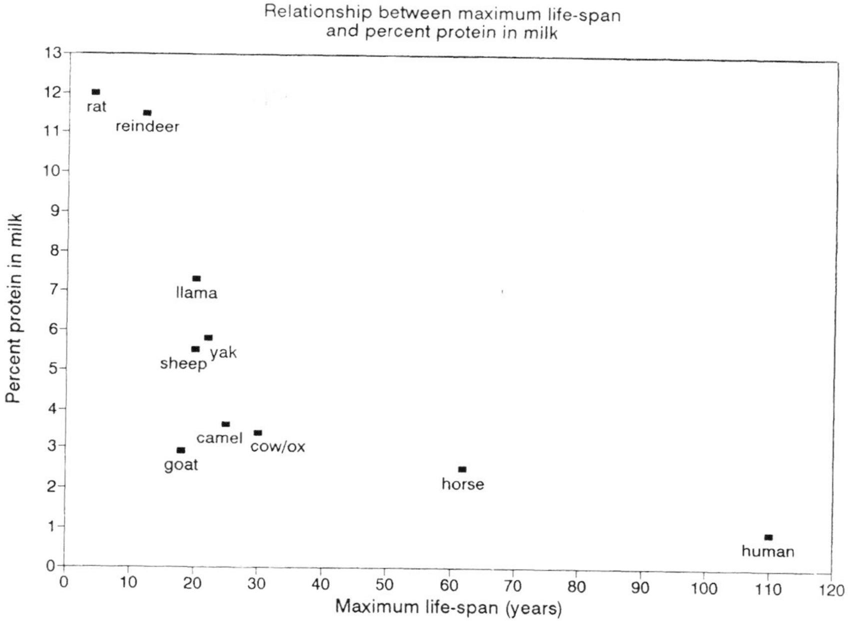

Figure 9.1. Relationship between maximum lifespan and percent protein in milk.

living species (Hambraeus, 1977; Jelliffe and Jelliffe, 1978; Spector, 1956). Feeding animal milk and formulas to human infants accelerates their physical growth, but as illustrated from the foregoing, it also leads to infections, intellectual deficits, and chronic disease. McCance (1962) observed that the growth of young animals is a race against time, but longevity is a feat of endurance. Like Aesop's tortoise, human milk is adapted for the long run, and we must be wary of the modern trends that have conspired against it (Vahlquist, 1975).

This recitation of the diseases that result from bottle-feeding and from the omission of breastfeeding is incomplete and, given the limitations of knowledge, always will be. Not mentioned are recently discovered and provisional associations of bottle-feeding with paralytic poliomyelitis (Pisacane, Grillo, Cafiero, Simeone, Coppola, Scarpellino and Mazzarella, 1992b), deaths from liver disease (Udall, Dixon and Newman, 1985), reduced bone mass in young women (Hirota, Nara, Ohguri, Manago and Hirota, 1992), and increased exposure to radioactivity (Lindemann and Christensen, 1987). Time will tell us more about the long-term effects of early nutrition (György, 1960).

In all circumstances, breastfeeding continues to be highly adaptive behavior.

REFERENCES

Acheson, E. D., and S. C. Truelove
1961 Early weaning in the aetiology of ulcerative colitis. *British Medical Journal* 4:929–933.
Arnon, S. S., K. Damus, B. Thompson, T. F. Midura, and J. Chin
1982 Protective role of human milk against sudden death from infant botulism. *Journal of Pediatrics* 100:568–573.
Bancroft, J., and M. B. Cohen
1993 Intracranial hemorrhage due to vitamin K deficiency in breastfed infants with cholestasis. *Journal of Pediatric Gastroenterology and Nutrition* 16:78–80.
Barker, D. J. P., and C. Osmond
1986 Childhood respiratory infection and adult chronic bronchitis in England and Wales. *British Medical Journal* 293:1271–1275.
Bauchner, H., J. M. Leventhal, and E. D. Shapiro
1988 Studies of breastfeeding and infections: How good is the evidence? *Journal of the American Medical Association* 256:889–892.
Björksten, B.
1983 Does breastfeeding prevent the development of allergy? *Immunology Today* 4:215–217.
Blythe, D. G., and D. B. de Sylva
1990 Mother's milk turns toxic after fish feast. *Journal of the American Medical Association* 264:2074.
Bode, H. H., W. J. Vanjonack, and J. D. Crawford
1978 Mitigation of cretinism by breastfeeding. *Pediatrics* 62:13–16.
Burr, M. L., E. S. Limb, M. J. Maguire, L. Amarah, B. A. Eldridge, J. C. Layzell, and T. G. Merrett
1993 Infant feeding, wheezing and allergy: A prospective study. *Archives of Disease in Childhood* 68:724–728.
Carpenter, R. G., A. Gardner, M. Jepson, E. M. Taylor, A. Salvin, R. Sunderland, J. L. Emery, E. Pursall, and J. Roe
1983 Prevention of unexpected infant death. *Lancet* 1:723–727.
Chasnoff, I. J., D. E. Lewis, and L. Squires
1987 Cocaine intoxication in a breastfed infant. *Pediatrics* 80:836–838.
Coppa, G. V., O. Gabrielli, P. Giorgi, C. Catassi, M. P. Montanari, P. E. Varaldo, and B. L. Nichols
1990 Preliminary study of breastfeeding and bacterial adhesion to uroepithelial cells. *Lancet* 335:569–571.
Cunningham, A. S.
1976 Lymphomas and animal protein consumption. *Lancet* 2:1184–1186.
1979 Morbidity in breastfed and artificially fed infants. *Journal of Pediatrics* 95:685–689.

1981 Breastfeeding and morbidity in industrialized countries: An update. In *Advances in Maternal and Child Health,* Vol. 1, edited by D. B. Jelliffe and E. F. P. Jelliffe, pp. 128–168. Oxford: Oxford University Press.
1986 Letter to the editor. *Lancet* 2:520.
Cunningham, A. S., D. B. Jelliffe, and E. F. P. Jelliffe
1991 Breastfeeding and health in the 1980s: A global epidemiologic review. *Journal of Pediatrics* 118:659–666.
Cutting, W. A.
1992 Breastfeeding and HIV infection. *British Medical Journal* 305:788–789.
Dahl-Jørgensen, K., G. Joner, and K. F. Hanssen
1991 Relationship between cow's milk consumption and incidence in IDDM in childhood. *Diabetes Care* 14:1081–1083.
Damus, K., J. Pakter, E. Krongrad, S. J. Standfast, and H. J. Hoffman
1988 Postnatal medical and epidemiological risk factors for the sudden infant death syndrome. In *Sudden Infant Death Syndrome: Risk Factors and Basic Mechanisms,* edited by R. M. Harper and H. J. Hoffman, pp. 187–201. New York: PMA Publishing Corporation.
Davis, M. K., D. A. Savitz, and B. I. Graubard
1988 Infant feeding and childhood cancer. *Lancet* 2:365–368.
Duffy, L. C., M. Riepenhoff-Talty, T. E. Byers, L. J. La Scolea, M. A. Zielezny, D. M. Dryja, and P. L. Ogra
1986 Modulation of rotavirus enteritis during breastfeeding. Implications on alterations in the intestinal bacterial flora. *American Journal of Diseases of Children* 140:1164–1168.
Edidin, D. V., L. L. Levitsky, W. Schey, N. Dumbovic, and A. Campos
1980 Resurgence of nutritional rickets associated with breastfeeding and special dietary practices. *Pediatrics* 65:232–235.
Fall, C. H., D. J. Barker, C. Osmond, P. D. Winter, P. M. Clark, and C. N. Hales
1992 Relation of infant feeding to adult serum cholesterol concentration and death from ischaemic heart disease. *British Medical Journal* 304:801–805.
Fallot, M. E., J. L. Boyd, III, and F. A. Oska
1980 Breastfeeding reduces incidence of hospital admission for infections in infants. *Pediatrics* 65:1121–1124.
Farquharson, J., F. Cockburn, W. A. Patrick, E. C. Jamieson, and R. W. Logan
1992 Infant cerebral cortex phospholipid fatty-acid composition and diet. *Lancet* 340:810–813.
Fredrickson, D. D., J. P. Sorenson, A. K. Biddle, and M. Kotelchuck
1993 Relationship of sudden infant death syndrome to breastfeeding duration and intensity. *American Journal of Diseases in Children* 147:460.
Freudenheim, J. L., J. R. Marshall, S. Graham, R. Laughlin, J. E. Vena, E. Bandera, P. Muti, M. Swanson, and T. Nemoto
1994 Exposure to breastmilk in infancy and the risk of breast cancer. *Epidemiology* 5(3):324–331.
Freundlich, M., G. Zilleruelo, C. Abitbol, J. Strauss, M. C. Faugere, and H. H. Malluche
1985 Infant formula as a cause of aluminum toxicity in neonatal uraemia. *Lancet* 2:527.

Goldblum, R. M., R. J. Schanler, C. Garza, and A. S. Goldman
1989 Human milk enhances the urinary excretion of immunologic factors in low birth weight infants. *Pediatric Research* 25:184–188.
Golding, J., M. Paterson, and L. J. Kinlen
1990 Factors associated with childhood cancer in a national cohort study. *British Journal of Cancer* 62:304–308.
Goldman, A. S., L. W. Thorpe, R. M. Goldblum, and L. A. Hanson
1986 Anti-inflammatory properties of human milk. *Acta Paediatrica Scandinavica* 75:689–695.
Greco, L., S. Auricchio, M. Mayer, and M. Grimaldi
1988 Case-control study on nutritional risk factors in celiac disease. *Journal of Pediatric Gastroenterology and Nutrition* 7:395–399.
György, P.
1960 The late effects of early nutrition. *American Journal of Clinical Nutrition* 8:344–345.
Haddock, R. L., J. N. Cousens, and C. C. Guzman
1991 Infant diet and salmonellosis. *American Journal of Public Health* 81:997–1000.
Hallman, M., K. Bry, K. Hoppu, M. Lappi, and M. Pohjavuori
1992 Inositol supplementation in premature infants with respiratory distress syndrome. *New England Journal of Medicine* 326(19):1233–1239.
Hambraeus, L.
1977 Proprietary milk versus human milk in infant feeding. *Pediatric Clinics of North America* 24:17–36.
Higginbottom, M. C., L. Sweetman, and N. L. Nyhan
1978 A syndrome of methylmalonic aciduria, homocystinuria, megaloblastic anemia and neurologic abnormalities in a vitamin B_{12}-deficient breastfed infant of a strict vegetarian. *New England Journal of Medicine* 299:317–323.
Hirota, T., M. Nara, M. Ohguri, E. Manago, and K. Hirota
1992 Effect of diet and lifestyle on bone mass in Asian young women. *American Journal of Clinical Nutrition* 55:1168–1173.
Ho, M. S., R. I. Glass, P. F. Pinsky, N. C. Young-Okoh, W. M. Sappenfield, J. W. Buehler, N. Gunter, and L. J. Anderson
1988 Diarrheal deaths in American children. *Journal of the American Medical Association* 260:3281–3285.
Hoefer, C., and M. C. Hardy
1929 Later development of breastfed and artificially fed infants. *Journal of the American Medical Association* 92:615–619.
Holmes, G. K., P. Prior, M. R. Lane, D. Pope, and R. N. Allan
1989 Malignancy in coeliac disease—effect of a gluten free diet. *Gut* 30:333–338.
Høst, A., S. Husby, and O. Østerballe
1988 A prospective study of cow's milk allergy in exclusively breastfed infants. *Acta Paediatrica Scandinavica* 77:663–670.
Infante-Rivard, C.
1993 Childhood asthma and indoor environmental risk factors. *American Journal of Epidemiology* 137:834–844.

Jarrett, E. E., and E. Hall
1986 Perinatal-maternal relationships in the regulation in IgE antibody responsiveness. *Journal of Allergy and Clinical Immunology* 78:1000–1003.
Jayanthi, V., C. S. J. Probert, and J. F. Mayberry
1991 Epidemiology of inflammatory bowel disease. *Quarterly Journal of Medicine* 78:5–12.
Jelliffe, D. B., and E. F. P. Jelliffe (eds.)
1978 Biochemical considerations. In *Human Milk in the Modern World*, pp. 26–58. Oxford: Oxford University Press.
Kaleita, T. A., M. Kinsbourne, and J. H. Menkes
1991 A neurobehavioral syndrome after failure to thrive on chloride-deficient formula. *Developmental Medicine and Child Neurology* 33:626–635.
Karjalainen, J., J. M. Martin, M. Knip, J. Ilonen, B. H. Robinson, E. Savilahti, H. K. Akerblom, and H. M. Dosch
1992 A bovine peptide as a possible trigger of insulin-dependent diabetes mellitus. *New England Journal of Medicine* 327:302–307.
Kato, H., O. Inoue, T. Kawasaki, H. Fujiwara, T. Watanabe, and H. Toshima
1992 Adult coronary artery disease due to childhood Kawasaki disease. *Lancet* 340:1127–1129.
Kawasaki, T., F. Kosaki, S. Okawa, I. Shigematsu, and H. Yanagawa
1974 A new infantile acute febrile mucocutaneous lymph node syndrome (MLNS) prevailing in Japan. *Pediatrics* 54:271–281.
Khoshoo, V., J. Kjarsgaard, B. Krafchick, and S. H. Zlotkin
1992 Zinc-deficiency in a full-term breastfed infant: Unusual presentation. *Pediatrics* 89:1094–1095.
Koletzko, S., P. Sherman, M. Corey, A. Griffiths, and C. Smith
1989 Role of infant feeding practices in development of Crohn's disease in childhood. *British Medical Journal* 298:1617–1618.
Kramer, M. S.
1988 Does breastfeeding help protect against atopic disease? *Journal of Pediatrics* 112:181–190.
Lederman, S. A.
1992 Estimating infant mortality from human immune deficiency virus and other causes in breastfeeding and bottle-feeding populations. *Pediatrics* 89:290–296.
Lindmann, R., and G. C. Christensen
1987 Radioactivity in breastmilk after the Chernobyl accident. *Acta Paediatrica Scandinavica* 1987:981–982.
Lucas, A.
1990 Does early diet program future outcome? *Acta Paediatrica Scandinavica* 365:58–67.
Lucas, A., and T. J. Cole
1990 Breast milk and necrotizing enterocolitis. *Lancet* 336:1519–1523.
Lucas, A., O. G. Brooke, R. Morley, T. J. Cole, and M. F. Bamford
1990 Early diet of preterm infants and development of allergic or atopic disease: Randomized prospective study. *British Medical Journal* 300:837–840.

Lucas, A., R. Morley, T. J. Cole, G. Lister, and C. Leeson-Payne
1992 Breast milk and subsequent intelligence quotient in children born preterm. *Lancet* 339:261–264.
Macedo, C. G.
1988 Infant mortality in the Americas. *PAHO Bulletin* 22:303–312.
Madeley, R. J., D. Hull, and T. Holland
1986 Prevention of postneonatal mortality. *Archives of Disease in Childhood* 61:459–463.
Mamunes, P., P. E. Prince, N. H. Thornton, P. A. Hunt, and E. S. Hitchcock
1976 Intellectual deficits after transient tyrosinemia in the term neonate. *Pediatrics* 57:675–680.
Mårild, S., U. Jodal, and L. Mangelus
1989 Medical histories of children with acute pyelonephritis compared with controls. *Pediatric Infectious Disease Journal* 8:511–515.
Marmot, M. G., C. M. Page, E. Atkins, and J. W. B. Douglas
1980 Effect of breastfeeding on plasma cholesterol and weight in young adults. *Journal of Epidemiology and Community Health* 34:164–167.
Mayer, E. J., R. F. Hamman, E. C. Gay, D. C. Lezotte, D. A. Savitz, and G. J. Klingensmith
1988 Reduced risk of IDDM among breastfed children. The Colorado IDDM Registry. *Diabetes* 37:1625–1632.
McCance, R. A.
1962 Food, growth, and time. *Lancet* 2:621–626.
McConnochie, K. M., and K. J. Roghmann
1986 Breastfeeding and maternal smoking as predictors of wheezing in children age 6 to 10 years. *Pediatric Pulmonology* 2:260–268.
McJunkin, J. E., W. G. Bithoney, and M. C. McCornick
1987 Errors in formula concentration in an out patient population. *Journal of Pediatrics* 111:848–850.
Miskelly, F. G., M. L. Burr, E. Vaughan-Williams, A. M. Fehily, B. K. Butland, and T. G. Merrett
1988 Infant feeding and allergy. *Archives of Disease in Childhood* 63:388–393.
Mitchell, E. A., R. Scragg, A. W. Stewart, D. M. Becroft, B. J. Taylor, R. P. Ford, I. B. Hassall, D. M. Barry, E. M. Allen, and A. P. Roberts
1991 Results from the first year of the New Zealand cot death study. *New Zealand Medical Journal* 104:71–76.
Mok, J. Y. Q., and H. Simpson
1982 Outcome of acute lower respiratory tract infection in infants: Preliminary report of seven-year follow-up study. *British Medical Journal* 285:333–337.
Morbidity Mortality Weekly Reports (MMWR)
1993 *Salmonella* serotype Tennessee in powdered milk products and infant formula. *Journal of the American Medical Association* 270:432.
Muytjens, H. L., and L. A. Kollee
1990 *Enterobacter sakazakii* meningitis in neonates: Causative role of formula? 'letter'. *Pediatric Infectious Disease Journal* 9:372–373.
Narayanan, I., K. Prakash, N. S. Murthy, and V. V. Gujral
1984 Randomized controlled trial of effect of raw and holder pasteurized

human milk and of formula supplements on incidence of neonatal infection. *Lancet* 2:1111–1113.

Osborn, G. R.

1968 Stages in development of coronary disease observed from 1500 young subjects. Relationship of hypotension and infant feeding to aetiology. *Colloque international sur le role de la paroi arterielle dan l'atherogenese*, pp. 93–129. Paris.

Pisacane, A., L. Graziano, and G. Zona

1990 Breastfeeding and urinary tract infection. *Lancet* 336:50.

Pisacane, A., W. Buffolano, G. Grillo, and C. Gaudiosi

1992a Infant feeding and Schönlein-Henoch purpura. *Acta Paediatrica Scandinavica* 81:630.

Pisacane, A., G. Grillo, M. Cafiero, C. Simeone, A. Coppola, B. Scarpellino, and G. Mazzarella

1992b Role of breastfeeding in paralytic poliomyelitis. *British Medical Journal* 305:1367.

Pisacane, A., N. Impagliazzo, M. Russo, R. Valiani, A. Mandarini, C. Florio, and P. Vivo

1994 Breastfeeding and multiple sclerosis. *British Medical Journal* 308:1411–1412.

Pittard, W. B., III

1979 Breast milk immunology. *American Journal of Diseases of Children* 133:83–87.

Prentice, A.

1987 Breastfeeding increases concentrations of IgA in infants' urine. *Archives of Disease of Childhood* 62:792–795.

Rodgers, B.

1978 Feeding in infancy and later ability and attainments: A longitudinal study. *Developmental Medicine and Child Neurology* 20:421–426.

Rogan, W. J.

1989 Cancer from PCBs in breast milk? A risk benefit analysis. *Pediatric Research* 25:105A.

Rogan, W. J., and B. C. Gladen

1993 Breastfeeding and cognitive development. *Early Human Development* 31:181–193.

Saarinen, U.

1982 Prolonged breastfeeding as prophylaxis for recurrent otitis media. *Acta Paediatrica Scandinavica* 71:567–571.

Schlesselman, J. J.

1982 *Case-Control Studies*, pp. 40–45. New York: Oxford University Press.

Shannon, M. W., and J. W. Graef

1992 Lead intoxication in infancy. *Pediatrics* 89:87–90.

Slonim, A. E., P. R. Borum, K. Tanaka, C. A. Stanley, A. G. Kasselberg, H. L. Greene, and I. M. Burr

1981 Dietary-dependent carnitine deficiency as a cause on non-ketotic hypoglycemia in an infant. *Journal of Pediatrics* 99:551–555.

Spector, W. S.

1956 *Handbook of Biological Data*, pp. 182–184. Philadelphia: W.B. Saunders.

Sturman, J. A., G. Y. Wen, H. M. Wisniewski, and M. D. Neuringe
1983 Retinal degeneration in primates raised on human infant formula. *Pediatric Research* 17:202A.
Tanner, M. S., A. H. Kantarjian, S. A. Bhave, and A. N. Pandit
1983 Early introduction of copper-contaminated milk as a possible cause of Indian childhood cirrhosis. *Lancet* 2:992.
Timmermans, F. J. W., and S. Gerson
1980 Chronic granulomatous otitis media in bottle-fed Inuit children. *Canadian Medical Association Journal* 122:545–547.
Uauy, R., E. Birch, D. Birch, and P. Peirano
1992 Visual and brain function measurements in studies in n-3 fatty acid requirements of infants. *Journal of Pediatrics* 120:S168–S180.
Udall, J. N., Jr., M. Dixon, and A. P. Newman
1985 Liver disease in alpha-1-antitrypsin deficiency. A retrospective analysis of early breast- vs. bottle-feeding. *Journal of the American Medical Association* 253:2679–2682.
Vahlquist, B.
1975 Evolution of breastfeeding in Europe. *Environmental Child Health* 21:11–18.
Venkataraman, P. S., R. C. Tsang, F. R. Greer, A. Noguchi, P. Laskarzewski, and J. J. Steichen
1985 Late infantile tetany and secondary hyperparathyroidism in infants fed humanized cow milk formula. Longitudinal follow up. *American Journal of Diseases of Children* 139:664–668.
Victora, C. G., P. G. Smith, J. P. Vaughan, L. C. Nobre, C. Lombardi, A. M. Teixeira, S. M. Fuchs, L. B. Moreira, L. P. Gigante, and F. C. Barros
1987 Evidence for protection by breastfeeding against infant deaths from infectious diseases in Brazil. *Lancet* 2:319–322.
Wegman, M. E.
1991 Annual summary of vital statistics-1990. *Pediatrics* 88:1081–1092.
Wilcox, D. T., A. B. Fiorello, and P. L. Glick
1993 Hypovolemic shock and intestinal ischemia: A preventable complication of incomplete formula labeling. *Journal of Pediatrics* 122:103–104.
Wood, C. B. S., and J. A. Walker-Smith
1981 *Mackeith's Infant Feeding and Feeding Difficulties*, 6th ed., p. 105. Edinburgh: Churchill Livingstone.

10

Breastfeeding and Infant–Parent Co-Sleeping as Adaptive Strategies: Are They Protective against SIDS?

James J. McKenna and Nicole J. Bernshaw

INTRODUCTION

Breastfeeding and infant–parent co-sleeping are part of the same adaptive complex designed by natural selection over millions of years of human evolution. Because human infants are born neurologically immature, develop slowly, and remain nonambulatory for a long period of time, continuous contact and proximity to mother served specifically to maximize the chances of infant survival and, hence, parental reproductive success (see Konner, 1981). Only in the last 100 to 200 years, and only in Western industrialized societies, have we come to think of breastfeeding and infant sleep location as two separate phenomena. From an evolutionary viewpoint, so entwined are the biology of infant sleep development and breastfeeding that any study of one that neglects its connection to the other must be considered incomplete, inaccurate, or both (Bernshaw, 1991a; McKenna, 1993).

While changing cultural forces have facilitated the scientific documentation of the benefits derived by infants (and mothers) from breastfeeding, those same forces have not yet encouraged scientists to explore the other half of this adaptive system—the potential physiological benefits to infants sleeping in proximity to their caregivers, especially in the first year of life.

This may be changing. During the past 10 years, several major epidemiological studies conducted on risk factors associated with the sudden infant death syndrome (SIDS, also referred to as cot death, or crib death) have shown that in some populations, *not* breastfeeding increased risk. Moreover, recent laboratory and anthropological research on infants sleeping apart and together (same bed) with the mother have raised the possibility that for some infants, sleeping with a parent may change the physiological experiences of the infant in ways helpful in resisting a SIDS event. In situations where mothers breastfeed, do not smoke, and keep their infants next to them for nocturnal sleep, SIDS death rates appear to be extremely low (see Balarajan, Raleigh and Botting, 1989; Gantley, Davies and Murcott, 1993; Takeda, 1987).

This is not to suggest that the practices of breastfeeding and co-sleeping can eliminate SIDS. The circumstances within which SIDS occurs, and the clinical histories of SIDS victims, are much too diverse for any single explanation to apply to all cases, or for one preventive strategy to work for all infants. However, the extent to which SIDS rates covary across cultures with rates of breastfeeding and co-sleeping is important and raises important questions. For example, in societies where co-sleeping is the norm and SIDS rates are low, do parents have a different understanding of infant needs, including when infants should "sleep through the night"? How do mothers interpret their own sleep patterns while co-sleeping? Coupled with recent research on the physiological effects of co-sleeping (see Mosko et al., n.d.; McKenna and Mosko, 1993), and the dramatic reduction in SIDS rates in England and New Zealand following public health campaigns recommending that infants be placed in the supine position (on their back) for sleep rather than in the prone position (on their stomach), the idea that other child care practices could also affect SIDS rates assumes more credibility.

This chapter reviews what is known about SIDS and, more specifically, the epidemiological studies that suggest that breastfeeding may be protective against the condition. Laboratory-based research on social and solitary sleeping infants is also reviewed. These data show how breastfeeding and infant–parent co-sleeping can be considered an integrated adaptive complex changing the physiological status of the sleeping infant in potentially beneficial ways.

WHAT IS SIDS?

Responding to the increasing need for more in-depth, on-the-scene environmental data and family history as part of the pathologist's criteria for a SIDS diagnosis, the National Institutes of Child Health and Human Development recently modified the definition of SIDS to read as follows: "The sudden death of an infant under one year of age that remains unexplained after a thorough case investigation, including performance of a complete autopsy, examination of the death scene, and a review of the clinical history" (Willinger, 1989:73). In brief, "SIDS" is diagnosed when everything else has been excluded. It remains a "protean" (catch-all) category into which all unexplained infant deaths fall. It is a "diagnosis by exclusion," which, in reality, is no diagnosis at all. It remains, after 30 years of intensive national and international research, and the expenditure of millions of dollars of research money, a human malady for which current research paradigms have proven inadequate.

CAN INFANTS AT RISK FOR SIDS BE IDENTIFIED?

No single, consistent criterion or pathological marker can be used to either predict potential SIDS victims or identify them upon postmortem autopsy. What we do know is that SIDS research, both epidemiological and in the laboratory, continues to suggest a multifactorial origin for the syndrome and to find an impressive amount of heterogeneity among SIDS victims (see Hoffman, Damus, Hillman and Krongrad, 1988). Table 10.1 summarizes the most important SIDS research findings through 1993, some of which will be discussed in more detail below. Comprehensive reviews of all aspects of SIDS research can be found in Bergman (1986), who reports on the history of SIDS research in the United States, in Golding, Limerick and MacFarlane (1985), Guntheroth (1989), McKenna (1986), Schwartz, Southall and Valdes-Dapena (1988), and Valdes-Dapena (1980a, b, 1988). As Table 10.1 illustrates, one of the most frustrating aspects of SIDS research continues to be the inability of researchers to replicate each other's findings.

In a major epidemiological study conducted in the United States (see Hoffman et al., 1988), about 90% of SIDS victims were less than 24 weeks old. Most SIDS victims generally had low birth weights (less than 2500 g), experienced slower overall (postnatal) growth rates than controls, and were more frequently born to unmarried and poor women, women who smoked during their pregnancies, and women who were less than 20 years of age. This is true especially in Western industrialized countries. In one study, "the reported incidence of SIDS in the population of low socioeconomic status served by the Kings County Hospital Center is 4.2 per 1000 live births, which is about 10 times higher than that of the more affluent areas of New York City" (see Bass, Kravath and Glass, 1986). Interestingly, when only maternal risk factors were analyzed, socioeconomic and behavioral factors, rather than maternal medical or health factors, were more significant predictors of SIDS risks (Hoffman

Table 10.1. Suspected or Implicated Causes of Suddent Infant Death Syndrome[a]

Observed Abnormality or Condition	*Investigators (Selected Studies)*	*Additional Studies or Critiques*
Neurological, Neurochemical, Respiratory, or Sleep Dysfunction		
Decrease in maturation of quiet sleep	Gould et al. 1988	
Premature maturation of sleep and arousal mechanisms	Sterman and Hodgman 1988	
Hypoxia or hypoxemia	Steinschneider 1972 Naeye 1974, 1976, 1980 Guntheroth 1982, 1983a Kelly 1983	Singer 1984 Tildon et al. 1983 Merritt and Valdes-Dapena 1984 Beckwith 1988
Protracted periods of apnea or increased breathing pauses	Steinschneider 1972 Guilleminault et al. 1975 Guilleminault, Tilkian and Dement 1976 Guilleminault, Souquet et al. 1976 Guntheroth 1982, 1983a Read and Jeffrey 1983 Kelly et al. 1980 Naeye 1974, 1980	Weinstein et al. 1983 Peterson 1983 Bagg et al. 1981 Hodgman et al. 1982 Hodgman and Hoppenbrouwers 1983 Southall et al. 1985 Hoffman et al. 1988 Beckwith 1988 Schwartz 1987 Southall and Talbert 1988 Southall et al. 1982
Deficiency of arousal response to increased CO_2 (hypercapnia) and decreased CO_2	Hunt et al. 1981 Sullivan 1984	Ariagno et al. 1980
Deficiency of arousal system; abnormal arousal levels in brain stem	Guilleminault, Ariagno, Forno et al. 1979 Guntheroth 1977, 1982, 1983a Guilleminault, Ariagno, Korobkin et al. 1979 Harper et al. 1981 Hunt et al. 1981 McCulloch et al. 1982 McGinty 1984	Guilleminault and Coons 1983

(continued)

Table 10.1. (Continued)

Observed Abnormality or Condition	*Investigators (Selected Studies)*	*Additional Studies or Critiques*
Petechiae (broken blood vessels) on surface of lungs and general interthoracic vegim caused by central apnea	Guntheroth 1983b	Tildon et al. 1983
Intrathoracic petechiae owing to upper respiratory obstruction	Beckwith 1988 Werne and Garrow 1953	
Respiratory vulnerability during REM sleep	Henderson-Smart and Read 1978 Phillipson 1978	Johnson et al. 1983 Orr et al. 1985
Small, constricted, thickened pulmonary arterioles; increased muscle mass	Naeye 1973 Mason et al. 1975 Williams et al. 1979	Beckwith 1983 Singer 1984
Inability to maintain homeostasis during the developmental period wherein NREM sleep is prolonged and predominates	Gould 1983 Salk et al. 1974	
Respiratory muscle failure owing to muscular immaturity or respiratory paralysis	Jansen and Chernick 1983 Stanton 1984	Beckwith 1988
Overcompliant lung or defective surfactant	Southall et al. 1985 Southall and Talbert 1988	
Leukomalacia or cerebral white matter lesions caused by hypoxemia and inadequate blood circulation to brain (ischemia)	Takashima, Armstrong, and Becker 1978	Beckwith 1983 Haddad and Mellins 1983 Pearson and Brandeis 1983

(continued)

Table 10.1. (Continued)

Observed Abnormality or Condition	Investigators (Selected Studies)	Additional Studies or Critiques
Neck-Throat Abnormalities		
Hypertrophy of laryngeal mucous glands or increased number of mucous glands	Fink and Beckwith 1980 Haddad et al. 1980, 1981	
Hypermobility of mandible causing suffocation, pharyngeal upper airway collapse, or occlusion exacerbated by smaller upper airway	Tonkin 1974, 1975, 1983 Colton and Steinschneider 1980 Thach 1983 Sullivan 1984 Guilleminault et al. 1975 Guilleminault et al. 1986	Guntheroth 1982, 1983a
Elongated uvula	Harpey and Renault 1984	Guilleminault 1984 Guilleminault et al. 1986
Cardiac Abnormalities		
Right ventricular hypertrophy (enlarged right ventricle), indicating hypoxia	Naeye 1973	Beckwith 1983 Williams et al. 1979 Valdes-Dapena 1980a
Prolonged QT interval (time between ventricular contraction and relaxation)	Schwartz 1983, 1987 Southall et al. 1982 Froggatt and James 1973 Verrier and Kirby 1988	Kukolich et al. 1977 Steinschneider 1978 Haddad et al. 1979 Guntheroth 1982
Cardiac and autonomic inactivity leading to arrhythmias	Church et al. 1967	Gunteroth 1983a
Lethal arrhythmias	Schwartz 1976	
Lack of maturational synchrony in right and left sympathetic nerves, leading to increased heart rate	Schwartz 1983	

(continued)

Table 10.1. (Continued)

Observed Abnormality or Condition	*Investigators (Selected Studies)*	*Additional Studies or Critiques*
Lack of breast-feeding and contact with mother during night; co-sleeping, microenvironment	McKenna 1986 Konner and Super 1987 Hoffman et al. 1988 Sears 1985 Maxwell and Maxwell 1979 Davies 1985 Lee et al. 1989 Damus et al. 1988	Cunningham 1976 Beckwith 1979
Overheating	Fleming et al. 1990 Nelson et al. 1989 Stanton 1984	
Carbon monoxide poisoning	Cleary 1984	
Infant botulism *(Clostridium botulinum)*	Arnon 1983 Sonnabend et al. 1985 Cornblath and Schwartz 1976	Cunningham 1976 Valdes-Dapena and Felipe 1971
Sleeping position (prone)	Nelson et al. 1989	Beal 1988 Emery 1988 Brennan et al. 1988
Risks from Diptheria-Tetanus-Pertussis vaccine	Bernier et al. 1982	Griffin et al. 1988 Hoffman et al. 1988
Suffocation in water beds	Bass 1988 Ramanthan et al. 1988	Filardo 1988
Startle disease (hyperplexia)	Vigevano et al. 1989 Kaada 1986 Franciosi 1987	
Suffocation owing to co-sleeping	Luke 1978 Thach et al. 1988 Bass et al. 1986	
Breath-holding or fear, paralysis reflex	Southall, Talbert, Johnson et al. 1985 Kaada 1986	
Intrauterine perturbations	Hoffman et al. 1988	

[a] Adapted from McKenna and Mosko (1990). References cited in this table appear in References to Table 10.1 following the text references.

et al., 1988). Postnatal risk factors in a small population of SIDS victims included mothers' reports that prior to their deaths their infants experienced a "stop breathing episode" or turned blue, an "apparent life threatening event" (ALTE). About 7% of ALTE infants have died of SIDS (Willinger, 1989). Most frequently, these especially prolonged apnea episodes occurred when the infant was awake. Mixed apneas continued to be associated with some infants before their deaths from SIDS, but more frequently apneic periods were markers for low-birth-weight infants. Apnea proved not to be a specific risk factor for SIDS (McKenna and Mosko, 1990), although the inability to arouse during apnea to reinitiate breathing, which is controlled by a different set of neurological structures, may be a significant SIDS risk factor, as we will discuss later.

A significant number of infants who died of SIDS had bouts with diarrhea and/or vomiting and colds within 2 weeks of death. They also experienced droopiness and listlessness during the last 24 hours, as well as increased irritability, respiratory distress, and tachycardia (rapid heartbeat) (Hoffman et al., 1988). According to the investigators, all of these factors acted in "secondary fashion" rather than as primary or causal agents. About 18% of all SIDS deaths involve premature infants, while as few as 10% of all SIDS victims had any symptoms associated with a potential SIDS event before their deaths (Ariagno and Glotzbach, 1991).

Some SIDS victims may differ from surviving healthy babies not so much in kind but in degree. It is suspected that many SIDS infants suffered from subtle deficits that developed during intrauterine life and were not apparent in the neonate. Researchers believe that the actual expression of the fatal deficit is likely to be influenced by, if not dependent on, a number of cofactors that converge at a vulnerable moment in the infant's life. As of the present, however, many of these cofactors remain unknown.

BREASTFEEDING AS PROTECTION AGAINST SIDS

Several studies indicate that breastfeeding does not guarantee protection from SIDS, only reduced risk (Hoffman et al., 1988; Mitchell, Scragg, Stewart, Becroft, Taylor, Ford, Hassall, Barry, Allen and Roberts, 1991), and the protective effect is not universally established. But calculating the relationship between breastfeeding practices and SIDS risks has been problematic because epidemiological studies do not differentiate between the various *forms* that breastfeeding can take. That is, epidemiological studies note simply the presence or absence of breastfeeding at the time of the infant's death, making comparisons between studies difficult, and a complete understanding of the relationship between SIDS risks and breastfeeding less precise. It could be, for example, that SIDS risk decreases the more an infant breastfeeds. In other words, the degree of increased protection may be dose-specific.

In an effort to increase exactitude and comparability in research on breastfeeding worldwide, an ad hoc group called the Interagency Group for Action on Breastfeeding (IGAB) worked out clearer definitions for breastfeeding patterns (see Labbok and Krasovec, 1990). They divide breastfeeding into categories: full, partial, and token breastfeeding. They further subdivide full breastfeeding into exclusive and almost exclusive breastfeeding, and partial breastfeeding into high, medium, and low. Each category and subcategory is specifically defined. If every researcher precisely defines breastfeeding using this schema, comparisons and meta-analyses would be improved and conclusions about the protective role of breastfeeding might be strengthened.

Over a decade ago, for example, Arnon reviewed studies performed mostly in Western countries that reported SIDS incidences (see Arnon, 1983). Although all studies agreed that the incidence of SIDS was highest in the same social strata where use of artificial baby milks was highest, they did not agree on the rate of occurrence of breastfeeding, which ranged from 61 to 97%. These discrepancies were attributed to differences in study design, and to the absence of standard definitions for breastfeeding. A similar lack of standardization was observed in a recent much publicized New Zealand study (see Mitchell et al., 1991). It could well be that details of the protective role of breastfeeding in future population studies will become more clear as dose–response definitions for breastfeeding are used, and recruitment strategies are followed that will ensure adequate sampling of populations with low breastfeeding rates.

To date, only one study of the link between breastfeeding and SIDS has used dose–response definitions and appropriate recruitment strategies. Fredrickson, Sorenson, Biddle and Kotelchuck (1993) utilized data from the National Maternal and Infant Health Survey of 10,000 births and 6000 deaths of babies born during 1988–1989. Their final sample included 7102 controls, 499 SIDS deaths, and 584 non-SIDS deaths. Their analysis used a consistent dosage-definition of breastfeeding and controlled for major confounders (birth weight, maternal age/race/education/postnatal smoking/prenatal cocaine use/lack of private insurance, household smoking, day care, and household size). They found that "the risk of SIDS for black infants increased by 1.19 for every month of not breastfeeding, and 2.13 for every month of not exclusively breastfeeding. Among white infants, the risk increased by 1.19 and 2.0 times, respectively. These associations remained even when deaths within the first month of life were excluded. A similar protective association existed also for non-SIDS deaths" (Fredrickson et al., 1993:460).

SIDS, INFANT BOTULISM, AND IMMUNITY

Infant botulism is an infectious disease that, according to Arnon (1983), can sometimes masquerade as SIDS. It results when the ingested spores of the bacterium *Clostridium botulinum* germinate, multiply, and produce their toxin in the baby's intestine (see Arnon, 1983:539). The toxin, one of the most potent poisons known, can be carried anteriorly to motor nerve endings, causing irreversible respiratory muscle paralysis and death, strikingly resembling SIDS deaths. The age distribution of infant botulism also matches closely that of SIDS. It is estimated that 5% of SIDS cases may be attributed to infant botulism (Arnon, 1984).

With regard to the immunological benefits, it may be noted that SIDS rates peak at between 2 and 4 months postpartum (90% of all SIDS deaths occur before 6 months) supposedly when maternal antibodies, abundant in the first and second months of life, are declining, "generally reaching the lowest level at three months of age before the infant builds up its own immunoglobulin to achieve immunological independence" (Huang, 1983:593; see also Arnon, 1983). Such a statement can be misleading, however. It has been shown, indeed over two decades ago, that the *concentration* of IgA decreases rapidly after birth (17 mg/ml in initial colostrum, 4.1 mg/ml in 2- to 4-day colostrum, 1.8 mg/ml in milk from 2 to 20 weeks) (Mata and Wyatt, 1971). These figures take an entirely different meaning when we take into account the volume of milk that exclusively breastfed babies ingest daily (between 7 and 137 ml colostrum on day 1, 500 ml on day 5, 750 ml at 3 to 5 months) (Riordan and Auerbach, 1993). Multiplying the IgA concentration by the volume of ingested milk per day yields a relatively constant intake of 1500 to 2000 mg IgA/day, reinforcing the concept of a protective role of breastfeeding through immunity. The same concentration/volume phenomenon has been shown recently in the investigation of gliadin-specific and cow's milk-specific IgA in human milk (Juto and Holm, 1992).

A more plausible explanation for the protective role of breastfeeding in infant botulism may depend in part on "the presence, the specificity, and the titer of the antibodies in human milk" (see Arnon, 1984). Human milk contains secretory A (S-IgA) antibody that can specifically agglutinate vegetative cells of C. botulinum. However, "not every woman's milk contained S-IgA against all strains of *C. botulinum* tested, and among those whose milk had agglutinating antibody, substantial variations in titers of antibody against a given strain was found" (Arnon, 1984:549). These variations in titers (or concentrations) of S-IgA would be due to the "mucosal immune system" (Arnon, 1984), also called the "enteromammary immune system" (Arnon, 1983). Briefly, lymphocytes in maternal gut-associated lymphoid tissue become sensitized to *indigenous* antigens, and migrate to the breast where they produce antigen-specific S-IgA as early as 3 days after the mother's ingestion of the antigen. Therefore, the mother's sensitization to a specific strain is only one component of the protection. Assuming the specific sensitization has occurred, the level of protection conferred to her infant is then a matter of degree: the higher the titer of S-IgA in her milk, the greater the protection, and vice versa.

The toxicity of the botulism toxin is so great that it is estimated that as few as 10 to 100 spores may be sufficient to infect an infant (Arnon, 1986). This, together with variable IgA titers in milk, make it conceivable that a single exposure to a foreign antigen (e.g., a drop of *Clostridium*-containing honey) could seriously compromise the health of infants breastfed to various degrees. The relative protective property of human milk against sudden death from infant botulism is illustrated by the fact that "all 10 SIDS positive at autopsy for *C. botulinum* occurred in infants who had been formula-fed, whereas 50 hospitalized patients were primarily (but not exclusively—author's emphasis) breast-fed" (Arnon, 1984). This deserves emphasis: all dead infants were artificially fed; all surviving infants were breastfed. It follows that if "botulism can be prevented by proper handling of food and utensils and avoidance of foods implicated in harboring spores," breastfeeding is the easiest, cheapest, and most effective way to do so (Bernshaw, 1991b). It also emphasizes the importance of exclusive breastfeeding that precludes exposure of the infant to any food potentially containing *C. botulinum* spores or the botulism toxin.

Other factors relating to some components of human milk have been implicated in theories on SIDS. For example, ß-casomorphins are short opiate-like acting peptide fragments that result from the digestion of the milk protein casein. It has been proposed (Ramabadran and Bansinath, 1988) that this small peptide would cross the blood–brain barrier where it would exert depressing effects on respiration and autonomic nervous system of susceptible infants. Although ß-casomorphins have been isolated from human milk, breastfeeding makes sense in the light of the fact that casein accounts for 80% of the total protein in cows' milk-based infant artificial milks as opposed to 30% in human milk (Kunz and Lönnerdal, 1989).

CO-SLEEPING, INFANT SLEEPING POSITION, AND BREASTFEEDING

From current data, it is not possible to disentangle the individual roles of breastfeeding and co-sleeping in SIDS rates. However, it is interesting that in countries where co-sleeping occurs as a favored and elected child care pattern, the rates of SIDS are the lowest in the world and dramatically lower than in Western industrialized countries. For example, in Japan, where co-sleeping and breastfeeding continue to be the norm (see Takeda, 1987), current published rates for SIDS are 0.15/1000 births in Tokyo, 1978, 0.053/1000 in Fukuoka, 1986, and 0.22/1000 births in Saga (Tasaki, Yamashita and Miyazaki, 1988). These findings do not, in themselves, prove that either co-sleeping or breastfeeding is protective against SIDS. It may well be that SIDS is underreported in Japan, or that it is misdiagnosed as infantile suffocation. Japanese medical scientists have not participated in international SIDS research studies to the extent that American and European scientists have, so the postmortem procedures they employ to identify SIDS may not be comparable to Western standards. Nevertheless, these low SIDS rates deserve explanation and further research.

In 1985, Davies reported a very low incidence of 0.036 per 1000 live births in Hong Kong (see Davies, 1985). Davies speculated that crowded living conditions and the practice of placing babies supine in their cot could contribute. The author asked "whether the possible influences of lifestyle and caretaking practices in cot death are being underestimated in preference for more exotic and esoteric explanations" (Davies, 1985:1348). This viewpoint is shared by Taylor and Emery (1988) and Emery (1983), who also implicate the importance of caregiving environments and other behavioral–socioeconomic factors. The fact that multiple cofactors are involved in understanding the ultimate "causes" of SIDS, and hence its prevention, is made abundantly clear by the fact that while co-sleeping is the norm among city-dwelling Hong Kong Chinese, breastfeeding is not. Out of 175 infants at 2, 4, and 6 months of age, the percentage of infants nursing was 9, 4, and 2%, respectively. Clearly, neither breastfeeding alone nor breastfeeding with co-sleeping is necessarily the most important SIDS cofactor for all populations.

Using postmortem diagnostic protocols that were judged by John Emery, a renowned SIDS researcher from Great Britain, to be comparative to Western diagnostic standards Lee, Chan, Davies, Lau and Yip (1989) confirmed the low incidence of SIDS in Hong Kong, although they found an incidence higher (0.3 per 1000 births) than previously reported. Commenting that "the syndrome did not seem so influenced by social deprivation as in many Western countries," they speculated that "greater environmental stimulation arising from crowded living conditions and a tradition of using a supine sleeping posture" might play a role (Lee et al., 1989:721).

The two studies above share one factor with the practice of breastfeeding: frequent physical closeness. The crowded living conditions in Hong Kong appear not to allow an infant to remain alone, a situation that is comparable to that of breastfed infants. This argument is even clearer if breastfeeding rates in Hong Kong are as low as the works of Davies and Lee claim: one key to the SIDS enigma may be that the protective role of breastfeeding resides in the frequent contact between the infant and its mother initiated by the need for frequent feedings. Its link with sleeping positions is explored below.

Much attention has been devoted to the relationship between SIDS and sleeping position. The two studies above are but a small sample of the work published about this concern (see Guntheroth and Spiers, 1992 for review). A more recent epidemiological study conducted in New Zealand identified and pointed out that infants sleeping in the prone position were at significantly higher risk for SIDS (Mitchell et al., 1991), although sleeping position was not the only significant factor.

Comparing ethnic differences in sleeping position and in the risks for SIDS reveals a lower SIDS rate in Asian babies born to Asian mothers in the Indian subcontinent where the supine position is favored as well as co-sleeping (see Farooqi, Perry and Beevers, 1991). This risk has been shown to increase when Asian mothers born in the U.K. adopted the "Western ways" of placing the baby in the prone position. The authors conclude, "It would be tragic if adoption of "Western ways" promoted by health care professionals were to place babies born in the Asian community in Britain at higher risk of SIDS" (Farooqi, 1991:1455).

PRONE VS. SUPINE SLEEP POSITION AND SIDS: RECENT RECOMMENDATIONS

The connection between breastfeeding and the prone sleeping position is far from clear, and a study of baby sleeping position when breastfed babies sleep with their mothers might shed some light on this point. In the United States in 1992 the American Academy of Pediatrics reluctantly, and only following intense international pressure from SIDS researchers around the world, recommended that American babies should be placed on their backs for sleep. The committee established to investigate the issue was reluctant to change the long-standing recommendation for infants to be placed in the prone position because, as of the present, there are no U.S. data suggesting that SIDS risks would be reduced by a change in the infant's sleep position. Yet, following public campaigns recommending that parents place their infants on their backs for sleep, SIDS rates have dropped dramatically in Great Britain, Ireland, Scandinavia, Tasmania, and New Zealand. Indeed, sometimes these decreases in the number of SIDS deaths were as much as one-half the annual rate (see Guntheroth and Spiers, 1992)! As of the present, large-scale systematic research on whether this change in recommendations has affected SIDS rates in the United States is just getting under way, as requests for grant proposals sponsored by the National Institutes of Health have just been promulgated.

Interestingly, if one considers that infant–parent co-sleeping and breastfeeding are the biologically more stable experiences for both mothers and infants, it is very clear that the supine (back, and not prone) position is the logical position for infants to assume while sleeping at night. It is difficult, if not impossible, for infants to nurse on their stomachs while lying next to their mothers. McKenna and Mosko's on-going studies of co-sleeping mother–infant pairs reveal quite dramatically that while co-sleeping (and breastfeeding), mothers consistently place their infants on their backs to lie next to them. But when some of these same mothers placed their infants "down" to sleep during the experimental night (when they slept in separate rooms), some of these mothers placed their infants on their stomachs. The researchers presume, though they did not ask, that the mothers do so because of the presumed "soothing effects" derived from the infants lying ventrally against the mattress, clinging to it—a soothing effect that in the co-sleeping context is provided by the mother's presence. In this way, it is clear that co-sleeping and breastfeeding directly mediate other SIDS risk factors as, for example, infant sleep position. Perhaps this behaviorally preferred co-sleeping position (i.e., the stomach or supine position also found among the Asian infants who die less frequently from SIDS), confers other heretofore undefined protective benefits, as the European SIDS epidemiological data suggest. However, more research is needed.

SLEEP MATURATION, CO-SLEEPING, AND BREASTFEEDING

The sleep–wake patterns of infants have been a matter of much research and a concern of parents for many years. The norms in infant sleep were developed in the 1950s and 1960s when breastfeeding rates were at their lowest in the United States. Parents have come to expect their infants to "sleep through the night" at a very young age and can get plenty of advice from experts both in the professional (see Pinilla and Birch, 1993) and lay (Brody, 1986) literature on how to "train" their infants to sleep to meet their expectations. Indeed, "sleeping through the night" and the ability of infants to soothe themselves back to sleep without parental intervention are considered major developmental milestones and signs of infant maturity, at least in cultures that define solitary sleeping infants as "normal."

During the early weeks, the type of sleep (called REM sleep) of infants is characterized by rapid eye movement, body movements, rapid and irregular cardiac and respiratory rates, and absent antigravity muscle tone. At 2 to 3 months of age, REM sleep gives way to a dramatic increase in quiet sleep time with brain waves that begin to resemble adult patterns. This period of sleep maturation coincides with the peak occurrence of SIDS (Gould, 1983).

It has been known for some time that both adults (Guilleminault, Eldridge and Dement, 1973) and infants terminate apneas by awakening or arousing to reinitiate breathing. Awakening (i.e., arousal) is a defensive response and has been described as a "stimulus for breathing" (Hoppenbrouwers and Hodgman, 1986). Though definitions vary, apneas refer to delays between breaths. If an infant's arousal mechanisms are immature, or somehow inefficient in awakening the infant during a respiratory crisis, that infant could be in danger. It has been hypothesized that some SIDS victims may exhibit some kind of arousal deficiency (Harper, Leake, Hoffman, Walter, Hoppenbrouwers, Hodgman and Sterman, 1981). Breastfed infants usually awaken more frequently to feed than do bottle-fed infants (Elias, Nicholson, Bora and Johnston, 1986). Their sleep–wake patterns have been shown to be dependent on the frequency of breastfeeding and sleep arrangement (i.e., whether sleeping alone or with a parent): breastfed infants slept in shorter bouts than the weaned infants and slept less overall; infants sleeping with their mothers slept in shorter bouts than those who slept alone; infants who both breastfed and shared beds with their mothers slept in shorter bouts and less overall; those who neither nursed nor shared beds slept longest; sharing the same bed but not breastfeeding rarely occurred (Elias et al., 1986) (in stark contrast to the situation in Hong Kong described by Davies, 1985). Since breastfed infants awaken more frequently, the risk for these infants of spending too much time in deep quiet stages of sleep is reduced. McKenna and Mosko's (1993) preliminary research on solitary and co-sleeping healthy 3 month olds raises this issue as a possibility. Their preliminary study showed that, on average, solitary sleeping infants spent more time in deep states of sleep (about 7 to 12% of their total sleep time) than they did on the nights they slept in their mothers' bed (see also McKenna, Thoman, Anders, Sadeh, Schechtman and Glotzbach, 1993; and Mosko, McKenna, Dickel and Hunt, 1993).

The fact that some SIDS victims may have had an arousal deficiency before they died lends support to this speculation. For example, a recent study showed that in a sample of 24 victims, the behavior with the greatest predictive probability for SIDS was the degree of difficulty these infants exhibited in awakening (Einspieler,Widder, Holzer and Kenner, 1988). Similarly, Hoppenbrouwers, Hodgman, Kazuko and Sterman (1989) compared the sleep patterns of subsequent siblings of SIDS victims with infants of a control group. Although they found that similarities between the two study groups "outweighed" the differences, the siblings of SIDS victims tended to awaken less frequently and, once asleep, "exhibited a higher probability of remaining asleep than the controls" (1989:269).

Reaction by infants to isolation has been referred to as "maternal deprivation syndrome," a state resembling depression. In describing Rene Spitz's study of institutionalized London orphans, Guntheroth (1989:109) points out that maternal deprivation syndrome can develop in infants despite favorable physical conditions such as "excellent nutrition, impeccable sanitary conditions, good health care, and the absence of overt abuse . . . 37% of orphans confined in one institution under such regimen died before reaching their first birthday!" Co-sleeping may be the path of least resistance for a breastfeeding mother, interrupting her sleep to a minimum while providing for her infant's needs. The obvious need for frequent feedings determined by the dilute nature of human milk may mask the more subtle (yet important) need of the infant for close contact. The sensory stimulation during co-sleeping could potentially increase numbers of arousals, interrupting prolonged nocturnal sleep bouts of both the infant and the mother (Konner, 1981; Short, 1984). This pattern of interrupted sleep, we argue later, is more compatible with the infant's evolutionary past (McKenna, Mosko, Dungy and McAninch, 1990; McKenna and Mosko, 1990).

It was pointed out earlier that in the United States, where present SIDS rates are about 1.5 per 1000 live births, many SIDS victims had low birth weights, experienced slower overall postnatal growth rates than controls, and were more frequently born to unmarried and poor women who smoked during their pregnancies and who were less than 20 years of age. Let us compare these conditions with those in Hong Kong (0.4 per 1000 live births) where "there is greater social stability than in many western countries, with fewer very young marriages and unwanted babies and a strong supporting extended family. Smoking in mothers is uncommon and the overall standard of antenatal and infant care is excellent" (Davies, 1985:1347). These observations indicate that the social environment is critical in the well-being of both the infant and the mother. Although the infant may not be conscious of the mother's destitute living conditions, breastfeeding may make the difference between thriving and not thriving. However, the state of mind and the attitudes of the mother toward breastfeeding should be considered because of the emotional involvement linked to the practice of breastfeeding. It is speculated that an unhappy or depressed mother, such as an unmarried mother with an unwanted pregnancy, may unconsciously find it difficult to nurture her baby in a loving manner, and this may preclude breastfeeding (see Guntheroth, 1989). We suggest that breastfeeding is the "support system" to the infant as the extended family and adequate health care are the support system to the mother.

CO-SLEEPING FROM AN EVOLUTIONARY STANDPOINT

Although the findings that some SIDS victims may have difficulty arousing are not new (see Guntheroth, 1989; Harper et al., 1981; McGinty, 1984), until recently there has been no theoretical context within which this issue could be analyzed further. Nor have there been any behavioral mechanisms known that might contribute to our understanding of how infantile constitutional deficits involving arousal might be affected by the infants' microenvironment, either to increase or decrease the role of arousal in some SIDS pathologies.

From an anthropological perspective that incorporates both cross-cultural and evolutionary data, it is particularly significant that no physiological studies of parent–infant co-sleeping exist outside of our lab's published reports (see McKenna and Mosko, 1990). Without question, co-sleeping is an evolutionarily ancient arrangement. Co-sleeping is the "environment of adaptedness," to use Bowlby's (1969) description, within which the human infant's nocturnal feeding, sleeping, breathing, and arousal patterns evolved. Infant sleep patterns, and the neurophysiological patterns that underlie them, coevolved under conditions of a high degree of dependence on the caregiver, including low levels of fat and protein in human breast milk, infantile neurological immaturity at birth, and slow postnatal growth. All of these characteristics necessitated constant physical contact with a caregiver, especially while the infant was sleeping. Far from being a speculation, this statement emerges from studies of our closest living relatives, the nonhuman primates (see Anderson, 1984), from cross-cultural studies of nonindustrialized peoples who continue to sleep with their children (Konner, 1981 for review), and from recent archaeological and paleontological models of hominid evolution (Lancaster and Lancaster, 1982).

Even though the absence of co-sleeping data in the context of SIDS research represents a serious gap in existing knowledge, the issue has only recently been raised. Especially in urban, Western, industrialized societies, parent–infant co-sleeping is not conceptualized as being either natural or even desirable (see Lozoff, Wolf and Davis, 1984). Co-sleeping is ordinarily discussed in the context of its potential for spoiling or endangering the infant, or for causing parent–child sleep struggles (see Schacter, Fuchs, Bijur and Stone, 1989). Overlying is the most common concern raised to discourage co-sleeping, despite the fact that as mammals, our species most certainly would not be here today had co-sleeping ever been dangerous or maladaptive for infants, although this does not, of course, preclude the possibility under unusual or unsafe conditions.

A death-scene investigation (independent of other agencies) has revealed maternal factors such as "drug abuse, seizure disorder, obesity, and extreme fatigue" as the cause of death of some diagnosed SIDS victims (Bass et al., 1986). Nevertheless, while no sleep environment is risk-free, the dangers of overlying are exaggerated. Fear of jeopardizing the primacy of the conjugal (husband-wife) bond, of violating concepts of parental sexual privacy (Spock and Rothenberg, 1985), of promoting incest or parental sexual arousal (Ferber, 1985), and of violating popular United States values of infant independence (Brazelton, Koslowski and Main, 1974) are all factors negatively influencing the opinions of both medical and lay communities concerning parent–infant co-sleeping.

Given our cultural context, it is not surprising that normative data on the development of infant sleep behavior are derived exclusively from studies of infants sleeping alone, either in sleep laboratories or at home in their cribs (see Anders, 1979). Together with the experiences of the Western urban middle-class, who are discouraged from sleeping with their infants (see Lozoff et al., 1984), these data have given rise to a conceptualization of infant sleep that may be at odds with the more universal and ancient human (species-specific) pattern.

Ethnographic data from preindustrial societies in which parent–infant co-sleeping and breastfeeding are the norm suggest that among infants less than 1 year old, the development of long periods of consolidated sleep with minimal numbers of arousals is unusual. Super and Harkness (1982) monitored 10 Kipsigis infants living in the Kenyan highlands who regularly slept with their mothers and were breastfed, and found major differences in sleep patterns when compared with those of typical middle-class U.S. infants. For example, while American babies increase their longest sleep episode from 4 to about 8 hours during the first 4 months (satisfying their parent's own desire to sleep through the night), the Kipsigis babies do not show this change. Their longest sleep episode increases very little for at least the first 8 months.

The studies of !Kung San Bushman infants by Konner (1981) and Konner and Worthman (1980) support these findings, as does the research by Elias et al. (1986) and Elias, Nicholson and Konner (1987), who studied La Leche League women in the United States who slept with their infants.

PHYSIOLOGICAL EFFECTS OF CO-SLEEPING/BREASTFEEDING: LABORATORY STUDIES

One of us (J.M.) has been studying, with Dr. Sarah Mosko at the University of California, Irvine, Sleep Disorders Laboratory, the physiological effects on infants in and out of contact with their mothers (same bed vs. adjacent rooms) (see Mosko et al., 1993; McKenna et al., 1993). The first two studies did not require mothers to be breastfeeding (although most were), but their current work makes this a requirement. Their first two preliminary studies revealed that mothers and infants have significant effects on the progression of each other's sleep stages as well as on the timing of their arousals. They found, for example, that mother–infant pairs spent more time in the same sleep stage or awake state while co-sleeping than while sleeping alone. They also noted an impressive amount of arousal overlap, in which each partner induced simultaneous arousals on the other, mostly without the other awakening (see McKenna et al., 1993).

Breastfeeding bouts occur more frequently when mothers and infants share the same bed, compared with when they sleep in separate rooms. For example, based on six mother–infant pairs sleeping apart and together over three consecutive nights in the sleep laboratory, mothers nursed their 3-month-old babies an average of 5.3 times per night (range 3–10 sessions) while sleeping together in the same bed, with an average duration of 12.2 (range 3.3–28) minutes per nursing session. When sleeping in adjacent rooms, however, mothers fed their infants an average of only 2.3 times per night (range 1–4), with an average duration of 23.4 (range 19.5–32) minutes per nursing episode (McKenna et al., 1994.

Preliminary data suggest that co-sleeping and breastfeeding infants may spend less time in deep stages of sleep. If this is sustained in subsequent work it could be an important finding, since this stage of sleep is the most difficult stage from which infants must arouse to reinitiate breathing following an apnea (McKenna and Mosko, 1993).

In addition, McKenna and Mosko found that co-sleeping creates more variable physiological experiences for the infant. For example, infants moved from one stage of sleep to another more frequently while co-sleeping than while sleeping alone. When their mothers moved or somehow startled them during sleep, they would occasionally look up, hold their breath for a second or two (thereby increasing heart and breathing rates), then resettle. It is possible that this increased physiological variation may lead to greater maturational synchrony among the infant's various developing subsystems—systems that essentially must "learn" to respond in unison to the respiratory system's internally based challenges. Again, the idea is that practice makes perfect: the more the infant arouses, the better he or she becomes at it (see McKenna et al., 1993). Although our study does not prove an association between the environmental factors and SIDS, it documents the physiological changes infants experience as they move from a solitary sleep environment to a more natural, ecological one (McKenna, 1992).

CONCLUSION AND COMMENTARY: BREASTFEEDING/CO-SLEEPING AS A WAY OF LIFE

If natural selection designed the developing human infant's sleeping, breathing, nursing, and arousal patterns in association with parental contact, this perspective gives us an initial basis for postulating and understanding better how and why related control systems might function less efficiently when infant caregiving practices diverge from the evolutionarily stable ones (Figure 10.1). If, as we contend here, infant–parent co-sleeping and breastfeeding are part of the same adaptive complex, separate sleep arrangements of mothers and infants that break and interrupt its fluidity should lead to both short- and long-term developmental effects. The question that McKenna and Mosko's sleep and breastfeeding research is attempting to shed light on is whether the kinds of physiological changes that infants experience when isolated from the parent increase the chances that cardiorespiratory or immunological control systems function less efficiently, thereby making some infants more vulnerable to certain forms of SIDS. As work progresses during the next few years, we will be in a better position to answer this question.

Up to about one hundred years ago, infant feeding and infant nurturing were inseparably performed through breastfeeding. Since the turn

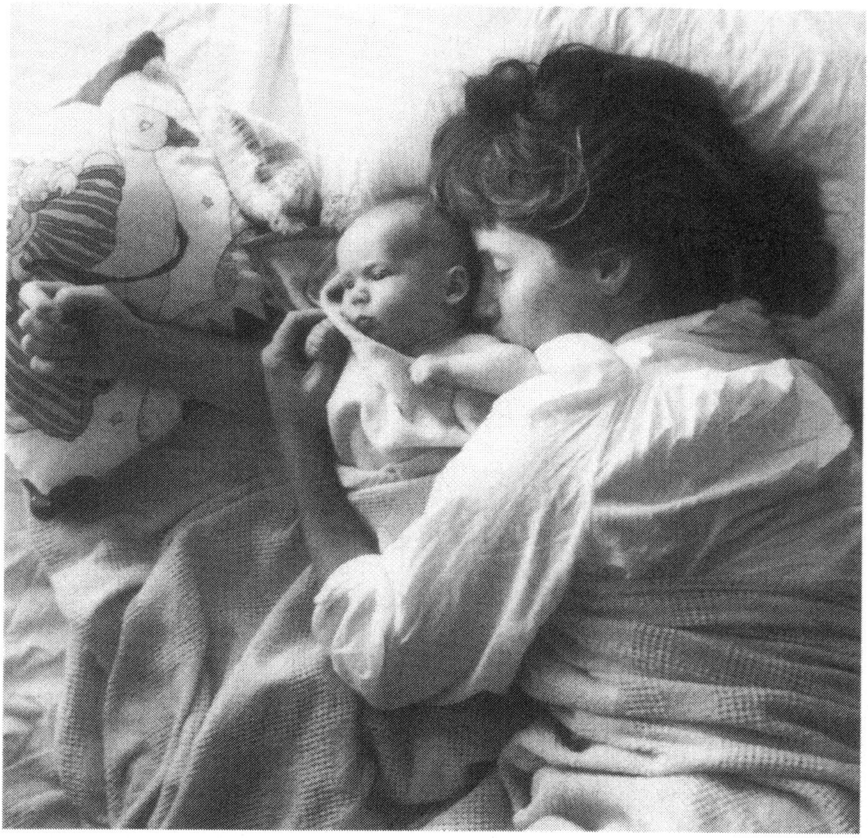

Figure 10.1 As shown here, infants experience multiple sensory stimuli (touch, gas-heat exchange, movement, breathing sounds) while sleeping (or awakening) in proximity and contact with a parent. Such sensory signals emitted from a co-sleeping partner may assist or help regulate the infant's immature nervous system. Photo © Don Milici, all rights reserved.

of this century, technology has created a means to separate infant feeding from nurturing (including the creation of separate sleep environments) through artificial baby milks and multiple rooms in the living environment (see Apple, 1987). But, at the same time, this same technology has revealed information about the nutritive content of breast milk and its immunological properties. Although this knowledge has been helpful in understanding, among other things, some nutrition and immunological needs of the infant, it sheds little light on the infant's emotional needs, except for those needs we can infer from movements of ink-filled needles on a polysomnograph, which reveal responsiveness and sensitivities of the infant's physiology to its co-sleeping parent's touch, sounds, and movements. An evolutionary perspective on parenting and infancy suggests, however, that the overall emotional and, hence, physiological needs of infants are larger than the sum of their parts, and no matter how powerful a polysomnographic machine may be, it cannot fully document the collective, transactional nature of infant–parent interactions that altogether shape infant health and development.

Despite the fact that breastfed infants have been shown to enjoy a definite biological and social advantage over their artificially fed counterparts, there does not appear to be any sense of urgency to promote breastfeeding, especially as one of several possible weapons against certain forms of SIDS. After over two decades of intense research, the cause(s) of SIDS remain(s), for the most part, intractable, although infants sleeping on their backs may further reduce SIDS incidences in Europe and the United States. What we do know is that breastfeeding and the closeness it fosters between infant and mother, whether it be during the night for sleep, or during the day to continue frequent feedings, affects a variety of known SIDS risk factors in positive ways. That is, if SIDS is thought to be caused by immunological immaturity of the infant, breast milk provides the most effective immunization schedule on a daily basis with no additional stress. If SIDS is thought to be caused by hypersensitivity to certain components of certain foods recently forced on him or her despite the infant's slow adaptation capability, time-tested breast milk contains every nutrient the infant needs in the right proportions. If SIDS is thought to be caused by the infant's immaturity in sleep or breathing functions, frequent contact of the infant with its mother because of the need for frequent feedings provides the sensory stimulation he or she needs to thrive, and places the mother in a better position to arouse the infant should it be necessary to do so. If the supine sleep position is thought to reduce the risk of SIDS, co-sleeping with breastfeeding practically ensures that the infant will assume the presumed safer position.

There appears to be no single component of breastfeeding (or co-sleeping, for that matter) that protects infants against SIDS, possibly because the breastfeeding/co-sleeping adaptive system may be just as complex as SIDS and we understand neither well. Yet, breastfeeding as a way of life, that is, including both the feeding, sleeping, and nurturing components, should provide some protection against SIDS—at least if we assume that natural selection designed this system (which we must) to maximize the chances of survival for the greatest number of infants. And even if it proves to be just "some" protection and not complete protection, it is still important to describe the practice of breastfeeding and co-sleeping as a critical adaptive strategy. Four million years of hominid evolution cannot be all wrong.

It may well be that one of the greatest problems in our technology-driven world is our nonconscious cultural ideologies that underlie and inform research, and that we mistake for "truth" supposedly established by scientific studies. For example, until the work of McKenna et al. (1991), not one study on infant–parent co-sleeping existed because the prevailing scientific assumption was simply, and without question, that solitary infant sleep is "normal" and always the most desirable form of infant sleep. An evolutionary research perspective, however, can make us aware not only which assumptions are false, but also that they exist! An evolutionary perspective also provides a way to transcend our own ethnocentrism. For example, it probably is not coincidental that infant care (such as breastfeeding and co-sleeping) practiced by peoples considered "exotic" or "primitive" are suspect, and thought to be inferior to our own Western practices. Infant care exhibited especially by nonindustrialized societies is thought to need improvement, including the use of any or all Western technological devices (undulating water beds, Fisher-Price Baby Monitors, Breathing Teddy-Bear Sleep Companions, etc.), which, by virtue of their technological nature, render their use superior to natural parenting.

Even though SIDS seems almost infinitely complex, the experience of other cultures can remind us of the ways in which industrialized societies have restructured even the most fundamental aspects of infancy and parenting, perhaps pushing both parents and infants beyond their adaptive limits. By "borrowing back" patterns of infant care that maximized the chances of infant survival and, hence, parental reproductive success throughout millions of years of human evolution, it is possible to take advantage of the best that medical technology and insight can offer while also accepting the benefits of time-tested, universal, species-wide patterns of infant care. When infants are fed and nurtured the way their evolutionary histories suggest is ideal—through exclusive breastfeeding for the first 4 to 6 months of life and increased contact between parents and infants both day and night—we might also be able to better understand important aspects of the SIDS enigma and work more effectively toward eliminating it.

REFERENCES

Anders, T. F.
1979 Night-waking in infants during the first year of life. *Pediatrics* 63:860–868.
Anderson, J. R.
1984 Ethology and ecology of sleep in monkeys and apes. In *Advances in the*

Study of Behavior, Vol. 14, edited by J. S. Rosenblatt, C. Beer, M. C. Busnel, and P. J. Slater, pp. 166–229. Orlando, FL: Academic Press.

Apple, R. D.
1987 *Mothers in Medicine: A Social History of Infant Feeding, 1890–1950*. Madison, WI: University of Wisconsin Press.

Ariagno, R. L., and S. F. Glotzbach
1991 Sudden infant death syndrome. In *Pediatrics*, 19th ed., edited by A. M. Rudolph, pp. 850–858. Norwalk, CT: Appleton and Lange.

Arnon, S. S.
1983 Breast-feeding and toxigenic intestinal infections: Missing links in SIDS. In *Sudden Infant Death Syndrome*, edited by J. T. Tildon, L. M. Roeder, and A. Steinschneider, pp. 539–556. New York: Academic Press.
1984 Breast feeding and toxigenic intestinal infections: Missing links in crib death. *Reviews of Infectious Diseases* 6(Suppl. 1):S193–S201.
1986 Infant botulism: Anticipating the second decade. *Journal of Infectious Disease* 154:201–206.

Balarajan, R., V. S. Raleigh, and B. Botting
1989 Sudden infant death syndrome and postneonatal mortality in immigrants in England and Wales. *British Medical Journal* 298:716–720.

Bass, M., R. E. Kravath, and L. Glass
1986 Sudden infant death: Death scene investigation. *New England Journal of Medicine* 315:100–105.

Bergman, A.
1986 *The Discovery of Sudden Infant Death Syndrome: Lessons in the Practice of Political Medicine*. New York: Praeger.

Bernshaw, N. B.
1991a Does breastfeeding protect against sudden infant death syndrome? *Journal of Human Lactation* 7(2):73–79.
1991b Breastfeeding and SIDS—Reply to Bruen (letter). *Journal of Human Lactation* 7(4):176.

Bowlby, J.
1969 Attachment and loss. *Attachment*, Vol. 1. London: Hogarth Press.

Brazelton, T. B., B. Koslowski, and M. Main
1974 The origins of reciprocity: The early mother–infant interactions. In *The Effect of the Infant on Its Caregiver*, edited by M. Lewis and L. A. Rosenblum, pp. 167–183. New York: John Wiley.

Brody, J. E.
1986 Helping a baby learn to sleep through the night. *New York Times*, Nov. 12, pp. 15 and 17.

Davies, D. P.
1985 Cot death in Hong Kong: A rare problem? *Lancet* 2:1346–1348.

Einspieler, C., J. Widder, A. Holzer, and T. Kenner
1988 The predictive value of behavioral risk factors for sudden infant death. *Early Human Development* 18:101–109.

Elias, M. F., N. Nicholson, C. Bora, and J. Johnston
1986 Sleep-wake patterns of breast-fed infants in the first two years of life. *Pediatrics* 77(3):322–329.

Elias, M. F., N. Nicholson, and M. Konner
1987 Two subcultures of maternal care in the United States. In *Current Perspectives in Primate Social Dynamics*, edited by D. Taub and F. King, pp. 31–36. New York: Van Nostrand Reinhold.
Emery, J. L.
1983 A way of looking at the causes of crib death. In *Sudden Infant Death Syndrome*, edited by J. T. Tildon, L. M. Roeder, and A. Steinschneider, pp. 123–132. New York: Academic Press.
Farooqi, S, I. J. Perry, and D. G. Beevers
1991 Ethnic differences in sleeping position and in risk of cot death. *Lancet* 338:1455.
Ferber, R.
1985 Sleep disorders in infants and children. In *Clinical Aspects of Sleep and Sleep Disorders*, edited by T. Riley, pp. 113–146. Boston: Butterworth Press.
Fredrickson, D. D., J. R. Sorenson, A. K. Biddle, and M. Kotelchuck
1993 Relationship of sudden infant death syndrome to breast-feeding duration and intensity (abstract). *American Journal of Diseases of Children* 147:460.
Gantley, M., D. P. Davies, and A. Murcott
1993 Sudden infant death syndrome: Links with infant care practices. *British Medical Journal* 306:16–20.
Golding, J., S. Limerick, and A. MacFarlane
1985 *Sudden Infant Death: Patterns, Puzzles, and Problems*. Shepton Mallet, London: Open Books.
Gould, J. B.
1983 SIDS—A sleep hypothesis. In *Sudden Infant Death Syndrome*, edited by J. T. Tildon, L. M. Roeder, and A. Steinschneider, pp. 443–452. New York: Academic Press.
Guilleminault, C., F. L. Eldridge, and W. C. Dement
1973 Insomnia with sleep apnea: A new syndrome. *Science* 181:856–858.
Guntheroth, W. G.
1989 *Crib Death: The Sudden Infant Death Syndrome*. Mount Kisko, NY: Futura.
Guntheroth, W. G., and P. Spiers
1992 Sleeping prone and the risk of the sudden infant death syndrome. *Journal of the American Medical Association* 267:2359–2362.
Harper, R. M., B. Leake, H. Hoffman, D. O. Walter, T. Hoppenbrouwers, J. Hodgman, and M. B. Sterman
1981 Periodicity of sleep states is altered in infants at risk for the SIDS. *Science* 213:1030–1032.
Hoffman, H., K. Damus, L. Hillman, and E. Krongrad
1988 Risk factors for SIDS: Results of the National Institute of Child Health and Human Development SIDS Cooperative Epidemiological Study. In *Sudden Infant Death Syndrome: Cardiac and Respiratory Mechanisms and Interventions*, Annals of the New York Academy of Sciences, Vol. 533, edited by P. Schwartz, D. Southall, and M. Valdes-Dapena, pp. 13–30. New York: New York Academy of Sciences.
Hoppenbrouwers, T., and J. Hodgman
1986 Commentary on "An anthropological perspective on the Sudden Infant

Death Syndrome (SIDS): The role of parental breathing cues and speech breathing adaptations," by James J. McKenna. *Medical Anthropology* (special issue) 10(1):61–65.

Hoppenbrouwers, T., J. Hodgman, A. Kazuko, and M. B. Sterman
1989 Polysomnographic sleep and waking states are similar in subsequent siblings of SIDS and control infants during the first six months of life. *Sleep* 12(3):265–276.

Huang, S.
1983 Infectious diseases, immunology, and SIDS: An overview. In *Sudden Infant Death Syndrome*, edited by J. T. Tildon, L. M. Roeder, and A. Steinschneider, pp. 593–606. New York: Academic Press.

Juto, P., and S. Holm
1992 Gliadin-specific and cow's milk-specific IgA in human milk. *Journal of Pediatric Gastroenterology and Nutrition* 151:159–162.

Konner, M. J.
1981 Evolution of human behavior development. In *Handbook of Cross-Cultural Human Development*, edited by R. Monroe and B. Whiting, pp. 3–52. New York: Garland Press.

Konner, M. J., and C. Worthman
1980 Nursing frequency, gonadal function and birthspacing among !Kung hunters and gatherers. *Science* 207:788–791.

Kunz, C., and B. Lönnerdal
1989 Casein micelles and casein subunits in human milk. In *Protein and Non-Protein Nitrogen in Human Milk*, edited by S. A. Atkinson and B. Lönnerdal, pp. 9–27. Boca Raton, FL: CRC Press.

Labbok, M., and K. Krasovec.
1990 Toward consistency in breastfeeding definitions. *Studies in Family Planning* 21(4):226–230.

Lancaster, J. B., and C. S. Lancaster
1982 Parental investment: The hominid adaptation. In *How Humans Adapt: A Biocultural Odyssey*, edited by D. Ortner, pp. 33–56. Washington, DC: Smithsonian Institution Press.

Lee, N. Y., Y. F. Chan, D. P. Davies, E. Lau, and D. C. P. Yip
1989 Sudden infant death syndrome in Hong Kong: Confirmation of low incidence. *British Medical Journal* 298:721.

Lozoff, B., A. W. Wolf, and N. S. Davis
1984 Co-sleeping in urban families with young children in the United States. *Pediatrics* 74(2):171–182.

Mata, L. J., and R. G. Wyatt
1971 Host resistance to infection. *American Journal of Clinical Nutrition* 24:976–986.

McGinty, D. J.
1984 Reticular formation modulation of state physiology. Paper presented at the International Symposium on Sudden Infant Death Syndrome, 17th Annual Intra-Science Symposium, February 22–24, 1984, Santa Monica, California.

McKenna, J. J.
1986 An anthropological perspective on the sudden infant death syndrome

(SIDS): The role of parental breathing cues and speech breathing adaptations. *Medical Anthropology* (special issue) 10(1):9–53.
1992 SIDS research. *Mothering* 62:45–51.
1993 Rethinking healthy infant sleep. *Breastfeeding Abstracts* 12(3):27.
1994 Behavior and behavioral interactions of solitary and cosleeping mother-infant pairs: Implications for SIDS. Annual meeting of the Association of Professional Sleep Societies. Boston, MA: June 2–7, 1994.

McKenna, J. J., and S. Mosko
1990 Evolution and the sudden infant death syndrome (SIDS). Part III: Infant arousal and parent-infant co-sleeping. *Human Nature* 1:291–330.
1993 Evolution and infant sleep: An experimental study of infant-parent co-sleeping and its implications for SIDS. *Acta Paediatrica Supplement* 389:31–36.

McKenna, J. J., S. Mosko, C. Dungy, and J. McAninch
1990 Sleep and arousal patterns of co-sleeping human mother/infant pairs: A preliminary physiological study with implications for the study of sudden infant death syndrome (SIDS). *American Journal of Physical Anthropology* 83:331–347.

McKenna J. J., E. B. Thoman, T. F. Anders, A. Sadeh, V. L. Schechtman, and S. F. Glotzbach
1993 Infant-parent co-sleeping in evolutionary perspective: Imperatives for understanding infant sleep development and SIDS. *Sleep* 16(3):263–282.

Mitchell E., R. Scragg, A. W. Stewart, D. M. Becroft, B. J. Taylor, R. P. Ford, I. B. Hassall, D. M. Barry, E. M. Allen, and A. P. Roberts
1991 Results from the first year of the New Zealand Cot Death Study. *New Zealand Medical Journal* 104:71–76.

Mosko, S., J. McKenna, M. Dickel, and L. Hunt
1993 Parent–infant co-sleeping: The appropriate context for the study of infant sleep and implications for sudden infant death syndrome (SIDS) research. *Journal of Behavioral Medicine* 16(6):589–610.

Mosko, S., C. Richard, J. McKenna, S. Drummond, and D. Mukai
1995 CO_2 environment of the cosleeping infant: The parents' contribution. *Journal of Pediatric Research*, submitted.

Pinilla, T., and L. L. Birch
1993 Help me make it through the night: Behavioral entrainment of breast-fed infants' sleep patterns. *Pediatrics* 91(2):436–444.

Ramabadran, K., and M. Bansinath
1988 Opioid peptides from milk as a possible cause of sudden infant death syndrome. *Medical Hypotheses* 27:181–187.

Riordan, J., and K. G. Auerbach
1993 *Breastfeeding and Human Lactation*. London: Jones and Bartlett.

Schacter, F. F., M. L. Fuchs, P. E. Bijur, and R. K. Stone
1989 Cosleeping and sleep problems in Hispanic-American urban young children. *Pediatrics* 84:522–530.

Schwartz, P. J., D. Southall, and M. Valdes-Dapena, eds.
1988 *Sudden Infant Death Syndrome: Cardiac and Respiratory Mechanisms and Interventions*. Annals of the New York Academy of Sciences, Vol. 533. New York: New York Academy of Sciences.

Short, R.
1984 Breast feeding. *Scientific American* 250(4):35–41.
Spock, B., and M. Rothenberg
1985 *Dr. Spock's Baby and Child Care*. New York: Pocket Books.
Super, C. M., and S. Harkness
1982 The infant's niche in rural Kenya and metropolitan America. In *Cross-Cultural Research at Issue*, edited by L. L. Adler, pp. 47–55. New York: Academic Press.
Takeda, K.
1987 A possible mechanism of sudden infant death syndrome (SIDS). *Journal of Kyoto Prefecture Medical University* 96:965–968.
Tasaki, H., M. Yamashita, and S. Miyazaki
1988 The incidence of SIDS in Saga prefecture (1981–1985). *Journal of the Pediatric Association of Japan* 92:364–368.
Taylor, E., and J. Emery
1988 Trends in unexpected infant deaths in Sheffield. *Lancet* 2:1121–1122.
Valdes-Dapena, M. A.
1980a Sudden infant death syndrome: A review of the medical literature, 1974–1979. *Pediatrics* 66(4):567–614.
1980b *Sudden Infant Death Syndrome*. U.S. Department of Health, Education, and Welfare Publication No. 80-5255. Washington, D. C.
1988 A pathologist's perspective on possible mechanisms in SIDS. In *Sudden Infant Death Syndrome: Cardiac and Respiratory Mechanisms and Interventions*, Annals of the New York Academy of Sciences, Vol. 533, edited by P. Schwartz, D. Southall, and M. Valdes-Dapena, pp. 31–37. New York: New York Academy of Sciences.
Willinger, M.
1989 SIDS: A challenge. *Journal of National Institutes of Health Research* 1:73–80.

REFERENCES TO TABLE 10.1

Ariagno, R. L., L. Nagel, and C. Guilleminault
1980 Waking and ventilatory responses during sleep in infants with near miss for sudden infant death syndrome. *Sleep* 3:351–359.
Arnon, S. S.
1983 Breast-feeding and toxigenic intestinal infections: Missing links in SIDS. In *Sudden Infant Death Syndrome*, edited by J. T. Tildon, L. M. Roeder, and A. Steinschneider, pp. 539–556. New York: Academic Press.
Aynsley-Green, A., J. M. Polak, J. Keeling, M. H. Gough, and J. D. Baum
1978 Averted sudden neonatal death due to pancreatic nesidioblastosis. *Lancet* 1:550–551.
Baba, N., J. Quattrochi, C. Reiner, W. Adrion, P. T. McBride, and A. J. Yates
1983 Possible role of the brain stem in sudden infant death syndrome. *Journal of the American Medical Association* 249:2789–2791.
Bagg, A. R., G. G. Haddad, G. M. Walsh, and R. B. Mellins
1981 Respiratory pauses in aborted SIDS infants during sleep. *American Review of Respiratory Disorders* 123:157.

Barker, J. N., F. Jordan, D. E. Hillwar, and O. Barlow
1982 Phrenic thiamin and neuropathy in sudden infant death. *Annals of the New York Academy of Science* 378:449–452.
Bass, M.
1988 Sudden infant death syndrome and water beds (letter to editor). *New England Journal of Medicine* 319(21):1415.
Bass, M., R. E. Kravath, and L. Glass
1986 Sudden infant death: Death scene investigation. *New England Journal of Medicine* 315:100–105.
Beal, S. M.
1988 Sleeping position and SIDS. *Lancet* 2:512.
Becker, L. E.
1983 Neuropathological bases for respiratory dysfunction in sudden infant death syndrome. In *Sudden Infant Death Syndrome,* edited by J. T. Tildon, L. M. Roeder, and A. Steinschneider, pp. 99–114. New York: Academic Press.
Beckwith, J. B.
1983 Chronic hypoxemia in the sudden infant death syndrome: A critical review of the data base. In *Sudden Infant Death Syndrome,* edited by J. T. Tildon, L. M. Roeder, and A. Steinschneider, pp. 145–160. New York: Academic Press.
1988 Intrathoracic petechial hemorrhages: A clue to the mechanism of death in sudden infant death syndrome? In *Sudden Infant Death Syndrome: Cardiac and Respiratory Mechanisms and Interventions,* edited by P. Schwartz, D. Southall, and M. Valdes-Dapena, pp. 62–78. Annals of the New York Academy of Sciences 533. New York: New York Academy of Sciences.
Beckwith, L.
1979 Prediction of emotional and social behavior. In *Handbook of Infant Development,* edited by J. D. Osofsky, pp. 671–706. New York: John Wiley.
Bernier, R. H., J. A. Frank, Jr., T. J. Dondero, Jr., and P. Turner
1982 Diptheria-tetanus-toxoids-pertussis vaccinations and sudden infant deaths in Tennessee. *Journal of Pediatrics* 101:419–421.
Brown, M.
1987 Fetal hemoglobin in SIDS. *New England Journal of Medicine* 317(17):607–613.
Church, S. C., B. C. Morgan, T. K. Oliver, and W. G. Guntheroth
1967 Cardiac arrhythmias in premature infants: An indication of autonomic immaturity. *Journal of Pediatrics* 71:542.
Cleary, J. T.
1984 *Cot Deaths CO_2 Deaths?* Obtainable from Cleary/SIDS Data, Box 1, Builth Wells, Powys, Wales, United Kingdom.
Colton, R. H., and A. Steinschneider
1980 Acoustic relationships of infant cries to the sudden infant death syndrome. In *Infant Communication: Cry and Early Speech,* edited by T. Murry and J. Murry, pp. 183–209. Houston: College-Hill Press.
Coombs, R. R. A., and P. McLaughlan
1983 The modified anaphylactic hypothesis for SIDS. In *Sudden Infant Death Syndrome,* edited by J. T. Tildon, L. M. Roeder, and A. Steinschneider, pp. 531–538. New York: Academic Press.

Cornblath, M., and R. Schwartz
1976 *Disorders of Carbohydrate Metabolism in Infancy.* Philadelphia: W.B. Saunders.
Cunningham, A. S.
1976 Infant feeding and SIDS. *Pediatrics* 58:467.
Damus, K., J. Pakter, E. Krongrad, S. J. Standfast, and H. J. Hoffman
1988 Postnatal medical and epidemiological risk factors for the sudden infant death syndrome. In *Sudden Infant Death Syndrome: Risk Factors and Basic Mechanisms,* edited by R. M. Harper and H. J. Hoffman, pp. 41–62. New York: PMA.
Davies, D. P.
1985 Cot death in Hong Kong: A rare problem? *Lancet* 2:1346–1349.
Davis, R. E., G. C. Icke, and J. M. Hilton
1983 Sudden infant death and abnormal thiamin metabolism. In *Sudden Infant Death Syndrome,* edited by J.T. Tildon, L.M. Roeder, and A. Steinschneider, pp. 201–210. New York: Academic Press.
Dinsdale, F., J. C. Emery, and D. R. Gadson
1977 The carotid body—A quantitative reassessment in children. *Histopathology* 1:179–187.
Emery, J., and F. Dinsdale
1978 Structure of periadrenal brown fat in childhood in both expected and cot deaths. *Archives of Diseases in Children* 53:154.
Emery, J. L.
1988 Sleeping position, cot mattresses and cot deaths. *Lancet* 2:738.
Filardo, T.
1988 sudden infant death syndrome and water beds (letter to editor). *New England Journal of Medicine* 319(21):1415.
Fink, B. R., and J. B. Beckwith
1980 Laryngeal mucous gland excess in victims of sudden infant death. *American Journal of Diseases of Children* 134:144–146.
Fleming, P. J., R. E. Gilbert, Y. Azaz, P. J. Berry, P. Rudd, A. Stuart, and E. Hall
1990 The interaction between bedding and sleeping position in the sudden infant death syndrome: A population based control study. *British Medical Journal* 341:85–89.
Franciosi, R. A.
1987 Hypothesis: Sudden infant death syndrome is a disorder of entrainment. *Medical Hypotheses* 22:443–446.
Froggatt, P., and T. N. James
1973 Sudden unexpected death in infants: Evidence on a lethal cardiac arrhythmia. *Ulster Medical Journal* 42:136–152.
Gadson, D. R., and J. L. Emery
1976 Fatty change in the brain in perinatal and unexpected death. *Archives of Diseases of Children* 51:42–48.
Giulian, G. G., E. F. Gilbert, and R. L. Moss
1987 Elevated fetal hemoglobin levels in sudden infant death syndrome. *New England Journal of Medicine* 316:1122–1126.

Gould, J.B.
1983 SIDS—A sleep hypothesis. In *Sudden Infant Death Syndrome*, edited by J. T. Tildon, L. M. Roeder, and A. Steinschneider, pp. 443–452. New York: Academic Press.
Gould, J., A. F. S. Lee, and S. Morelock
1988 The relationship between sleep and sudden infant death. In *Sudden Infant Death Syndrome: Cardiac and Respiratory Mechanisms and Interventions*, edited by P. Schwartz, D. Southall, and M. Valdes-Dapena, pp. 62–78. Annals of the New York Academy of Sciences 533. New York: New York Academy of Sciences.
Griffin, M., W. A. Ray, J. R. Livengoon, and W. Schaffner
1988 Risk of sudden infant death syndrome after immunization with the diptheria-tetanus-pertussis vaccine. *New England Journal of Medicine* 319(10):618–623.
Guilleminault, C.
1980 Sleep apnea syndromes: Impact of sleep and sleep states. *Sleep* 3:227–234.
1984 Reply to Harpey and Renault. *Pediatrics* 74:319.
1988 SIDS, near-miss SIDS and cardiac arrhythmia. In *Sudden Infant Death Syndrome: Cardiac and Respiratory Mechanisms and Interventions*, edited by P. Schwartz, D. Southall, and M. Valdes-Dapena, pp. 358–368. Annals of the New York Academy of Sciences 533. New York: New York Academy of Sciences.
Guilleminault, C., and S. Coons
1983 Sleep states and maturation of sleep: A comparative study between full-term normal controls and near miss SIDS infants. In *Sudden Infant Death Syndrome*, edited by J. T. Tildon, L. M. Roeder, and A. Steinschneider, pp. 401–411. New York: Academic Press.
Guilleminault, C., R. L. Ariagno, L. S. Forno, L. Nagel, R. Baldwin, and M. Owen
1979 Obstructive sleep apnea and near-miss for SIDS: 1. Report of an infant with sudden death. *Pediatrics* 63:837–843.
Guilleminault, C., R. L. Ariagno, R. Korobkin, L. Nagel, R. Baldwin, S. Coons, and M. Owen
1979 Obstructive sleep apnea and near-miss for sudden infant death syndrome: 2. Comparison of near miss and normal control infants by age. *Pediatrics* 64:882–891.
Guilleminault, C., G. Heldt, N. Powell, and R. Riley
1986 Small upper airway in near-miss sudden infant death syndrome infants and their families. *Lancet* 1:402–407.
Guilleminault, C., M. Peraita, M. Souquet, and W.C. Dement
1975 Apneas during sleep in infants: Possible relationship with sudden infant death syndrome. *Science* 190:6.
Guilleminault, C., M. Souquet, R. Ariagno, and W.C. Dement
1976 Abnormal polygraphic findings in near miss and sudden infant death. *Lancet* 1:1326–1327.
Guilleminault, C., A. Tilkian, and W.C. Dement
1976 The sleep apnea syndrome. *Annual Review of Medicine* 27:465–484.

Gunby, P.
1978 Brainstem abnormalities may characterize SIDS victims. *Journal of the American Medical Association* 240:2138–2144.
Guntheroth, W. G.
1977 sudden infant death syndrome (crib death). *American Heart Journal* 93:784.
1982 *Crib Death: The Sudden Infant Death Syndrome*. New York: Futura.
1983a Arrhythmia, apnea, or arousal? In *Sudden Infant Death Syndrome*, edited by J. T. Tildon, L. M. Roeder, and A. Steinschneider, pp. 268–270. New York: Academic Press.
1983b The pathology of petechiae. In *Sudden Infant Death Syndrome*, edited by J. T. Tildon, L. M. Roeder, and A. Steinschneider, pp. 271–278. New York: Academic Press.
Gupta, P. R., C. Guilleminault, and L. J. Dorfman
1981 Brain stem auditory evoked potentials in near miss sudden infant death syndrome. *Journal of Pediatrics* 98:791–794.
Haddad, G. G., and R. B. Mellins
1983 Cardiorespiratory aspects of SIDS: An overview. In *Sudden Infant Death Syndrome*, edited by J. T. Tildon, L. M. Roeder, and A. Steinschneider, pp. 357–374. New York: Academic Press.
Haddad, G. G., R. A. Epstein, M. A. F. Epstein, M. L. Leistner, P. A. Marino, and R. B. Mellins
1979 Maturation of ventilation and ventilatory pattern in normal sleeping infants. *Journal of Applied Physiology* 46:998–1002.
Haddad, G. G., H. L. Leistner, R. A. Epstein, M. A. F. Epstein, W. K. Grodin, and R. B. Mellins
1980 CO_2 induced changes in ventilation and ventilatory pattern in normal sleeping infants. *Journal of Applied Physiology* 48:684–688.
Haddad, G. G., H. L. Leistner, T. L. Lai, and R. B. Mellins
1981 Ventilation and ventilatory patterns during sleep in aborted sudden infant death syndrome. *Pediatric Research* 15:879–883.
Harper, R. M., B. Leake, H. Hoffman, D. O. Walter, T. Hoppenbrouwers, J. Hodgman, and M. B. Sterman
1981 Periodicity of sleep states is altered in infants at risk for the SIDS. *Science* 213:1030–1032.
Harpey, J. P., and F. Renault
1984 The uvula and sudden infant death syndrome. *Pediatrics* 74:319.
Henderson-Smart, D. J., and D. J. Read
1978 Depression of intercostal and abdominal muscle activity and vulnerability to asphyxia during active sleep in the newborn. In *Sleep Apnea Syndrome*, edited by C. Guilleminault and W. Dement, pp. 213–229. New York: Alan Liss.
Hillman, L. S., M. Erickson, and G. G. Haddad
1980 Serum 25-hydroxy vitamin D concentrations in sudden infant death syndrome. *Pediatrics* 65:1137–1139.
Hodgman, J., and T. Hoppenbrouwers
1988 Home monitoring for the sudden infant death syndrome: The case against. In *The Sudden Infant Death Syndrome: Cardiac and Respiratory Mechanisms and Interventions*, edited by P. Schwartz, D. Southall, and M. Valdes-

Dapena, pp. 164–175. Annals of the New York Academy of Sciences 533. New York: New York Academy of Sciences.

Hodgman, J. E., T. Hoppenbrouwers, S. Geidel, A. Hadeed, M. B. Sterman, R. Harper, and D. McGinty
1982 Respiratory behavior in near-miss sudden infant death syndrome. *Pediatrics* 69:785–792.

Hoffman, H., K. Damus, L. Hillman, and E. Krongrad
1988 Risk factors for SIDS: Results of the National Institute of Child Health and Human Development SIDS Cooperative Epidemiological Study. In *Sudden Infant Death Syndrome: Cardiac and Respiratory Mechanisms and Interventions*, edited by P. Schwartz, D. Southall, and M. Valdes-Dapena, pp. 13–31. Annals of the New York Academy of Sciences 533. New York: New York Academy of Sciences.

Hunt D., K. McCulloch, and R. Brovillette
1981 Diminished hypoxia ventilatory responses in near-miss SIDS. *Journal of Applied Physiology* 50:1313–1317.

Jansen, A. H., and V. Chernick
1983 Development of respiratory control. *Physiological Reviews* 63:437–483.

Jeffrey, H. E., B. V. McCleary, W. J. Hensley, and D. J. C. Read
1985 Thiamine deficiency—A neglected problem of infants and mothers—Possible relationships to sudden infant death syndrome. *Australia-New Zealand Journal of Obstetrics and Gynaecology* 25:198–202.

Johnson, P., J. E. Fewel, L. M. Fedako, and J. C. Wollner
1983 The vagal control of breathing in postnatal life: Implications for sleep-related respiratory failure. In *Sudden Infant Death Syndrome*, edited by J. T. Tildon, L. M. Roeder, and A. Steinschneider, pp. 467–490. New York: Academic Press.

Kaada, B.
1986 *Sudden Infant Death Syndrome: The Possible Role of the Fear Paralysis Reflex.* Oslo: Norwegian University Press and New York: Oxford University Press.

Kelly, D. H.
1983 Incidence of severe apnea and death in infants identified as high risk for sudden infant death. In *Sudden Infant Death Syndrome*, edited by J. T. Tildon, L. M. Roeder, and A. Steinschneider, pp. 607–614. New York: Academic Press.

Kelly, D. H., A. M. Walker, L. Cohen, and D. C. Shannon
1980 Periodic breathing in siblings of sudden infant death syndrome victims. *Pediatrics* 66:515–520.

Kemp, J. S., and B. G. Thach
1991 Sudden death in infants sleeping on polystyrene-filled cushions. *New England Journal of Medicine* 324:1858–1864.

Konner, M. J., and C. M. Super
1987 Sudden infant death: An anthropological hypothesis. In *The Role of Culture in Developmental Disorder*, edited by C. M. Super and S. Harkness, pp. 60–80. New York: Academic Press.

Kukolich, M. K., A. Telsey, J. Oh, and A. G. Motulsky
1977 Sudden infant death syndrome: Normal QT interval on ECGs of relatives. *Pediatrics* 60:51.

Lee, N. Y., Y. F. Chan, D. P. Davies, E. Lau, and D. C. P. Yip
1989 Sudden infant death syndrome in Hong Kong: Confirmation of low incidence. *British Medical Journal* 298:721.

Luke, J.L.
1978 Sleeping arrangements of sudden infant death syndrome victims in the District of Columbia—A preliminary report. *Journal of Forensic Science* 23:379–383.

Mason, J. M., L. H. Mason, J. Jackson, J. S. Bell, J. T. Francisco, and B. R. Jennings
1975 Pulmonary vessels in SIDS. *New England Journal of Medicine* 292:479.

Maxwell, W., and M. Maxwell
1979 52 ways to raise the I. Q. of a child. Appendix to: *The Forces of Achievement: A Systems Approach to Schooling and Society*. Privately published. Address available from James McKenna.

McCulloch, K., R. T. Brouillette, A. J. Guzetta, and C. E. Hunt
1982 Arousal responses in near-miss sudden infant death syndrome and in normal infants. *Journal of Pediatrics* 101:911.

McGinty, D. J.
1984 Reticular formation modulation of state physiology. Paper presented at the International Symposium on Sudden Infant Death Syndrome, 17th Annual Intra-Science Symposium, February 22–24, Santa Monica, California.

McKenna, J. J.
1986 An anthropological perspective on the sudden infant death syndrome (SIDS): The role of parental breathing cues and speech breathing adaptations. *Medical Anthropology* (special issue) 10(1):9–53.

Merritt, A. T., and M. A. Valdes-Dapena
1984 SIDS research update. *Pediatric Annals* 13(3)195–216.

Mitchell, E. A., R. Scragg, A. W. Stewart, D. M. O. Becroft, B. J. Taylor, and R. P. K. Ford
1991 Results from the first year of the New Zealand Cot Death Study. *New Zealand Medical Journal* 104:71–76.

Morley, C. J., C. M. Hill, B. O. Brown, A. J. Barson, D. Southall, and J. Davis
1984 Surfactant and sudden infant death (SIDS). *Pediatric Research* 18:810.

Naeye, R. L.
1973 Pulmonary arterial abnormalities in sudden infant death syndrome. *New England Journal of Medicine* 289:1167–1170.
1974 Hypoxia and the sudden infant death syndrome. *Science* 186:837–838.
1976 Brainstem and adrenal abnormalities in SIDS. *American Journal of Clinical Pathology* 66:526–529.
1980 Sudden infant death. *Scientific American* 242:556–562.

Naeye, R. L., B. Ladis, and J. S. Drage
1976 Sudden infant death syndrome—A prospective study. *American Journal of Diseases of Children* 130:1207–1210.

Nelson, E. A. S., B. J. Taylor, and I. L. Weatherall
1989 Sleeping position and infant bedding may predispose to hyperthermia and the sudden infant death syndrome. *Lancet* 1:199–200.

Orlowski, J. P., R. H. Nodar, and D. Lonsdale
1979 Abnormal brainstem auditory evoked potentials in infants with threatened sudden infant death syndrome. *Cleveland Clinic Quarterly* 46(3):77–81.
Orr, W. C., M. L. Stahl, J. Duke, M. A. McLaffree, P. Torbas, C. Maltice, and H. Krauss
1985 Effect of sleep state and position on the incidence of obstructive and central apnea in infants. *Pediatrics* 75(5):832–835.
Patrick, J. R., and S. T. Patrick
1982 Adrenal chromaffin tissue in sudden infant death syndrome. *Lab Investigation* 46:12.
Pearson, J., and L. Brandeis
1983 Normal aspects of morphometry of brain stem astrocytes, carotid bodies and ganglia in SIDS. In *Sudden Infant Death Syndrome*, edited by J. T. Tildon, L. M. Roeder, and A. Steinschneider, pp. 115–122. New York: Academic Press.
Perrin, D. G., L. E. Becker, A. Madapallimatum, E. Cruz, A. C. Bryan, and M. J. Sole
1984 Sudden infant death syndrome: Increased carotid body dopamine and noradrenaline content. *Lancet* 2:535–537.
Peterson, D.
1983 Epidemiology of the sudden infant death syndrome: Problems, progress, prospects—A review. In *Sudden Infant Death Syndrome*, edited by J. T. Tildon, L. M. Roeder, and A. Steinschneider, pp. 89–98. New York: Academic Press.
Peterson, D., E. Sabotta, and D. Strickland
1988 Sudden infant death syndrome in epidemiological perspective: Etiologic implications of variation with season of the year. In *Sudden Infant Death Syndrome: Cardiac and Respiratory Mechanisms and Interventions*, edited by P. Schwartz, D. Southall, and M. Valdes-Dapena, pp. 6–13. Annals of the New York Academy of Sciences 533. New York: New York Academy of Sciences.
Phillipson, E. A.
1978 Respiratory adaptation in sleep. *Annual Review of Physiology* 40:117–137.
Quattrochi, J. J., N. Baba, L. Liss, and W. Adrion
1980 Sudden infant death syndrome (SIDS): A preliminary study of reticular dendritic spines in infants with SIDS. *Brain Research* 181:245–249.
Quattrochi, J. J., P. T. McBride, and A. J. Yates
1984 Brainstem immaturity in sudden infant death syndrome: A quantitative rapid golgi study of dendritic spines in 95 infants. *Brain Research* 325:39–48.
Ramanthan, R., S. Chandra, E. Gilbert-Barness, and R. Franciosi
1988 Sudden infant death syndrome and water beds. *New England Journal of Medicine* 318(25):1700.
Read, D. J. C., and H. E. Jeffery
1983 Many paths to asphyxial death in SIDS—A search for underlying neurochemical defects. In *Sudden Infant Death Syndrome*, edited by J. T. Tildon, L. M. Roeder, and A. Steinschneider, pp. 183–200. New York: Academic Press.

Sachis, P. W., D. L. Armstrong, L. E. Becker, and A. C. Bryan
1981 The vagus nerve and sudden infant death syndrome: A morphometric study. *Journal of Pediatrics* 98:278–280.
Salk, L., B. A. Grellong, and J. Dietrich
1974 Sudden infant death: Normal cardiac habituation and poor autonomic control. *New England Journal of Medicine* 241:219–225.
Schwartz, P. J.
1976 Cardiac sympathetic innervation and the sudden infant death syndrome: A possible pathogenetic link. *American Journal of Medicine* 60:167.
1983 Autonomic nervous system, ventricular fibrillation and SIDS. In *Sudden Infant Death Syndrome*, edited by J. T. Tildon, L. M. Roeder, and A. Steinschneider, pp. 319–340. New York: Academic Press.
1987 The quest for the mechanisms of the sudden infant death syndrome: Doubts and progress. *Circulation* 75:677-683.
Schwartz, P. J., and A. Segantini
1988 Cardiac intervention, neonatal electrocardiography and SIDS: A key for a novel preventive strategy? In *Sudden Infant Death Syndrome: Cardiac and Respiratory Mechanisms and Interventions*, edited by P. Schwartz, D. Southall, and M. Valdes-Dapena, pp. 210–221. Annals of the New York Academy of Sciences 533. New York: New York Academy of Sciences.
Sears, W.
1985 *Nighttime Parenting*. Franklin Park, IL: La Leche League International.
Silverstein, R., D. L. Nelson, C. C. Lin, and A. B. Rawitch
1983 Enzyme stability and SIDS: Studies with phosphoenolpyruvate carboxykinase. In *Sudden Infant Death Syndrome*, edited by J. T. Tildon, L. M. Roeder, and A. Steinschneider, pp. 233–242. New York: Academic Press.
Singer, D.
1984 Pulmonary vasculature in SIDS. Paper presented at the International Symposium on Sudden Infant Death Syndrome, 17th Annual Intra-Science Symposium, February 22–24, Santa Monica, California.
Sonnabend, O. A., W. F. Sonnabend, U. Krech, G. Molz, and T. Sigrist
1985 Continuous microbiological and pathological study of 70 sudden and unexpected infant deaths: Toxigenic infection in 9 cases of sudden infant death syndrome. *Lancet* 1:237–242.
Southall, D. P., and D. G. Talbert
1988 Mechanisms for abnormal apnea of possible relevance to sudden infant death syndrome. In *Sudden Infant Death Syndrome: Cardiac and Respiratory Mechanisms and Interventions*, edited by P. Schwartz, D. Southall, and M. Valdes-Dapena, pp. 329–350. Annals of the New York Academy of Sciences 533. New York: New York Academy of Sciences.
Southall, D. P., J. M. Richards, and K. J. Rhoden
1982 Prolonged apnea and cardiac arrhythmias in infants discharged from neonatal care units: Failure to predict an increased risk for sudden infant death syndrome. *Pediatrics* 70:844–851.
Southall, D. P., D. G. Talbert, P. Johnson, C. J. Morley, S. Salmons, J. Miller, and P. J. Helms

1985 Prolonged expiratory apnea: A disorder resulting in episodes of severe arterial hypoxemia in infants and young children. *Lancet* 2:571–577.

Stanton, A. N.
1984 Overheating and cot death. *Lancet* 2:1199–1201.

Steinschneider, A.
1972 Prolonged apnea and the sudden infant death syndrome: Clinical and laboratory observations. *Pediatrics* 50:646–654.
1978 Sudden infant death syndrome and prolongation of the QT interval. *American Journal of Diseases of Children* 132:688–691.

Sterman, M. B., and J. Hodgman
1988 The role of sleep and arousal in SIDS. In *Sudden Infant Death Syndrome: Cardiac and Respiratory Mechanisms and Interventions,* edited by P. Schwartz, D. Southall, and M. Valdes-Dapena, pp. 48–62. Annals of the New York Academy of Sciences 533. New York: New York Academy of Sciences.

Stockard, J.J.
1981 *Brainstem Auditory Evoked Potentials in Adult and Infant Sleep Apnea Syndromes, Including Sudden Infant Death Syndrome and Near Miss for Sudden Infant Death.* Annals of the New York Academy of Sciences 522. New York: New York Academy of Sciences.

Sturner, W. Q., and J. B. Susa
1983 Sudden infant death and liver phosphoenol pyruvate carboxykinase analysis. *Forensic Science International* 16:19–26.

Sullivan, C.
1984 Upper airway function in sleep apnea. Paper presented at the International Symposium on Sudden Infant Death Syndrome, 17th Annual Intra-Science Symposium, February 22–24, Santa Monica, California.

Swift, P. G., E. Worthy, and J. L. Emery
1974 Biochemical state of the vitreous humor of infants at necropsy. *Archives of Diseases in Children* 49:680–685.

Takashima, S., D. L. Armstrong, and L. E. Becker
1978 Subcortical leukomalacia: Relationship to development of the cerebral sulcus and its vascular supply. *Archives of Neurology* 35:470–472.

Takashima, S., D. L. Armstrong, L. E. Becker, and C. Bryan
1978 Cerebral hypoperfusion in the sudden infant death syndrome? Brain stem gliosis and vasculature. *Annals of Neurology* 4:257–262.

Thach, B. T.
1983 The role of pharyngeal airway obstruction in prolonging infantile apnea spells. In *Sudden Infant Death Syndrome,* edited by J. T. Tildon, L. M. Roeder, and A. Steinschneider, pp. 279–292. New York: Academic Press.

Thach, T. H., A. M. Davies, and J. S. Koenig
1988 Pathophysiology of sudden upper airway obstruction in sleeping infants and its relevance for SIDS. In *Sudden Infant Death Syndrome: Cardiac and Respiratory Mechanisms and Interventions,* edited by P. Schwartz, D. Southall, and M. Valdes-Dapena, pp. 314–329. Annals of the New York Academy of Sciences 533. New York: New York Academy of Sciences.

Tildon, J. T., and L. M. Roeder
1983 Metabolic and endocrine aspects of SIDS: An overview. In *Sudden Infant*

Death Syndrome, edited by J. T. Tildon, L. M. Roeder, and A. Steinschneider, pp. 243–262. New York: Academic Press.

Tildon, J. T., L. M. Roeder, and A. Steinschneider, eds.
1983 *Sudden Infant Death Syndrome*. New York: Academic Press.

Tonkin, S.
1974 Airway occlusion as a possible cause of SIDS. In *SIDS 1974*, edited by R. R. Robinson, pp. 73–74. Toronto: Canadian Foundation for the Study of Sudden Infant Death.
1975 Sudden infant death: Hypothesis of causation. *Pediatrics* 55:650.
1983 Pharyngeal airway obstruction—Physical signs and factors in its production. In *Sudden Infant Death Syndrome*, edited by J. T. Tildon, L. M. Roeder, and A. Steinschneider, pp. 453–466. New York: Academic Press.

Valdes-Dapena, M. A.
1978 *Sudden Infant Death Syndrome, 1970–1975*. Washington, DC: U.S. Department of Health, Education and Welfare. Publication No. 78-5255.
1980 Sudden infant death syndrome: A review of the medical literature, 1974–1979. *Pediatrics* 66:(4):567–614.
1983 The morphology of the sudden infant death syndrome: An overview. In *Sudden Infant Death Syndrome*, edited by J. T. Tildon, L. M. Roeder, and A. Steinschneider, pp. 169–182. New York: Academic Press.
1988 Pathologist's perspective on possible mechanisms in SIDS. In *Sudden Infant Death Syndrome: Cardiac and Respiratory Mechanisms and Interventions*, edited by P. Schwartz, D. Southall, and M. Valdes-Dapena, pp. 31–37. Annals of the New York Academy of Sciences 533. New York: New York Academy of Sciences.

Valdes-Dapena, M. A., and R. P. Felipe
1971 Immunofluorescent studies in crib death: Absence of evidence of hypersensitivity to cows' milk. *American Journal of Clinical Pathology* 56:421.

Valimaki, I. A., T. Nieminen, K. J. Antila, and D.P. Southall
1988 Heart-rate variability and SIDS: Examination of heart-rate patterns using an expert system generator. In *Sudden Infant Death Syndrome: Cardiac and Respiratory Mechanisms and Interventions*, edited by P. Schwartz, D. Southall, and M. Valdes-Dapena, pp. 228–238. Annals of the New York Academy of Sciences 533. New York: New York Academy of Sciences.

Verrier, R., and D. Kirby
1988 Sleep and cardiac arrhythmias. In *Sudden Infant Death Syndrome: Cardiac and Respiratory Mechanisms and Interventions*, edited by P. Schwartz, D. Southall, and M. Valdes-Dapena, pp. 238–252. Annals of the New York Academy of Sciences 533. New York: New York Academy of Sciences.

Vigevano, F., M. Di Capna, and B. Dalla Bernardina
1989 Startle disease: An avoidable cause of sudden infant death. *Lancet* 1:216.

Weinstein, S., A. Steinschneider, and E. Diamond
1983 SIDS and prolonged apnea during sleep: Are they only a matter of state? In *Sudden Infant Death Syndrome*, edited by J. T. Tildon, L. M. Roeder, and A. Steinschneider, pp. 413–422. New York: Academic Press.

Werne, J., and I. Garrow
1953 Sudden apparently unexplained death during infancy: Pathological finding in infants found dead. *American Journal of Pathology* 29:633–652.
Williams, A. G., G. Walter, and L. Reed
1979 Increased muscularity of the pulmonary circulation in victims of sudden infant death syndrome. *Pediatrics* 63:18–23.

11

Breastfeeding, Fertility, and Maternal Condition

Peter T. Ellison

INTRODUCTION

In 1961, in a seminal contribution to the literature on human fertility, the French demographer Louis Henry ventured a bold suggestion: that the practice of lactation might act as the primary determinant of fertility variation in "natural fertility" populations (i.e., those without evidence of conscious limitation of family size) (Henry, 1961). The notion that breastfeeding lowers the likelihood of pregnancy, although long a part of Western cultural tradition, was still largely considered an "old wives' tale" among physicians and population scientists at the time Henry wrote. Indeed, in their landmark paper of 1956 purporting to exhaustively list the intermediate variables by which human fertility levels must be determined, Kingsley Davis and Judith Blake make no mention of lactation (Davis and Blake, 1956). Similarly, in the influential 1954 UNESCO volume, *Culture and Human Fertility*, edited by Frank Lorimer (Lorimer, 1954), cultural prohibitions on intercourse during lactation are presented as demographically significant, but no direct physiological effect of breastfeeding itself on female fecundity is mentioned.

Yet in 1988, less than 30 years since the publication of Henry's paper, an international conference was convened in Bellagio, Italy, jointly sponsored by the Rockefeller Foundation, the World Health Organization, and Family Health International, expressly to arrive at "a consensus about the conditions under which breastfeeding can be used as a safe and effective method of family planning" (Kennedy, Rivera and McNeilly, 1989:447). No longer classed as mere folk wisdom, the lactational suppression of female fecundity has now been exalted to the status of a virtual principle of human population biology and public health policy.

This small scientific revolution was achieved through a conjunction of research spanning an array of disciplines, including medicine, endocrinology, demography, and anthropology. The transdisciplinary nature of this area of human fertility research makes it at once fascinating and obscure. The purpose of this chapter is to review what we now think we know about the role of lactation in modulating female fecundity and how we came to know it, as well as to point out what we still do not know. To achieve this end, it is necessary to pick up the threads of the discourse that brought us from Henry's speculations to the Bellagio Consensus. It will also be useful to distinguish from the outset between three terms that are easily confused. Fertility refers to the actual production of offspring; fecundity refers to the biological capacity to produce offspring. A man or woman may be fully fecund and yet, if they have not yet had children, be technically infertile. Fecundability is a much more restricted aspect of female fecundity, referring to the monthly probability of conception in a woman engaged in unprotected intercourse. It does not include, for example, postconceptive variation in fecundity due to embryonic or fetal loss.

HENRY'S HYPOTHESIS

In his landmark paper, "Some data on natural fertility" (Henry, 1961), Louis Henry quite transformed both the nature of analytical approaches to the study of human fertility and the research agenda itself. Henry directed his attention toward variation in human fertility that is not a result of conscious control of family size by defining "natural fertility" precisely as absence of such control. He also confined his attention to marital fertility rates. By adopting these two conventions he eliminated *ab initio* the two sources of variation in human fertility that had dominated the attention of other investigators, such as Davis and Blake (1956): variation in contraceptive usage and variation in marriage patterns (both age at marriage and percentage of women ever married). The basic Malthusian assumption latent in most thinking on human population dynamics, that human fertility unconstrained by conventions of marriage or individual "moral restraint" would be constant and superprolific, was also laid bare by this approach and shown to be incorrect. Rather, the variation in total marital fertility rates manifest in even the small sample of 13 natural fertility populations that Henry assembled varied from 6 to 11 offspring over a woman's reproductive career, a range that has only been increased by subsequent research. He also found that the relative age pattern of fertility across his sample of 13 societies was remarkably constant, a result that has also been confirmed subsequently. Having produced these unexpected results, Henry asked the next logical question: what could account for such a range of fertility levels and yet produce such conformity of age pattern?

To pursue this question Henry introduced a new analytical framework that reflected the temporal nature of human reproduction as a physiological process. Having rejected interpopulation differences in the prevalence of sterility or in the ages at first or last birth as potential explanations, he focused attention on the time interval separating consecutive births. He subdivided this interbirth interval into three major components, the period of postpartum "nonsusceptibility" to conception, the period between the restoration of "susceptibility" and the next conception, and the period of gestation. In addition he noted the possibility of reproductive losses during gestation resulting in some of these subintervals occurring more than once in a given interbirth interval. Population level variation in natural marital fertility, he reasoned, must be traceable to population level variation in one or more of these components of the interbirth interval. Available evidence suggested that there was negligible variation in gestation length between populations, and only small variation in the waiting time to conception or the rate of gestational losses. The postpartum nonsusceptible period, on the other hand, appeared highly variable between populations. Two factors seemed potentially responsible for this variation: either variation must exist in the pace with which sexual intercourse resumes after childbirth, or variation must exist in the pace with which ovulation resumes. Anthropologists had been fond of citing variation in "postpartum taboos" on sexual intercourse, particularly in sub-Saharan Africa (Lorimer, 1954), and Davis and Blake had listed these as among the intermediate variables that generally suppress the fertility of nonindustrialized societies (Davis and Blake, 1956). Henry noted, however, that this explanation was not completely consistent with the information available on cultural practices and fertility in Africa, much less with the rest of the world. Rather, he suggested that variation in the resumption in ovulation, driven by variation in the practice of breastfeeding, might be the most important source of variation in interbirth intervals, and hence fertility, in natural fertility populations.

The data to support this contention in 1961 were still fairly thin, though there was evidence that women who never breastfed their offspring, e.g., because of neonatal death or stillbirth, usually resumed menstruating earlier than those who did breastfeed. Beyond that, however, lay a paradox.

> Ovulation is resumed very rapidly among some women even though they are suckling their babies. With others some time elapses after confinement before it is resumed but still before the infant is weaned; and with still others, it is resumed only after weaning. (Henry, 1961:90–91)

If we could ever understand how it is that women fall into these different categories, Henry reasoned, we would be well on our way to understanding variation in natural human fertility. He also noted that such an understanding would, in its essence, be "physiological" rather than sociological, another challenge to the basic Malthusian paradigm of human fertility.

> To accept the second explanation [of differing effects of lactation on the resumption of ovulation] is to admit that this physiological characteristic can be included among those which, for reasons of heredity or environment, vary from one population to another. Research in this field would help us to understand why there exists among populations such variability in natural fertility. (Henry, 1961:91)

In fact, although the phenomenon of postpartum amenorrhea was well known to clinicians and physiologists in Henry's day, it was not clear to what extent this suppression of ovarian cycling was a residual effect of pregnancy or a current effect of lactation. In one large study in the United States, for example, in which 2885 women were followed for a year postpartum, it was found that 71% resumed menstruating while still lactating at a median time of 4 months postpartum (Peckham, 1934). A smaller study a year later found a median time to resumption of menses among lactating mothers of less than 3 months (Booth, 1935), not much longer than the period of amenorrhea observed in nonlactating mothers. In both cases it was suggested that postpartum amenorrhea represented a variable refractory period on the part of the ovary and uterus after the stresses of pregnancy, and that the association with lactation was largely spurious.

In the years before the development of reliable chemical assays of ovarian hormones, the technique of endometrial biopsy provided more specific evidence of the resumption of ovarian activity than simple resumption of menses. Histological examination of endometrial tissue provides evidence of the action of progesterone, secreted by the corpus luteum of the ovary, which is, in turn, evidence of ovulation. Results generated from this technique indicated that the resumption of full postpartum fecundity in nursing women was an even more gradual process than the resumption of menses. In a study of 194 biopsies from 47 lactating women who had resumed menses, 45% showed evidence of ovulation while 55% did not (Lass, Smelser and Kurzrok, 1938). In 145 biopsies from 28 lactating women who were still amenorrheic, however, only 6% showed evidence of ovulation (Topkins, 1943). Udesky (1950) examined women at all stages of the postpartum resumption of ovarian function. In 200 biopsies from 85 lactating, amenorrheic women, only 1.5% showed evidence of ovulation; in 36 biopsies from lactating women performed from 2 weeks before to 4 weeks after their first postpartum menses, 14% showed evidence of ovulation; in a small sample of biopsies performed after at least three postpartum menses, 28% showed evidence of ovulation. The resumption of full ovarian function seemed to vary greatly between women, occurring early in some and much later in others. When pressed by colleagues to account for this variation, Udesky speculated, "It seemed to me that the intensity of the suckling and lactation process had a direct bearing upon the occurrence of ovulation" (Udesky, 1950:851).

This intuition regarding the "intensity" of lactation was not easily operationalized, however. The simplest distinction of levels of lactational intensity was to contrast "full" with "partial" or "supplemented" breastfeeding, and the results of such contrasts tended to support Udesky's notion. Sharman found that the median time of resumption of menses for British women practicing unsupplemented breastfeeding was 20 to 26 weeks, depending on parity, compared to 8 to 9 weeks for supplemented nursing (Sharman, 1951). McKeown and Gibson (1954) in a study of 943 lactating women found that 40% of mothers supplementing with formula and 57% of mothers supplementing breast milk with other foods were still amenorrheic at 4 months postpartum, compared to 95% of mothers practicing "full" breastfeeding. On the basis of such results Gioiosa suggested that one important function of lactation, besides its obvious nutritional role for the infant, might be to act as a "natural birth spacer," and advocated counseling mothers on the contraceptive benefits of lactation (Gioiosa, 1955).

It was not, then, an entirely radical proposition in 1961 for Henry to suggest that the practice of lactation could affect the fertility of individual women. What was daring was to suggest that the variation in natural human fertility, which Henry had shown to be so substantial, could be largely accounted for by this phenomenon. Two problems loomed as immediate obstacles to that idea, as judged from the perspective of Western clinical medicine. First was the fact that even where the data were good, lactational suppression of fertility appeared to be limited to the first 4 to 6 months postpartum, nowhere near enough of an effect to account for the variation in natural birth spacing Henry had documented. Second, after those first several months, the relationship between breastfeeding and ovarian function seemed too tenuous and unpredictable to bear the weight of such a hypothesis even if one imagined a less "modern" context.

OUT OF THE CLINIC AND INTO THE FIELD

The 1960s and 1970s produced an increasing number of reports from non-Western populations supporting and extending the relationships between the duration of lactation, postpartum amenorrhea, and interbirth intervals. Reports documented longer periods of postpartum amenorrhea among breastfeeding than nonbreastfeeding mothers in Nigeria (Martin, Morley and Woodland, 1964), India (Potter, New, Wyon and Gordon, 1965), Rwanda (Bonte and van Balen, 1969), Taiwan (Jain, 1969), the Philippines (Del Mundo and Adiao, 1970), Senegal (Cantrelle and Leridon, 1971), Egypt (El-Minawi and Foda, 1971), Alaskan Eskimos (Berman, Hanson and Hellman, 1972), Bangladesh and Pakistan (Chen, Ahmed, Gesche and Mosley, 1974; Chowdhury, Khan and Chen, 1976), and Zambia (Wenlock, 1977). Reviewing the data that had accumulated by the mid-1970s, Van Ginneken (1977) was able to show that the actual duration of postpartum amenorrhea was positively associated with the duration of lactation—the longer a woman breastfed her offspring the longer her period of amenorrhea, though for women who continued to nurse their children longer than 3 to 6 months, menses ordinarily resumed before weaning. Furthermore, periods of amenorrhea considerably longer than the median 3- to 4-month period in Western women were commonly observed, up to median durations of 20 months. But variance in the relationship, both within and between populations, was considerable. Even in populations like India, Taiwan, and South Korea, where lactation was prolonged and the median duration of amenorrhea about 12 months, 15–20% of women resumed cycling as early as 3 months after delivery, scarcely later than nonnursing mothers in the same populations. Henry's central problem, the explanation for this tremendous variability, remained unsolved.

Two clues to this puzzle appeared in print in the same year, and in the same journal, as Van Ginneken's review (*Journal of Biosocial Science*). The first was a summary of new information regarding the neuroendocrine control of lactation (Tyson, 1977). Tyson was able to assemble, at an astonishingly early date,[1] a quite accurate picture of the dynamics of neuroendocrine responses to nursing. At the center of attention was the hormone prolactin, produced by the pituitary throughout pregnancy and during lactation in response to physical stimulation of the nipple.

The primary physiological role of prolactin, from which it derives its name, is in promoting milk production. The system in which it functions is essentially self-regulating. Each time a baby draws milk from the nipple, the stimulation that the suckling provides signals the hypothalamus to trigger the release of prolactin, thus sustaining milk production. When a baby ceases to nurse, either because it has died or because it has been weaned, the absence of nipple stimulation allows prolactin levels to fall and milk production ceases. But the striking contribution of Tyson's 1977 paper was the depiction of moment-to-moment changes in prolactin over 8 hours in nursing mothers with infants of various ages. Although anecdotal in coverage (only five 8-hour series are shown), the dynamics of the relationship between prolactin concentrations and suckling are, at least in gross form, unmistakable (Figure 11.1). Each time the infant takes the nipple, prolactin levels shoot up within minutes, often to many times their baseline values. Then, soon after the infant stops sucking, the prolactin levels begin a slower, exponential decay.

Clinical data already had begun to suggest that prolactin itself might be linked to the suppression of ovarian function in lactating women, since women suffering from prolactin-secreting pituitary tumors also showed suppressed ovarian activity, activity that returned when the hyperprolactinemia was brought under pharmacological control (Delvoye, Desnoeck-Delogne and Robyn, 1976; Robyn et al., 1976). Tyson's graphic depiction of the temporal relationship between prolactin and suckling, by revealing the transient nature of the prolactin response, immediately suggested that the *frequency* of suckling might be of key importance in any effect of lactation in modulating ovarian function.

Delvoye, Demaegd, Delogne-Desnoeck and Robyn (1977) provided the second clue by demonstrating the empirical significance of this relationship in the field. Working with a natural fertility population in Zaïre where prolonged lactation was the norm, Delvoye et al. compared prolactin levels in plasma samples drawn *ad libitum* to self-reported nursing frequency in 97 women at various times postpartum. Separating these cross-sectional data by categories of nursing frequency showed clear differences in the trajectories of postpartum prolactin decline, with mothers nursing three times a day or less falling to the range of prolactin values typical of nonpregnant, nonlactating women within 6 months, while mothers who nursed more than six times a day maintained prolactin levels three times as high (Figure 11.2). In fact, among mothers nursing more than six times a day, there was no significant decline in prolactin over the first postpartum year! In a previous study of Western women Delvoye and colleagues had already shown that lactating women who were menstruating had lower prolactin levels than amenorrheic lactating women (Delvoye et al., 1976). So a tentative causal arrow could

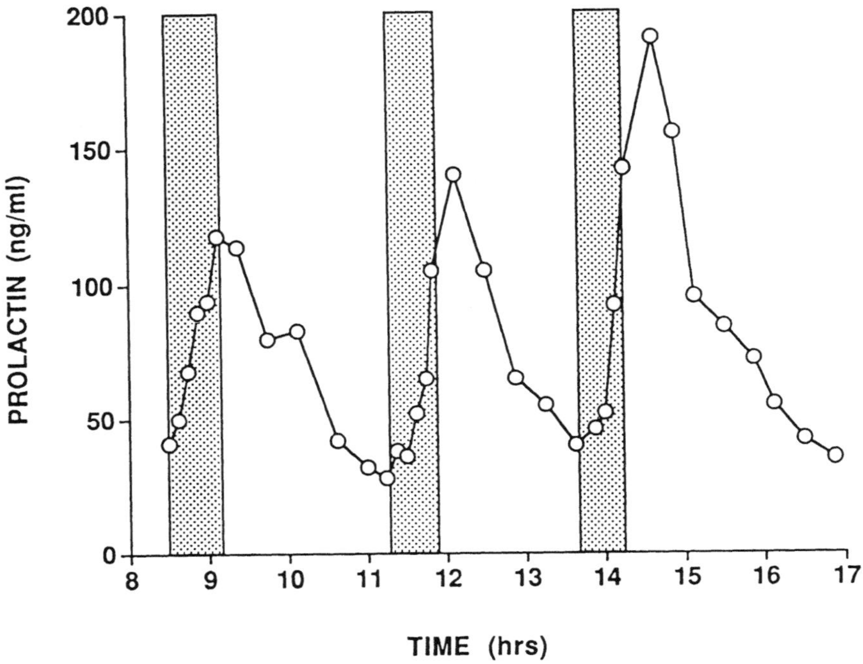

Figure 11.1. The time course of serum prolactin in relation to nursing episodes, designated by shaded bars, in one subject. Redrawn from Tyson (1977, Fig. 4, p. 29).

be established, from high nursing frequency, to higher average prolactin levels, to suppressed ovarian function, and the effectiveness of this mechanism could apparently extend for many months, or even years, postpartum.

The importance of this contribution is hard to overestimate. In the frequency of nursing could be found an apparently unambiguous, empirical quantification of Udesky's "intensity of suckling" with a clear physiological pathway linking it to the neuroendocrine mechanisms thought to govern the suppression of ovarian function. It at once seemed clear that the dichotomous analysis implicit in most preceding work, both clinical and demographic, contrasting lactating and nonlactating women had perhaps focused on the wrong variable. It might not be the *fact* of lactation but its *intensity*, as perhaps reflected in suckling frequency, that was key. In this new insight lay the promise of an answer to Henry's lingering problem: how to explain why some lactating women resume cycling rapidly postpartum while others remain amenorrheic for extended periods.

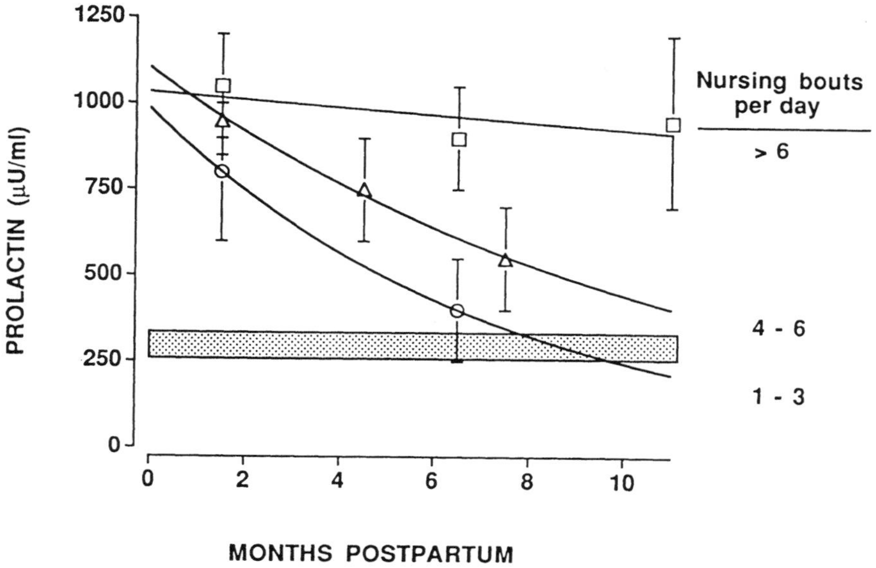

Figure 11.2. Plasma prolactin (mean ± SE) in random samples from lactating, amenorrheic Zaïrois women at various times postpartum, separated by the number of reported nursing episodes in the preceding 24 hours. Shaded area represents range of values in nonpregnant, nonlactating subjects. Redrawn from Delvoye et al. (1977, Fig. 2, p. 449).

Unfortunately, what seemed so promising in 1977 became problematic in 1978. A follow-up study in Zaïre of women in their second year of lactation found that prolactin levels, and hence nursing frequency, no longer discriminated significantly between menstruating and amenorrheic mothers (Delvoye, Demaegd, Uwayitu-Nyampeta and Robyn, 1978). Whatever caused extended amenorrhea during the second postpartum year could not be clearly linked to nursing frequency. By itself this observation did not negate the importance of nursing frequency as a proximate regulator of ovarian suppression during the first postpartum year. But it did mean that lactation might fall short of accounting for the full range of variation in interbirth intervals among natural fertility populations Henry had described.

A potential resolution to this problem appeared in 1980 when Konner and Worthman, two biological anthropologists, reported on nursing patterns and ovarian function among the !Kung San of the Kalahari Desert (Konner and Worthman, 1980). They documented a particularly intensive pattern of breastfeeding, extending well into the third year of a child's life and often beyond, and argued that such a pattern could extend the period of lactational suppression of ovarian function long enough to account for an interbirth interval of 44 months. The key to their analysis was to observe breastfeeding directly, rather than relying on mothers' retrospective self-reports. By following 17 mother–infant pairs for three 2-hour sessions on separate days, and 4 mother–infant pairs from dawn to dusk, recording all nursing activity to the nearest 30 seconds, they were able to provide an astonishingly detailed description of the choreography of suckling behavior, a choreography dramatically different from the Western norm, and even from that implied by the studies of Delvoye et al. (1976, 1977, 1978). Mothers nursed their children with a nearly uniform frequency across the day, averaging four bouts per hour of 2 minutes duration separated by 13 minute intervals. This high frequency was maintained even in children 18 to 24 months old. Such a pattern, they reasoned, might well maintain prolactin levels at a chronically high level and keep ovarian activity suppressed into the third year postpartum. Cross-sectional analyses of ovarian steroids in a subsample of !Kung mothers seemed to support the notion. Levels of the ovarian steroids estradiol and progesterone in randomly drawn blood samples from 16 nursing mothers rose with the age of the child, but in a pattern that was significantly correlated with the average length of the interval separating suckling bouts. Because the steroid levels were not correlated with the total time spent nursing, or with the average length of a bout, it seemed that the amount of milk being consumed was not an important factor. Rather the frequency of nipple stimulation, measured on a very fine time scale, emerged as the crucial determinant of lactational suppression of ovarian function among the !Kung.

The model that emerged from the seminal work of Tyson, Delvoye et al., and Konner and Worthman nicely integrated the behavioral and endocrinological aspects of human nursing into a story that seemed to make sense. When nursing bouts are widely spaced, as they often are in Western women who may be encouraged to train their infants to 4-hour feeding regimes, prolactin elevations are transient and separated by long periods of basal circulating levels of the hormone not significantly different from those in a nonpregnant, nonlactating woman. As the frequency of suckling increases, and the interval separating nursing bouts decreases, the fraction of time spent with elevated prolactin levels increases, until, at suckling frequencies as high as the !Kung's, the elevation of prolactin may become chronic (Figure 11.3). If, as the !Kung data suggested, this mechanism could be extended in time into the third year postpartum, it could well serve as an answer to Henry's original demographic conundrum. Interestingly, this solution derived not from demographic analyses, but from an improved understanding of the physiology of lactation and its hormonal correlates. As Henry had originally sus-

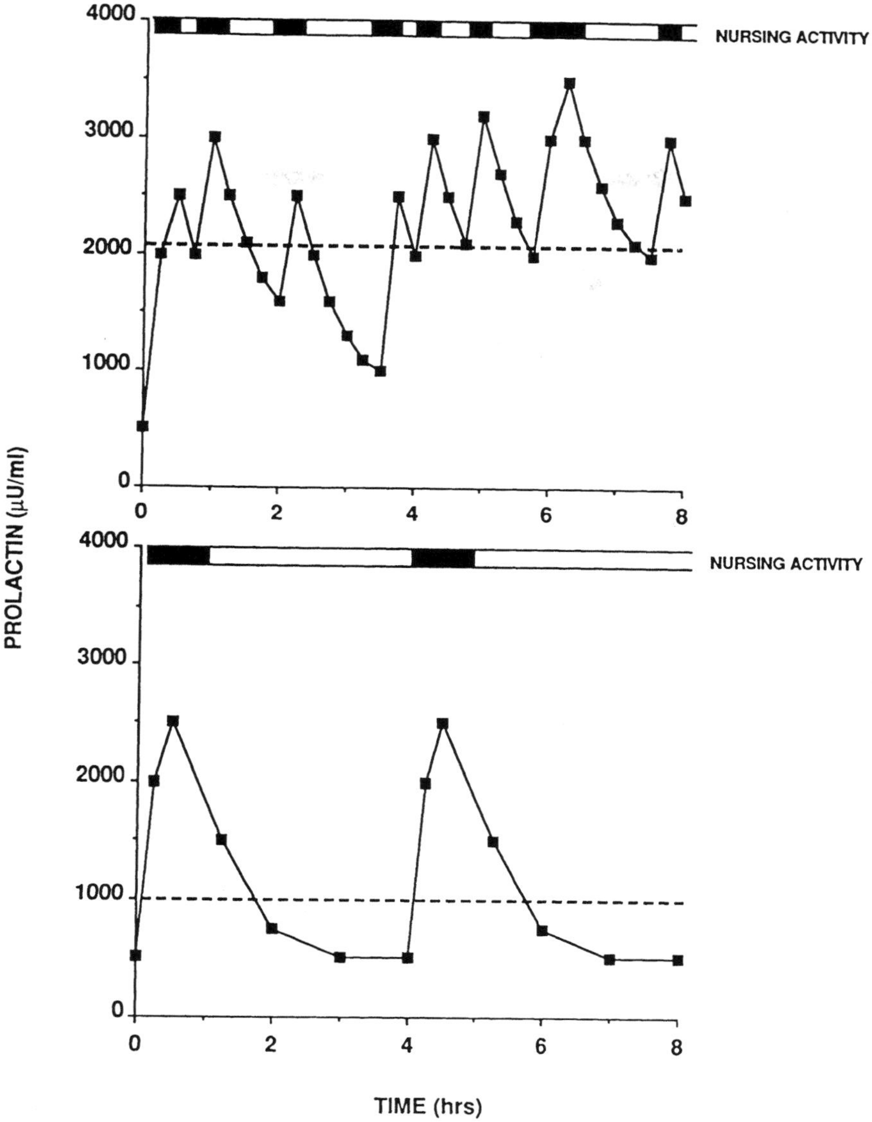

Figure 11.3. Schematic representation of the potential influence of nursing frequency and interbout interval on average circulating prolactin levels. Nursing bouts indicated by black portions of the nursing activity bar. Upper panel: A pattern of frequent, closely spaced nursing bouts results in chronically elevated prolactin with an average level above 2000 μU/ml. Lower panel: A pattern of infrequent, widely spaced nursing bouts, even if equivalent in total nursing time to the pattern of frequent bouts, results in prolactin levels that are only episodically elevated with average levels as low as 1000 μU/ml.

pected, natural fertility variation appeared to be a reflection of variation in biological functions, albeit an aspect of reproductive biology intimately connected with behavior. Indeed, it seemed that the high frequency of suckling among !Kung children was at least partly due to the nomadic lifestyle of their hunting and gathering parents. !Kung mothers had of necessity to spend long periods of time foraging for the vegetable foods that provided the bulk of their family's subsistence requirements and were accustomed to carry small children with them in a shoulder sling where they had continuous access to the breast. An indulgent cultural attitude toward children, together with a scarcity of good weaning foods, meant that toddlers were allowed to continue to nurse on demand well into their third year. Where cultural patterns regarding nursing and weaning differed, the neuroendocrine correlates of lactation would presumably vary as well, producing considerable variation in the modulation of ovarian function and hence fecundity.

Although compelling, this scenario was still largely hypothetical, and important questions remained. The precise definition of the "critical nursing variable" seemed to matter a great deal. Delvoye et al. had replaced the simple dichotomy of nursing/not nursing with "frequency of nursing." Konner and Worthman had refined the notion still further to "interbout interval." How could one be sure that some further refinement might not still be possible? The question of how long lactational suppression of ovarian function could be maintained remained open. Delvoye et al.'s (1978) data suggested that the effectiveness of nursing frequency in stimulating prolactin responses might decay with time postpartum, while Konner and Worthman's (1980) evidence suggested that some subtle change in the temporal pattern of nursing might be involved in that apparent decay. Was lactation *the answer* to variation in natural fertility, or only part of the answer?

THE CHOREOGRAPHY OF NURSING

Pursuing the relationship between temporal patterns of nursing behavior and either indices of ovarian function or resumption of postpartum menses has proved to be a difficult task. An extremely intensive investment of an investigator's time and effort is required in direct observation of nursing activity of individual mother–infant pairs. To date only a handful of studies have been published reporting such data, all with certain individual shortcomings, and with somewhat different results.

Wood and colleagues (Wood, Lai, Johnson, Campbell and Maslar, 1985) reported on breastfeeding patterns among Gainj women of highland Papua New Guinea, a group of subsistence horticulturalists, and their relationship to prolactin levels. Twenty-one mother–infant pairs were observed for one 8-hour day each, during which all suckling activity was recorded to the nearest second. These behavioral observations were matched with a single blood sample from which several reproductive hormones, including prolactin, were measured. Among the Gainj women, as among the !Kung, patterns of breastfeeding changed in a regular fashion with increasing infant age, older infants suckling less frequently and at wider intervals. Also like the !Kung, nursing activity was distributed rather uniformly across the day, in a pattern that suggested feeding on demand. Wood et al. (1985) compared the data on nursing patterns in a subset of 15 nursing mothers (those not already pregnant) to prolactin levels, rather than to steroid levels as Konner and Worthman (1980) had, but nonetheless with a similar result. Both age of the infant and the interval between suckling bouts emerged as strong determinants of maternal prolactin levels. Wood et al. (1985) pushed their analysis one step further, however, testing a particular causal model by path analysis, with the conclusion that the age of the infant (or time postpartum) made no significant independent contribution to the determination of prolactin levels over and above its effect on nursing patterns. That is, there was no evidence that the responsiveness of the pituitary to the stimulus of suckling decayed with time, at least into the third year.

Vitzthum (1989) studied nursing behavior among 10 rural Quechua women living at high altitude (4000 m) in Peru. A total of 86 hours of direct observation was carried out in 4-hour periods. As in Wood et al.'s study, suckling activity was recorded to the nearest second. Unlike previous investigators, however, Vitzthum recognized two levels of suckling behavior, "episodes" where intervals off the nipple are less than 5 seconds, and "sessions" that consist of groups of episodes separated by less than 1 minute. No hormonal data were collected to compare with observations of nursing activity, nor were these data analyzed by the menstrual status of the mothers. Rather, patterns of association were sought among the variables describing nursing behavior themselves and between those variables and characteristics such as infant's age, mother's age, and time of day. Although the Quechua women practice what is generally referred to as "demand feeding," Vitzthum described a structure to nursing activities that had been unreported in previous studies.

There is a distinct diurnal variation in the pattern of breastfeeding described by Vitzthum. More nursing occurred in the morning than in the afternoon, and whereas the total amount of suckling that occurred in the morning was a function of the infant's age, with older children nursing less, total time on the nipple in the afternoon was a function of the mother's age (or perhaps parity, closely associated with age in this population). Vitzthum notes at least two possible contributing factors to the afternoon nursing pattern. It might be that older women have a diminished capacity for milk production and curb suckling activity in response to a diminished supply. Alternatively, older women of higher parity may have more help available in the form of older daughters home from school in the afternoons able to assist in child care tasks.

A second important observation derived from the distinction of nursing "episodes" and "sessions," namely that total nursing time was primarily a function of the number of episodes per session, not the duration of individual episodes nor the frequency of sessions during the day, both of which remained fairly constant across both infant and maternal age. As a consequence, the average nonnursing interval did not change significantly in length with time postpartum and was considered unlikely to be an important determinant of the timing of menstrual resumption. What did change as offspring aged was the total amount of time spent on the nipple. Total nursing time declined as babies nursed for fewer episodes in each session as they grew older, even though the number of sessions per day stayed fairly constant.

Jones (1989) collected information on nursing patterns and menstruation by recall during monthly visits to 44 Indonesian women over 2 years. Three indices of nursing activity were derived from the data collected for each woman: number of minutes per nursing episode, number of episodes per day, and number of episodes per night. High values for all three measures of nursing activity were associated independently with a delay in the resumption of postpartum menses. The longest durations of amenorrhea were observed in conjunction with high scores on both the number of minutes per episode and the number of episodes per day or night. Some question, however, can be raised concerning the ability of the subjects in this study to recall nursing activity with sufficient accuracy and precision to permit adequate discrimination of the different aspects of nursing activity.

Panter-Brick (1991) trained local assistants to help her observe breastfeeding practices of 16 Tamang and 8 Kami mother–infant pairs at moderate altitude (2000 m) in Nepal as part of a larger study of time-allocation among these two ethnic/caste groups. The Tamang are agro-pastoralists of Tibetan origin who cultivate various crops and husband animals at a series of altitudes up and down the mountainside between 1350 and 2500 m. The Kami are low-caste blacksmiths of Aryan background who do little agricultural work. Observations of each woman's activities were carried out several occasions during the year from sunrise to sunset totaling 2202 hours of direct observation. Nursing activities were recorded to the nearest minute. Like Vitzthum, Panter-Brick did not analyze her data with respect to hormonal variables or menstrual status, but rather sought to understand how nursing behavior was structured in these two groups and how it varied with infant's age and season of the year. (Panter-Brick has, however, collected hormonal data in conjunction with observations of nursing behavior in a more recent field study among the Tamang and Kami. Preliminary results of this work were reported at the 1994 meeting of the American Association of Physical Anthropologists.)

An important contribution of these studies is an increased appreciation for the way in which individual women integrate their child care activities with other subsistence and household chores. Indeed, as Panter-Brick observes, women in her study followed nursing schedules "based 'on opportunity' as well as 'on demand.'" This was particularly evident in the comparison of nursing activities during agricultural labor versus husbandry, and during individual versus group labor. Where Tamang and Kami women have a greater opportunity to indulge their offspring and feed "on demand," they do. But such freedom is often constrained by the type of subsistence labor a woman may be engaged in on a given day.

Nevertheless, the results of this study are in some ways surprising. Among the Tamang agro-pastoralists, infant's age had a strong effect on the frequency and duration of nursing bouts (declining with age), the interval between bouts (increasing with age), and the total time spent nursing during the day (decreasing with age), but these relationships did not hold for the blacksmith-caste Kami. Conversely, breastfeeding activity showed strong seasonal variation among the Kami for children of all ages, with greater nursing activity during the monsoon and less in the winter, while no seasonal variation was apparent among Tamang children less than 3 years old. This latter result seems somewhat counterintuitive, in that Tamang subsistence activities are much more profoundly affected by season than are Kami activities. But it is the different relationships to infant age between the two ethnic groups that are most difficult to reconcile with the notion that the temporal pattern of breastfeeding is the primary determinant of lactational suppression of ovarian function. Although Panter-Brick did not collect hormonal data on her subjects in her original research, average interbirth intervals among the Kami (29.4 months) are significantly shorter than among the Tamang (37.7 months), despite the fact that the Kami maintain a pattern of frequent nursing as their offspring age while the Tamang taper off nursing activities with time postpartum.

The standard of data collection set by these studies is extremely high, and in fact presents something of a problem for those interested in rigorously testing the idea that breastfeeding practices significantly influence natural human fertility. As we shall see, the bulk of the work on this question has been carried out at a *macro* level of analysis where statistical analysis of interbirth intervals can be carried out on large populations. Yet the line of research that originated with Delvoye et al.'s work has led instead to a very fine-grained, *micro* level of analysis where hours must be spent watching single mother–infant pairs, and then controlling those observations by mother's age and parity, season, type of subsistence work, and general opportunity to nurse. Such few studies as have been conducted at this level are not in full agreement with each other, either. Konner and Worthman (1980) and Wood et al. (1985) stress the importance of interbout interval, but Vitzthum (1989) suggests that in her population, total time spent nursing seems more important while interbout interval is relatively invariant. Panter-Brick (1991, 1992a,b) finds that these two aspects of nursing behavior by and large covary, but that both are constrained by opportunity, caste, and season as much as by infant's age. In addition to the important differences in reported results, which may well be a reflection of the cultural diversity of the populations studied, there are important methodological differences among the investigators and their respective research designs. Exactly how a nursing "event" should be defined has an important impact on the quantitative results that will come from a given study. Setting the minimum separation between events at 1 second will result in many more events and much shorter interevent intervals than setting the minimum separation at 1 minute. Further, some studies have compared nursing variables to hormonal measures, while some have not. Konner and Worthman (1980) compared their nursing data to steroid values; Wood et al. (1985) compared theirs to prolactin values. It seems as if the "answer" to Henry's problem—the importance of the temporal pattern of breastfeeding as opposed to the simple dichotomous variable "nursing/not nursing"—has itself become a problem of enormous complexity.

All of the studies reviewed here share an additional limitation, in that they are all essentially cross-sectional in design. The biology of lactational suppression of ovarian function is essentially diachronic: what we would like to understand is the process by which a woman passes from a state of initial ovarian quiescence back to a state of full fecundity. Yet if the observation of the temporal patterning of nursing activities is labor intensive, how much more intensive is it to attempt to document longitudinal changes in breastfeeding patterns with time postpartum in individual women, and to complement that effort with hormonal data over the same period of time?

THE RETURN TO FULL FECUNDITY

As daunting as the task may seem, several researchers have documented various aspects of the return to full fecundity in the postpartum human female. The most thorough and influential of those studies was conducted by A. S. McNeilly, P. W. Howie, and their colleagues at the University of Edinburgh in the late 1970s, culminating in a series of publications in the early 1980s (Glasier, McNeilly and Howie, 1983; Howie, McNeilly, Houston, Cook and Boyle, 1982a,b; McNeilly, Howie, Houston, Cook and Boyle, 1982; McNeilly, Glasier, Howie, Houston, Cook and Boyle, 1983). A nice summary of many of those results is available in Howie and McNeilly (1982), which also discusses the policy implications of this line of research from the authors' perspective. A few other, less comprehensive studies have been carried out by other groups with results that by and large confirm those of the Edinburgh group, but with some differences worth noting. Among the most important results of the Edinburgh study are (1) the observation that ovarian function resumes more or less gradually in lactating women, not abruptly, and (2) the important influence of the introduction of supplemental foods into the infant's diet on subsequent nursing behavior.

The Edinburgh study involved 37 mothers, 27 of whom breastfed and 10 of whom bottle-fed their babies from birth. These mother–infant pairs were followed longitudinally from the birth of the baby through the resumption of ovarian activity and ovulation in the mother. Mothers kept daily records of the duration, timing, and number of suckling episodes (strict definition of a suckling episode is not given), the number of supplementary feeds (either formula or solid food), and periods of menstrual bleeding. Twenty-four hour urine samples were collected each week for estimation of ovarian steroid production. Every 2 weeks the mothers were visited by a researcher who collected the accumulated data and samples since the previous visit and drew a blood sample for prolactin determination, at least 2 hours after the most recent nursing bout. From these data an extremely detailed picture was compiled of the diachronic changes in mother–infant nursing behavior and its relationship to both the introduction of supplementary foods and the hormonal profile of the mother. The hormonal profile of the mother was itself resolved into changes in prolactin levels and changes in ovarian activity, and the relationship of these two dimensions to each other were explored. No other study has been as complete in the array of information collected.

The results of the Edinburgh study appeared in a series of five publications in *Clinical Endocrinology* in 1982 and 1983, each with the primary title "Fertility after childbirth." These papers dealt in sequence[2] with the relationship of breastfeeding patterns to ovulation and menstruation, prolactin profiles, luteal function, rates of conception, and patterns of gonadotropin secretion. The results presented in the first paper (Howie et al., 1982a) confirmed the generally suppressive effect of lactation on ovarian function, but presented that suppression in a diachronic framework. Lactating women resumed ovarian function later postpartum than those who bottle-fed, as indicated both by dates of first menstruation (32.5 ± 2.5 vs. 8.1 ± 1.0 weeks postpartum, mean $\pm$ standard error) and first ovulation (36.4 ± 2.5 vs. 10.8 ± 1.0 weeks postpartum). In breastfeeding mothers the frequency of ovulation (as determined from urinary steroid levels) increased with time and as lactation was phased out, occurring in 45% of the first cycles during lactation, 66% of subsequent cycles during lactation, 70% of first cycles after weaning, and 84% of subsequent cycles after weaning. This gradual resumption of full ovarian activity contrasted sharply with the rapid resumption of activity in bottle feeders, among whom 94% of second and subsequent cycles were ovulatory. Thus, not only was the initiation of postpartum ovarian activity significantly delayed by lactation, the pace of resumption of full ovarian function was significantly slowed.

The second paper (Howie et al., 1982b) focused on prolactin as the potential intermediate variable between nursing patterns and ovarian function in the 27 breastfeeding mothers. Thirteen of those mothers had their first ovulation while still lactating while the other 14 had suppressed ovarian function throughout the period of lactation. Those who resumed ovulating during lactation had all recently changed their pattern of breastfeeding, reducing nursing frequency to <6 bouts/day, total nursing time to <60 minutes/day, and introducing at least two supplementary feeds per day. In association with this change in feeding pattern, average prolactin levels had fallen to 367 ± 63 micro-International Units per liter (μU/liter),[3] well into the range of nonpregnant, nonlactating women, at the time of first ovulation. When the subjects were divided into three roughly equal groups—those who resumed ovulating before 30 weeks postpartum (early), between 30 and 40 weeks postpartum (middle), or later than 40 weeks postpartum (late)—different trajectories of prolactin and nursing behavior were apparent as well. The early-ovulation group nursed with equal frequency but for significantly less total time than the other two groups from the earliest weeks postpartum, introduced supplementary foods more rapidly, and abandoned nighttime nursing sooner. They also had prolactin levels that were consistently lower than those of the other groups, with average values reaching the nonpregnant, nonlactating level by 20 weeks postpartum. Members of the late-ovulating group, in contrast, were nursing more in total time at 20 weeks postpartum than the early-ovulating group had been at 4 weeks, maintained a high nursing frequency (>4 times/day on average) for over 30 weeks, and introduced supplementary foods much more slowly. In addition, 85% of the late-ovulating group continued the regime of nighttime nursing through 40 weeks postpartum, after all the infants of the early-ovulating mothers had been fully weaned. Prolactin levels in the late-ovulating group were nearly twice as high as those of the early-ovulating group at 4 weeks postpartum and did not fall into the nonpregnant, nonlactating range until between 30 and 40 weeks postpartum. The middle-ovulating group fell nicely in-between the early and late groups on all measures.

The third paper (McNeilly et al., 1982) provided a more detailed examination of the profiles of ovarian function in both breast and bottle feeders in the first postpartum cycles. In both groups of mothers, there was a transitional period in ovarian activity, with a high initial frequency of anovulatory cycles, followed by a lower frequency of anovulation but a high frequency of luteally deficient cycles, and finally a high frequency of fully competent cycles (Figure 11.4).

The fourth paper (McNeilly et al., 1983) dealt with the probability of conception during lactation. Twelve of the breastfeeding mothers used no other contraception during the study. Eight pregnancies occurred in this group during the study, seven during the period of lactation and one 2 weeks after weaning. Of the seven conceptions that occurred during lactation, one occurred prior to any postpartum menstruation. The other six were preceded by a total of 19 menstrual cycles, 4 of which

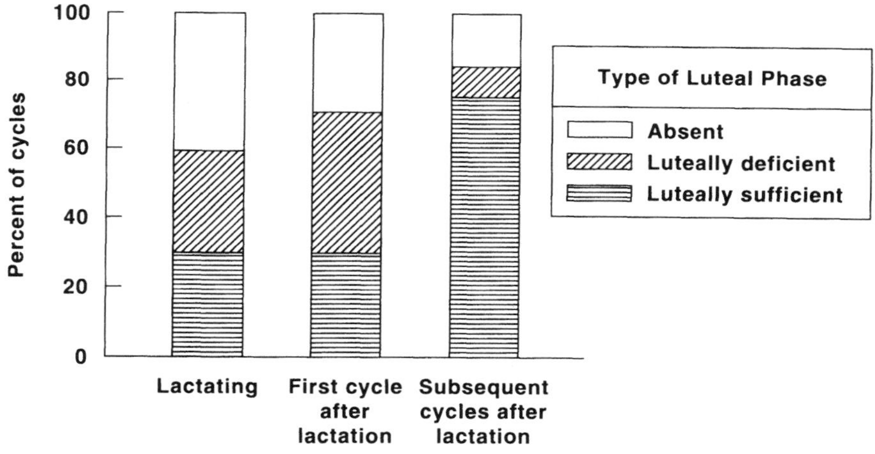

Figure 11.4. Observed quality of postpartum menstrual cycles before and after weaning in Edinburgh women. Data from McNeilly et al. (1982, Table 1, p. 611).

were anovulatory and 13 of which were luteally deficient. All of the mothers who conceived had recently decreased the frequency of their nursing activity to three or fewer times per day. All but one had decreased the total time spent nursing to ≤30 minutes/day.

The fifth paper (Glasier et al., 1983) sought to explore the mechanisms involved in lactational suppression of ovarian function, examining changes in gonadotropin levels in both breast and bottle feeders. The results were somewhat surprising, in that follicle-stimulating hormone (FSH) levels were normal from the earliest postpartum weeks in both groups while leutinizing hormone (LH) levels were initially suppressed and remained suppressed through the period of ovarian quiescence and luteal deficiency, not attaining normal levels until the appearance of fully competent cycles. The resumption of follicular activity thus remained unexplained by observed changes in serum gonadotropins.

The richness of this set of data is most apparent in the composite, longitudinal profiles that can be constructed for individual women, some of which demonstrate nicely the relationships analyzed separately in the five papers mentioned. For example, in Figure 11.5 one can easily see the shift in nursing patterns that accompanies the introduction of solid food. As suggested by Vitzthum's (1989) work, it is not the number of nursing episodes (Vitzthum's "sessions") that declines with the introduction of solid supplements as much as the amount of time spent suckling at each episode, resulting in a rapid decline in the total time spent nursing to less than half its previous value in the course of a month. Prolactin levels fall from their initially high late pregnancy and immediate postpartum levels over the first 3 months of the infant's life, and then stabilize at something over 1000 μU/liter. The introduction of solid foods is associated with a transient decline in prolactin levels that then recover and decline only slowly as suckling frequency declines. Soon after weaning, prolactin levels fall below 500 μU/liter into the normal range for nonpregnant, nonlactating women. Ovarian activity resumes at about this time as well, some 38 to 40 weeks postpartum, first with rising estrogen levels indicative of follicular maturation but with no luteal activity. The first postpartum menstruation occurs at about 47 weeks, or 2 months after the resumption of follicular activity, terminating an apparently anovulatory cycle. The subsequent cycle is rather long, about 6 weeks in length, ending with menses at about 53 weeks, but includes elevated pregnanediol levels indicating ovulation and a robust luteal phase. A year after the birth of her child, this subject has returned to full fecundity.

This picture of the longitudinal return to full fecundity has several noteworthy features. Perhaps the most influential general result of this study has been recognition of the importance of the introduction of

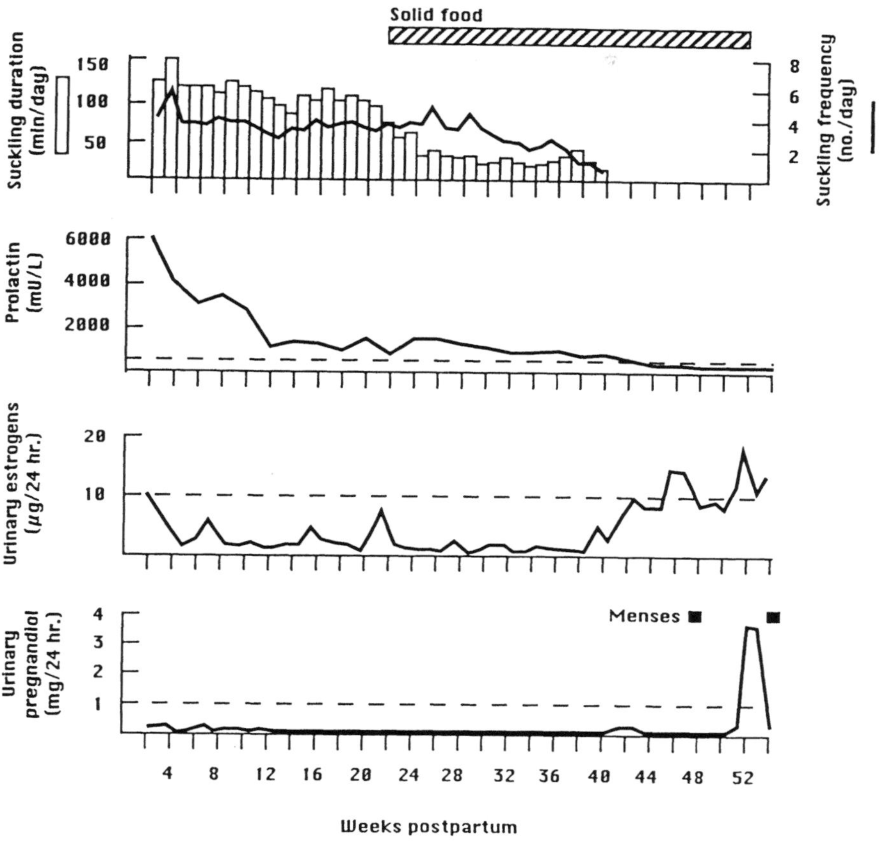

Figure 11.5. Postpartum time course of nursing activity, prolactin, and urinary ovarian steroid metabolites, and their responses to the introduction of solid foods in one Edinburgh subject. Redrawn from Howie and McNeilly (1982, Fig. 4, p. 548).

supplementary food as the key event in the course of lactation that seems to set all the others in motion. In some ways this observation released the demographic investigator from the dilemma that previous research on the temporal pattern of nursing had created. Detailed, minute-to-minute observations of nursing behavior are generally beyond the scope of most broad-scale, demographic research; yet the simple nursing/not nursing dichotomy is just as obviously inadequate to capture the important aspect of lactational suppression of ovarian function. The Edinburgh study, however, seemed to suggest that a full breastfeeding/partial breastfeeding dichotomy might succeed where the nursing/not nursing dichotomy failed. That is, documenting the date of the introduction of some certain amount of solid food into the infant's diet might provide a good index of the duration of lactational suppression of ovarian function, better, perhaps, than the ultimate date of weaning, which often happens long after ovarian function has resumed. In one influential summary article, for example, Howie and McNeilly (1982) align their data on the date of introduction of supplementary foods rather than on the date of birth of the baby, stressing the interpretation of this as the key event in the longitudinal process of lactation.

In general, however, this possibility must be entertained with skepticism. Western mothers, whether Scottish or American, may guide their babies through a more abrupt transition to solid foods than mothers in other societies. With a vast array of easily digestible, palatable, convenient "weaning foods" at their disposal on supermarket shelves, Western mothers may find it easy to satisfy the growing appetites of their children to a significant degree with solid foods soon after their initial introduction, whereas mothers in other societies, under extremely different subsistence regimes, may have far fewer suitable foods available, or may have to invest much more time and energy in their preparation. The tempo of introduction of solid foods in Western societies may also be influenced more by pediatricians' advice rather than by the child's appetite. Certainly it is true that the introduction of supplementary foods in many societies in the developing world is a period of heightened risk for the children, with "weanling diarrhea" causing a significant elevation in rates of morbidity and mortality (Gordon, Chitkara and Wyon, 1963; Weaver and Beckerleg, 1993). This fact may contribute in more than one way to a cultural pattern of gradual transition to solid foods: sick babies may have less appetite for solid foods and receive more nursing time whether for nutritional reasons or simply for comfort; mothers may have additional motivation to delay the introduction of and full transition to solid foods and to continue breastfeeding for the sake of their children's health, whether this motivation is conscious or merely "cultural wisdom" (Dettwyler, 1989). To date we have nothing approaching the data of the Edinburgh study for any society in the developing world, and we must certainly refrain from generalizing too liberally, even from so excellent a study, on points where there is likely to be great cultural heterogeneity.

Another important generalization emerging from the Edinburgh study concerns the gradual pace of the resumption of full ovarian activity. Resumption of menses is not synonymous with the resumption of full fecundity. Rather, within each individual woman, ovarian activity seems to be reestablished in a series of steps along a set trajectory: follicular activity resumes first, evidenced by cyclically rising and falling

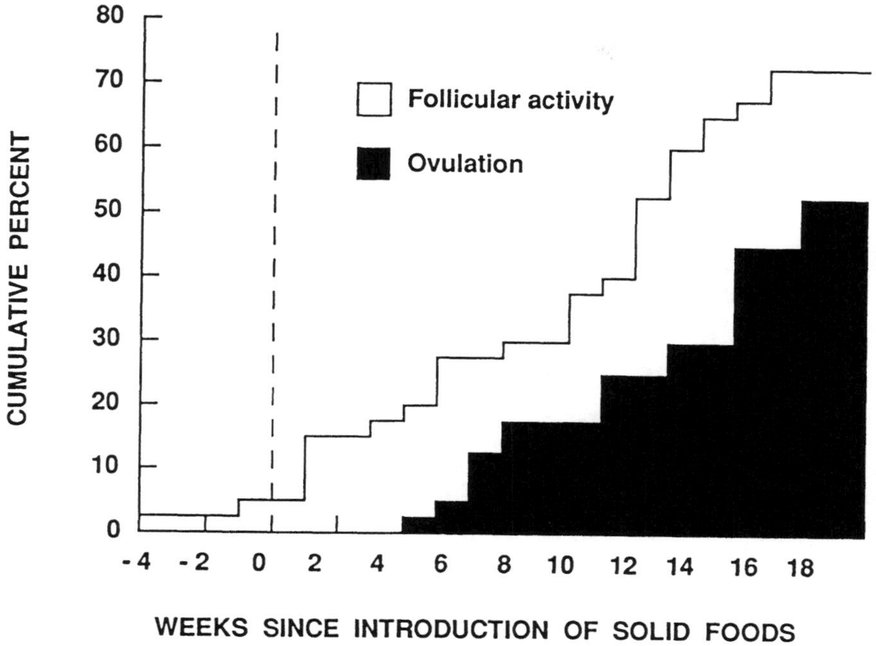

Figure 11.6. Cumulative resumption of ovarian activity in relation to the introduction of solid foods in Edinburgh women. Redrawn from Howie and McNeilly (1982, Fig. 9, p. 553).

estrogen levels; menses resume as a result of the stimulation of endometrial proliferation that occurs when estrogen titers reach sufficient levels; ovulation, evidenced by a significant rise in progesterone or its metabolites, resumes when estrogen levels become high enough to trigger a positive feedback LH surge, levels that are generally much higher than those required to stimulate endometrial development; finally, full luteal competence is established when the postovulatory rise in progesterone attains an elevation and duration comparable to that in regularly cycling women who have not recently been pregnant or lactating. This transitional sequence may be relatively compressed or drawn out in individual women. The fact that a few percent of women become pregnant without ever experiencing postpartum menses is evidence that the full transition may occur very quickly, while in the Edinburgh study some women took many months to pass completely from the stage of initial follicular activity to that of full luteal competence (Figure 11.6).

A comparable description of the process of postpartum resumption of ovarian function has emerged from a more limited study in Santiago,

Chile (Diaz, Cardenas, Brandeis, Miranda, Salvatierra and Croxatto, 1992). Yet, in the absence of comparable data from societies with distinctly different socioeconomic and cultural circumstances, it is probably well to refrain from further extrapolating the Edinburgh results on this point. It is possible, for example, that under different conditions this period of transition may have a much broader range of variation than it does in Scotland. Indeed, the range of duration of postpartum suppression of ovarian function in the Edinburgh study is much less than what appears to be the case on a worldwide basis. It is possible and even likely that the variation in duration of the various components of this longitudinal process will be much greater under other circumstances as well.

A handful of other studies have investigated aspects of the longitudinal return to full postpartum fecundity, though none so fully as the Edinburgh study. Two have focused on populations of women who, although drawn from Western societies, practice patterns of breastfeeding that are more intensive and prolonged than the pattern of the Scottish mothers. Brown and colleagues at the University of Melbourne reported in 1985 on a study, actually conducted in 1971–1972, of 55 Australian women (Brown, Harrisson and Smith, 1985). Many of the subjects were members of the Australian Nursing Mothers' Association (an association promoting the practice of breastfeeding). All of the subjects used a method of natural family planning based on monitoring cervical mucus changes (though not all were actively trying to avoid pregnancy during the study). The original intention of the study, which included nonlactating women as well, was to aid in the development of a reliable method of birth control based on monitoring two physical signs of ovulation, elevation of basal body temperature and thinning of cervical mucus. All the lactating subjects recorded daily information on times and durations of nursing sessions, the introduction of solid and supplementary foods, nighttime nursing, and comfort nursing. Menses were recorded as well as cervical mucus scores. Weekly urine samples were collected for measurement of estrogen and progesterone metabolites. Because the focus of the original study was on predicting the return of fecundity from physical symptoms rather than on the relationship between breastfeeding patterns and the return of fecundity (note that the study was carried out 5 years before Delvoye et al., 1977), no information is provided coupling changes in nursing patterns with changes in ovarian function. Nevertheless, the results of the Australian study do corroborate those of the Edinburgh study in several important areas.

Most importantly, like the Edinburgh study, the Australian data also depict a graded progression to the return of full fecundity through stages of follicular activity without menstruation, menstruation without ovulation, ovulation without luteal competence, and finally fully competent cycles. The subjects in the Australian study did tend to nurse their children for a longer time postpartum than the Scottish subjects, with a median weaning age of about 46 weeks. Interestingly, their progress through the stages of resumption of ovarian activity was also slower than the Scottish group. Among women who resumed initial signs of ovarian activity between 6 and 12 months postpartum, 75% of cycles were fully competent at a date 7 to 12 months after the resumption of menses. Among women who initially resumed signs of ovarian activity between 12 and 24 months, only 85% of cycles were fully competent 7 to 12 months after resumption of menses. This frequency of fully competent cycles was significantly lower than that in a nonlactating control group assessed by the same criteria (96%), suggesting that lactation maintained a suppressive effect on ovarian function, at least in some women, well into the second year postpartum and long after menstrual cycles had resumed. Twenty-two pregnancies occurred during the study, 14 of them unplanned, and their distribution supports the interpretation that full fecundity returns only with fully competent cycles. The 22 conceptions occurred between the second and the thirteenth postpartum menstrual cycles, preceded in 17 cases by at least one fully competent cycle. Many of the women recorded acts of intercourse during the study, yet no conceptions occurred during luteally deficient cycles even when coitus was close in time to ovulation. As a whole, the results of this study confirm the picture provided by the Edinburgh study of a gradual process of return to full fecundity, and add weight to the possibility that the period of transition from initial to full ovarian activity may be particularly drawn out when breastfeeding is intense and prolonged.

Elias, Teas, Johnston and Bora (1986) reported on a study of 30 Boston area women, half of whom were members of La Leche League (an international association promoting the practice of breastfeeding) and highly motivated to nurse their infants on demand. The other half were solicited from newspaper birth announcements and nursed their babies on a less frequent schedule. Although no hormonal data were collected in this study, various aspects of the pattern of nursing activity were examined with respect to the timing of the resumption of postpartum menstruation. The most important predictors of prolonged amenorrhea were full breastfeeding (i.e., without any supplements) and nursing at night. For the League mothers, who nursed their offspring an average of 10 times per day, the occurrence of nighttime nursing was particularly important in maintaining postpartum amenorrhea; for the non-League mothers, who nursed an average of 5 times a day, full breastfeeding was a more important predictor. The importance of full breastfeeding among the non-League mothers is in line with the importance of the introduction of solid foods in the Edinburgh study. The importance of nighttime nursing among the League mothers is intriguing as it suggests a potential circadian variation in the suppressive effect of suckling on ovarian activity.

One longitudinal study of lactation and the resumption of ovarian function has been carried out in a rural community of a developing country. Roberto Rivera and his colleagues (Rivera, Ortiz, Barrera, Kennedy and Bhiwandiwala, 1985) followed 29 breastfeeding mothers and 8 bottle-feeding controls from a rural part of the Mexican state of Durango for up to a year postpartum, collecting information on nursing frequency, supplemental feeding, and menstruation by self-report, together with weekly urine samples for pregnanediol determinations and monthly serum samples for prolactin determinations. These researchers designed an elegant card on which women could record information, using pictures of nursing mothers and typical supplementary foods, grouped under simple symbols for daytime and nighttime. The results of the Mexican study broadly corroborate those of other studies. All of the bottle-feeders had resumed ovulation by 6 months postpartum while only 66% of the breastfeeders had. By 12 months postpartum 28% of the nursing mothers were still anovulatory. As in the Edinburgh study, nonovulators maintained a higher frequency of nursing than ovulators at the same point postpartum, and the earlier the introduction of supplementary food, the earlier the resumption of ovarian function. The cumulative pregnancy rate had reached 50% among bottle-feeders by 9 months postpartum, while the comparable rate among breastfeeding mothers was only 7%. This study provides the most complete information of the postpartum return of fecundity in a developing country, though it must be noted that the Mexican government has a vigorous family planning program.

The detailed evidence of the Edinburgh study together with the more limited results of other studies allow us to identify those aspects of the longitudinal return to full fecundity postpartum in individual women that at this time seem most certain and generalizable. First, the timing of the transition to full ovarian function appears to be related to changes in the temporal pattern and intensity of nursing. Second, the transition to full ovarian function passes through an identifiable sequence of phases with measurable hormonal correlates. Third, these phases represent some intermediate level of fecundity between the infecund, amenorrheic state and the state of full ovarian function. Fourth, the tempo of individual progress through these phases may vary greatly. Fifth, prolactin appears to provide a physiological index of those aspects of the pattern and intensity of nursing associated with the lactational suppression of ovarian function. We must be cautious, however, not to generalize other aspects of the Edinburgh data. It would seem particularly important to complement the Edinburgh data with additional data from natural fertility populations with different socioeconomic and cultural circumstances. In particular the key change in breastfeeding patterns that is associated with initiating the transition in ovarian function may vary across populations: it may be the introduction of solid food in some and the elimination of nighttime nursing in others.

LACTATION AND MATERNAL CONDITION

Abundant evidence thus now serves to link the behavioral choreography of breastfeeding with the lactational suppression of ovarian function. But there is also mounting evidence that nursing behavior is not the only modulator of postpartum fecundity. In particular, maternal condition seems an important part of the equation. Data from several sources show that as maternal condition is compromised, either by increasing age or poor nutritional status, lactational suppression of ovarian function is intensified and/or extended in time. For example, World Fertility Survey (WFS) data from several countries (Hobcraft, McDonald and Rutstein, 1983; Retherford, Choe, Thapa and Gubhaju, 1989) indicate that closely spaced births have a negative impact on the survival probabilities not only of the first born child in a sequence (due, for example, to premature weaning) but also of the second. Hobcraft et al. (1983) found that a birth in the 2 years prior to the birth of the index child increased that child's risk of dying by over 50% in 13 of 23 countries. In addition they found in 9 of the countries that previous closely spaced births (2 or more births in the 2 to 6 years before the birth of the index child) further increased the risk of mortality for the index child. Retherford et al. (1989) observed a similar effect in Nepal that was not accounted for by the lactational status of the child preceding the index child, that is, they found no indication that competition for the mother's breast was the cause of elevated mortality risk for the younger child. Rather it would seem that closely spaced births have a cumulative negative effect on maternal condition that affects the survivorship of subsequent offspring.

Although the mechanism producing this effect is unclear, one possibility is that closely spaced births in some way deplete maternal reserves, jeopardizing a mother's ability to invest in additional offspring. It has been shown in other studies that poor maternal nutritional status can negatively affect neonatal birth weight, increasing the prevalence of low birth weight babies and elevating infant mortality risk (Prentice, Cole, Foord, Lamb and Whitehead, 1987; Roberts, Paul, Cole and Whitehead, 1982). The phenomenon of maternal depletion was first described by Jelliffe and Maddocks in 1964 based on work in highland New Guinea. In 1966 Jelliffe extended the notion of a "maternal depletion syndrome," suggesting that it might have a broad distribution in the developing world, especially where the energetic drain of pregnancy and lactation is compounded by high female workloads and patterns of domestic food consumption that undermine a woman's nutritional status (Jelliffe, 1966). Subsequent efforts to document maternal depletion through a relationship between female body composition and parity have been equivocal (Thapa, Short and Potts, 1988), though the most careful studies seem to verify the existence of a depleting effect of closely spaced births on maternal tissue reserves (Tracer, 1991).

It seems at least a reasonable assumption, then, that poor maternal condition compromises reproductive success probability in a way that is compounded by closely spaced births. If the function of lactational subfecundity is to help avoid such negative consequences, we can generate the qualitative prediction that poor maternal condition should be associated with an intensification and/or extension of the suppressive effect of lactation on ovarian function. Other things being equal, the optimal birth spacing for a woman in poor condition should be wider than the optimum for a woman in good condition. This prediction is supported for at least two important aspects of maternal condition: increasing age and poor nutritional status.

After the age of 35 or so, increasing age can be interpreted as a correlate of generally poorer reproductive condition. Infant mortality rates, maternal mortality rates, and rates of pregnancy and delivery complications all rise with increasing age independently of parity (Pebley, Huffman, Chowdhury and Stupp, 1985).[4] For these reasons, as a woman ages, the evolutionary cost/benefit balance between increasing investment in a current offspring versus initiating investment in a new offspring shifts in favor of the current child. Ever since Henry's original analysis (Henry, 1961), evidence has mounted showing that natural fertility declines with advancing maternal age. Henry was able to show that this decline was not solely a product of increasing rates of sterility with age, but that fertility declined among fecund couples as well, implicating an increase in birth spacing. Although some fraction of this increase could presumably be attributed to declining frequency of intercourse, Henry was convinced that most of the difference was in an extended period of lactational infecundability. Potter et al. (1965), in studying birth interval dynamics in the Punjabi villages, found that maternal age was related both to the duration of lactation and the duration of amenorrhea. Jain, Hsu, Freedman and Chang (1970), through a multiple regression analysis of Taiwanese data, found that maternal age affected the period of lactational amenorrhea both through its influence on the period of lactation and independently. That is, in the Taiwanese data, women over 30 years of age had longer periods of lactational amenorrhea than women under age 30, even when the length of the period of lactation was the same. Habicht, Davanzo, Butz and Meyers (1985) found that the duration of postpartum anovulation is linearly related to maternal age among Malaysian women 20 years and older, after controlling for duration of lactation. Santow (1987) also found that older Javanese women were slower to resume menses postpartum than younger women after controlling for the period of lactation. In Bangladesh, Huffman, Chowdhury, Allen and Nahar (1987) found that mothers aged 13 to over 45 had similar periods of full and total breastfeeding, but the duration of postpartum amenorrhea increased steadily with age. Chen et al. (1974) had previously reported this effect from Bangladesh based on a smaller sample and a broader age grouping of subjects. Similarly, in a recent study in India, Srinivasan, Pathak and Pandey (1989) found no difference in the median duration of lactation between women over and under 30 years of age, but a significantly longer period of lactational amenorrhea in the older women. In a broad survey of WFS data from 20 countries with a worldwide distribution, Goldman, Westhoff and Paul (1987) found that the interval from delivery to next conception had a U-shaped relationship to age after controlling for parity, duration of marriage, and lactation. The interval for women over 35 years was 1 to 7 months longer on average than for women between 20 and 24 years of age (Figure 11.7). In this case, however, we cannot be sure, due to the nature of the dependent variable, that the observed effect is a consequence of an extended period of lactational amenorrhea rather than an extended waiting time to conception after the return of menses. (An extended waiting time to conception could itself be a function of physiological factors (slow resumption of fully fecund cycles), behavioral factors (lower frequency of intercourse), or male factors, or a combination of all three.) In all these studies, the effect of increasing age is small compared to the average duration of lactational amenorrhea, generally increasing the period of amenorrhea on the order of 20 to 25% in women 30 and over. It is, nevertheless, a significant shift in maternal reproductive physiology in the direction expected by an adaptationist paradigm.

The evidence for a modulating effect of maternal nutritional status is even more compelling. Two longitudinal field studies have produced the most relevant data, one in Bangladesh and one in The Gambia. A longitudinal study of birth interval dynamics has been conducted in the vi-

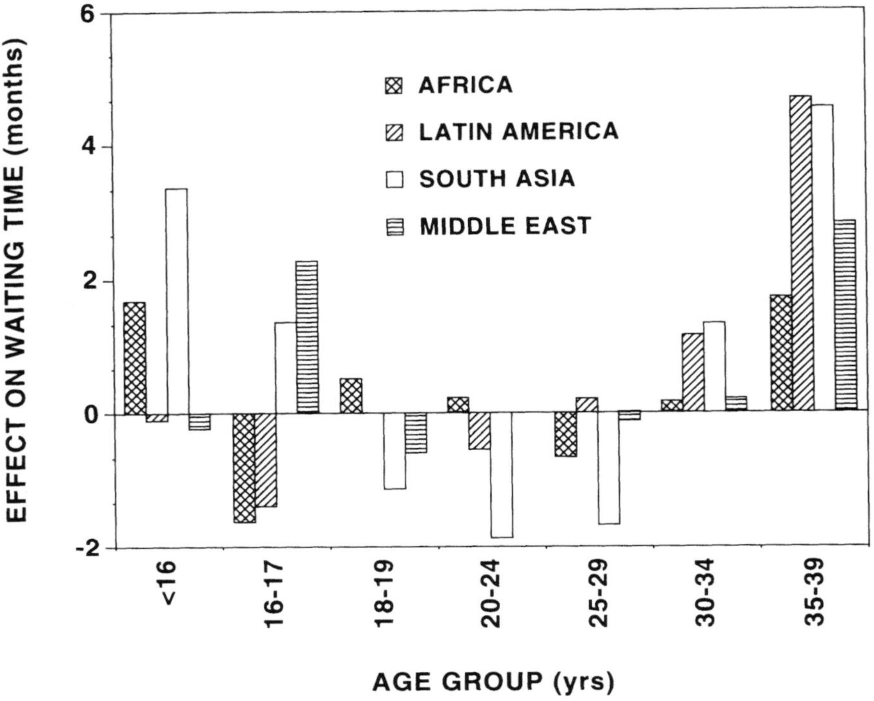

Figure 11.7. The effect of age on the average time between birth and the next conception in lactating women from 21 countries, after correction for average duration of lactation. Redrawn from Goldman et al. (1987, Fig. 5, p. 142).

cinity of Matlab, Bangladesh by the International Center for Diarrhoeal Disease Research (formerly the Cholera Research Laboratory) since 1966 involving a population of over a quarter of a million people (Huffman, Ford, Allen and Streble, 1987b). One of the significant early findings of the study, reported by Chen et al. in 1974, was a pronounced seasonality in several birth interval components. Not only was there a significant birth seasonality with an excess of births between October and February, corresponding to a conception peak between March and June (before the monsoon), but there was a distinct seasonality to the resumption of menses postpartum, peaking in November and continuing through March. The peak in resumption of menses coincides with and follows the major rice harvest in November. In seeking to explain their findings, the authors considered several possible influences on the timing of postpartum resumption of menstruation. Possibly the change in women's activity patterns associated with the November harvest could have led to some synchronized decrease in suckling intensity and/or frequency, causing a secondary synchronization in the resumption of menses. The more recent work of Panter-Brick in Nepal (1989, 1991, 1992a) certainly lends credence to such a scenario, although Chen et al. present no evidence to support such an argument. They do, however, speculate that maternal nutrition and "maternal depletion" (Chen et al., 1974:290) may play a role. The improvement in maternal nutritional status occasioned by the rice harvest might accelerate the resumption of postpartum cycles, either directly by decreasing the degree of lactational suppression of ovarian function, or indirectly by increasing the quantity and quality of maternal milk so that the intensity of suckling declines.

More recently the relationship between maternal nutritional status and lactational suppression of ovarian function has been explored more explicitly, using data from Matlab. In 1980, Huffman, Chowdury, Chakraborty and Simpson reported on a large study of breastfeeding patterns in the Matlab area. They were able to document a decline in time spent suckling during the harvest season that was not a function of maternal nutritional status, or maternal or infant morbidity. Yet when these data were analyzed to establish a relationship between the pattern of suckling and the timing of resumption of menses, no significant association was found (Huffman et al., 1987a). Obviously surprised at this result, Huffman and her colleagues speculate that some individual difference in the suppressive effect of lactation could account for their finding. In a separate analysis (Huffman et al., 1987b) of nutritional status and postpartum amenorrhea, they report a significant difference in the length of amenorrhea among women classified by their weight at pregnancy termination. Women who show evidence of poorer nutritional status in the months immediately following delivery eventually resume menses at a later postpartum date than those with better nutritional status. The median duration of postpartum amenorrhea for women in the lowest weight quartile after delivery (20.2 months) is longer by nearly a third than the duration of amenorrhea experienced by women in the highest weight quartile (15.5 months). When both maternal nutritional status (as maternal weight at pregnancy termination) and nursing pattern (as the presence or absence of supplementation) were used in a hazards model analysis, both were found to contribute significantly, and independently, to the monthly risk of resumption of menses (Ford and Huffman, 1988). Data from the same study also show that maternal nutritional status has a significant effect on the probability of intrauterine mortality (Becker, Chowdhury and Leridon, 1986; Ford, Huffman, Chowdhury, Becker, Allen and Menken, 1989; Pebley et al., 1985), again confirming the associated cost of attempting to reproduce when in poor condition. Similar results have also been reported for low-income urban women in India (Prema, Naidu, Neelakumari and Ramalakshmi, 1981).

Longitudinal research into the determinants of maternal and child health in The Gambia has a history as impressive as the Matlab Study, dating from 1949 (Weaver and Beckerleg, 1993). A central objective of the research in The Gambia was to measure the impact of nutritional intervention on reproductive health, child survival, and child growth in a marginally nourished population. As a part of that project Lunn and colleagues (Lunn, 1992; Lunn, Prentice, Austin, and Whitehead, 1980; Lunn, Austin, Prentice and Whitehead, 1984) examined the effect of maternal supplementation on the hormonal correlates of lactation. Other researchers had found that the effect of a significant supplementation of calories on the quantity and quality of breast milk produced by nursing mothers was very modest (Prentice, Whitehead, Roberts, Paul, Watkinson, Prentice and Watkinson 1980; Prentice, Prentice and Whitehead, 1981a,b). Lunn et al., however, found that the effect on prolactin levels was profound. Women supplemented during lactation showed prolactin levels that diverged from those of unsupplemented women almost immediately postpartum and fell with increasing infant age at a much steeper rate (Lunn et al., 1980, see Figure 11.8). When supplementation was extended to include the period of gestation, the effect was even more pronounced, with a shortening of the subsequent period of postpartum amenorrhea by 35 weeks compared to unsupplemented women. A similar effect of maternal nutritional status could be demonstrated by comparing mothers with infants of similar age nursing during the season of the year when nutritional status of all adult members of the population was at its lowest, versus mothers nursing during the season of highest food availability and highest nutritional status (Lunn et al., 1980). Prolactin levels were much higher in the former group for infants of the same age. Worthman, Jenkins, Stallings and Lai (1993) recently reported that among the Amele of Papua New Guinea, maternal nutritional status may actually attenuate the pituitary response to the suckling stimulus.

Recent attention has also been directed toward the fecundability of menstrual cycles during lactation. Physiological studies of the return to full fecundity postpartum, reviewed above, consistently have found evidence of continued suppression of ovarian function during lactation after the return of menstruation, suggesting that lactation may continue to constrain fertility after the end of lactational amenorrhea. John, Menken and Chowbhury (1987) use hazards model analysis to explore the determinants of the waiting time to conception in Matlab women after the postpartum resumption of menses. They find that lactation continues to suppress the monthly probability of conception in menstruating,

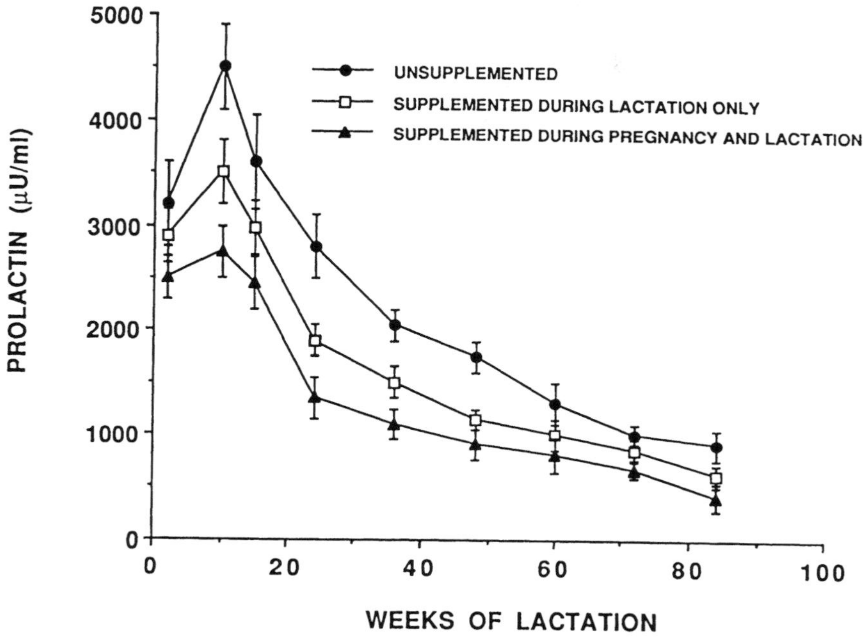

Figure 11.8. The time course of plasma prolactin by weeks postpartum in Gambian women categorized by the period during which they received nutritional supplements. Redrawn from Lunn et al. (1984, Fig. 1, p. 229).

lactating women to a degree that diminishes with time. They also find that "the longer a woman's postpartum amenorrhoea, the higher her fecundability when she resumes menses and the more rapidly she conceives" (1987:446). This inverse relationship between the duration of amenorrhea and subsequent fecundability has also been observed in other studies (Delgado, Martorell and Klein, 1982; Santow, 1987). Santow, for example, found among Javanese women that "women who were amenorrheic for at least eight months were subject to an instantaneous conception hazard twice as great as women who were amenorrheic for a shorter time" (Santow, 1987:157). While it is possible that such an effect could be mediated by increased coital frequency or some other intermediate variable, it is also consistent with the adaptationist view that the "function" of lactational suppression of fecundity is to allow for adequate maternal recovery between reproductive efforts. Other things being equal, longer periods of lactation should allow for more complete maternal recuperation and thus might be expected to be associated with higher fecundability when the period of lactational suppression of ovarian function ends.

CONCLUSION

The class Mammalia takes its name from the peculiarly intense form of maternal reproductive investment that lactation represents. The development of this form of maternal investment appears to have been a watershed in animal evolution to which many aspects of mammalian life history can be linked. The relationship of lactation to the regulation of natural human fertility should not then surprise us. Yet it was not until 1955 that Gioiosa first suggested that an important function of human lactation, over and above the nutritional and immunological benefits to the infant, might be its role as a "natural birth spacer." More recently, Short (1987) has elegantly presented this case to clinicians and population scientists. The negative effects of early weaning on child survival have been amply documented by WFS data from a broad range of populations (Adlakha and Suchindran, 1985; Cleland and Sathar, 1984; Hobcraft et al., 1983; Hobcraft, McDonald and Rutstein, 1985; Palloni and Millman, 1986; Palloni and Tienda, 1986; Retherford et al., 1989; Trussell and Hammerslough, 1983). By linking postpartum infecundability to the intensity of lactation, natural selection seems to have provided a mechanism to reduce the probability of a nursing mother, already energetically burdened by "metabolizing for two," being saddled with a concurrent pregnancy and the even more challenging task of "metabolizing for three." An alternative physiological "rule" that caused lactation to cease upon the next conception would also prevent simultaneous lactation and pregnancy, but with disastrous results for individual fitness. If ovarian function were not suppressed after birth, a typical 5 to 7 month waiting time to the next conception would produce a typical 14 to 16 month interbirth interval, well below the 2 year interval that WFS data associate with rapidly increasing rates of child mortality (Cleland and Sathar, 1984; Hobcraft et al., 1983, 1985; Palloni and Millman, 1986; Palloni and Tienda, 1986; Rutstein, 1983). By linking postpartum infecundability to maternal condition, natural selection seems also to scale this birth spacing mechanism to the individual woman's ability to bear the energy demands of another conception, and so helps to modulate natural reproductive effort over the life span of the individual.

In the present day, variation in breastfeeding behavior appears to be a more powerful determinant of variation in natural fertility than does variation in maternal condition. In some ways, this seems to undercut the notion of lactation as a natural birth spacer. As Vitzthum (1989, 1992) and Panter-Brick (1991, 1992b) have made clear, the pattern and intensity of lactation are often constrained by culture, opportunity, or even individual preference, hardly the foundation for a reliable mechanism to optimize reproductive histories. Yet under formative human conditions the situation may well have been quite different. The great latitude in breastfeeding patterns that women in today's world demonstrate is perhaps principally due to the availability of supplementary and weaning foods, which are themselves a product of agriculture and animal domestication. It is arguable that hunter–gatherer populations living before agriculture would have been constrained much more in their nursing patterns by the pace of infant maturation. In such a formative human context, then, maternal and infant physiology may have been much more important modulators of lactational suppression of ovarian function, while the impact of variation in maternal behavior may have been much less.

NOTES

1. The date was astonishingly early in the sense that prolactin was only isolated in 1970, with specific radioimmunoassays becoming available in the succeeding years (Hwang, Guyda and Friesen, 1971, 1972; Lewis, Singh and Seavey, 1971).

2. The first two papers, Howie et al. (1982a,b) appeared back-to-back in a single issue of *Clinical Endocrinology*, but were obviously printed in the inverse order from the authors' original intention, since the paper printed first states "the age and parity of the mothers and the method of their recruitment to the study have previously been described" (Howie et al., 1982b:316), citing the paper printed second. In my discussion I refer to the papers in their logical order as originally intended by the authors.

3. The units used in measurements of prolactin vary considerably. Many protein hormones have indeterminate molecular weights, due to variable conjugation with sugars and other smaller subcomponents. In such cases measurements are expressed in International Units based on a standard reference preparation. These standard reference preparations have themselves varied over the years. Because prolactin is less variable in its molecular weight than many larger protein hormones, there is a tendency for more recent measurements to be expressed in nanograms per milliliter. There is, however, no conversion factor to translate between International Units and units of mass per volume. Thus, it is necessary to quote measurements in the units used by each author in the original publications.

4. These changes are independent of any increase in rates of chromosomal anomalies and congenital malformations.

REFERENCES

Adlakha, A. L., and C. M. Suchindran
1985 Factors affecting infant and child mortality. *Journal of Biosocial Science* 17:481–496.

Becker, S., A. Chowdhury, and H. Leridon
1986 Seasonal patterns of reproduction in Matlab, Bangladesh. *Population Studies* 40:457–472.
Berman, M. L., K. Hanson, and I. L. Hellman
1972 Effect of breast-feeding on postpartum menstruation, ovulation, and pregnancy in Alaskan Eskimos. *American Journal of Obstetrics and Gynecology* 114:524–534.
Bonte, M., and H. van Balen
1969 Prolonged lactation and family spacing in Rwanda. *Journal of Biosocial Science* 1:97–100.
Booth, M.
1935 The time of reappearance and the character of the menstrual cycle following gestation. *Yale Journal of Biology and Medicine* 1935:215–216.
Brown, J. B., P. Harrisson, and M. Smith
1985 A study of returning fertility after childbirth and during lactation by measurement of urinary oestrogen and pregnanediol excretion and cervical mucus production. *Journal of Biosocial Science Supplement* 9:5–24.
Cantrelle, P., and H. Leridon
1971 Breast feeding, mortality in childhood and fertility in a rural zone of Senegal. *Population Studies* 25:505–533.
Chen, L. C., S. Ahmed, M. Gesche, and W. H. Mosley
1974 A prospective study of birth interval dynamics in rural Bangladesh. *Population Studies* 28:277–297.
Chowdhury, A., A. Khan, and L. Chen
1976 The effect of child mortality experience on subsequent fertility in Pakistan and Bangladesh. *Population Studies* 30:2.
Cleland, J. G., and Z. Sathar
1984 The effect of birth-spacing on childhood mortality in Pakistan. *Population Studies* 38:401–418.
Davis, K., and J. Blake
1956 Social structure and fertility: An analytic framework. *Economic Development and Cultural Change* 4:211–235.
Delgado, H., R. Martorell, and R. Klein
1982 Nutrition, lactation and birth interval components in rural Guatemala. *American Journal of Clinical Nutrition* 35:1468–1476.
Del Mundo, M. D., and A. C. Adiao
1970 Lactation and child spacing as observed among 2102 rural Filipino mothers. *Philippine Journal of Pediatrics* 19:128.
Delvoye, P., J. Desnoeck-Delogne, and C. Robyn
1976 Serum-prolactin in long-lasting amenorrhea. *Lancet* 2:288.
Delvoye, P., M. Demaegd, J. Delogne-Desnoeck, and C. Robyn
1977 The influence of the frequency of nursing and of previous lactation experience on serum prolactin in lactating mothers. *Journal of Biosocial Science* 9:447–451.
Delvoye, P., M. Demaegd, Uwayitu-Nyampeta, and C. Robyn
1978 Serum prolactin, gonadotropins, and estradiol in menstruating and amenorrheic mothers during two years' lactation. *American Journal of Obstetrics and Gynecology* 130:635–639.

Dettwyler, K. A.
1989 Interaction of anorexia and cultural beliefs in infant malnutrition in Mali. *American Journal of Human Biology* 1:683–695.
Diaz, S., H. Cardenas, A. Brandeis, P. Miranda, A. M. Salvatierra, and H. B. Croxatto
1992 Relative contributions of anovulation and luteal phase defect to the reduced pregnancy rate of breastfeeding women. *Fertility and Sterility* 58:498–503.
Elias, M. F., J. Teas, J. Johnston, and C. Bora
1986 Nursing practices and lactation amenorrhea. *Journal of Biosocial Science* 18:1–10.
El-Minawi, M. F., and M. S. Foda
1971 Postpartum lactation amenorrhea. *American Journal of Obstetrics and Gynecology* 111:17–21.
Ford, K., and S. Huffman
1988 Nutrition, infant feeding and post-partum amenorrhea in rural Bangladesh. *Journal of Biosocial Science* 20:461–469.
Ford, K., S. L. Huffman, A. K. Chowdhury, S. Becker, H. Allen, and J. Menken
1989 Birth-interval dynamics in rural Bangladesh and maternal weight. *Demography* 26:425–437.
Gioiosa, R.
1955 Incidence of pregnancy during lactation in 500 cases. *American Journal of Obstetrics and Gynecology* 70:162–174.
Glasier, A., A. S. McNeilly, and P. W. Howie
1983 Fertility after childbirth: Changes in serum gonadotrophin levels in bottle and breast feeding women. *Clinical Endocrinology* 19:493–501.
Goldman, N., C. F. Westhoff, and L. E. Paul
1987 Variations in natural fertility: The effect of lactation and other determinants. *Population Studies* 41:127–146.
Gordon, J. E., I. D. Chitkara, and J. B. Wyon
1963 Weanling diarrhea. *American Journal of Medical Science* March:129–161.
Habicht, J. -P., J. Davanzo, W. P. Butz, and L. Meyers
1985 The contraceptive role of breastfeeding. *Population Studies* 39:213–232.
Henry, L.
1961 Some data on natural fertility. *Eugenics Quarterly* 8:81–91.
Hobcraft, J., J. W. McDonald, and S. Rutstein
1983 Child-spacing effects on infant and early child mortality. *Population Index* 49:585–618.
1985 Demographic determinants of infant and early child mortality: A comparative analysis. *Population Studies* 39:363–385.
Howie, P. W., A. S. McNeilly, M. J. Houston, A. Cook, and H. Boyle
1982a Fertility after childbirth: Infant feeding patterns, basal PRL levels and post-partum ovulation. *Clinical Endocrinology* 17:315–322.
1982b Fertility after childbirth: Post-partum ovulation and menstruation in bottle and breast feeding mothers. *Clinical Endocrinology* 17:323–332.
Howie, P. W., and A. S. McNeilly
1982 Effect of breast feeding patterns on human birth intervals. *Journal of Reproduction and Fertility* 65:545–557.

Huffman, S. L., A. K. M. Chowdury, J. Chakraborty, and N. K. Simpson
1980 Breast-feeding patterns in rural Bangladesh. *American Journal of Clinical Nutrition* 33:144–154.

Huffman, S. L., A. Chowdhury, H. Allen, and L. Nahar
1987a Suckling patterns and post-partum amenorrhea in Bangladesh. *Journal of Biosocial Science* 19:171–179.

Huffman, S. L., K. Ford, H. A. Allen, and P. Streble
1987b Nutrition and fertility in Bangladesh: Breastfeeding and post partum amenorrhea. *Population Studies* 41:447–462.

Hwang, P., H. Guyda, and H. G. Friesen
1971 A radioimmunoassay for human prolactin. *Proceedings of the National Academy of Sciences of the U.S.A.* 68:1902.
1972 Purification of human prolactin. *Journal of Biological Chemistry* 247:1955.

Jain, A. K.
1969 Pregnancy outcome and the time required for the next conception. *Demography* 7:255.

Jain, A. K., C. Hsu, R. Freedman, and M. C. Chang
1970 Demographic aspects of lactation and postpartum amenorrhea. *Demography* 7:255–271.

Jelliffe, D. B.
1966 The assessment of the nutritional status of the community. *WHO Monograph Series*, No. 53. Geneva: World Health Organization.

Jelliffe, D. B., and I. Maddocks
1964 Notes on ecologic malnutrition in the New Guinea Highlands. *Clinical Pediatrics* 3:432–438.

John, A. M., J. A. Menken, and A. K. M. Chowdhury
1987 The effects of breastfeeding and nutrition on fecundity in rural Bangladesh: A hazards-model analysis. *Population Studies* 41:433–446.

Jones, R. E.
1989 Breast-feeding and post-partum amenorrhea in Indonesia. *Journal of Biosocial Science* 21:83–100.

Kennedy, K. I., R. Rivera, and A. S. McNeilly
1989 Consensus statement on the use of breastfeeding as a family planning method. *Contraception* 39:477–496.

Konner, M., and C. Worthman
1980 Nursing frequency, gonadal function, and birth spacing among !Kung hunter-gatherers. *Science* 207:788–791.

Lass, P. M., J. Smelser, and R. Kurzrok
1938 Studies relating to time of human ovulation. III. During lactation. *Endocrinology* 23:39–43.

Lewis, U. J., N. P. Singh, and B. K. Seavey
1971 Human prolactin: Isolation and some properties. *Biochemical and Biophysical Research Communications* 44:1169.

Lorimer, F. (ed.)
1954 *Culture and Human Fertility.* Paris: UNESCO.

Lunn, P. G.
1992 Breast-feeding patterns, maternal milk output and lactational infecundity. *Journal of Biosocial Science* 24:317–324.

Lunn, P. G., A. M. Prentice, S. Austin, and R. G. Whitehead
1980 Influence of maternal diet on plasma-prolactin levels during lactation. *Lancet* 1(8169):623–625.
Lunn, P. G., S. Austin, A. M. Prentice, and R. G. Whitehead
1984 The effect of improved nutrition on plasma prolactin concentrations and postpartum infertility in lactating Gambian women. *American Journal of Clinical Nutrition* 39:227–235.
Martin, W., D. Morley, and M. Woodland
1964 Intervals between births in a Nigerian village. *Journal of Tropical Pediatrics* 10:82–85.
McKeown, T., and J. R. Gibson
1954 A note on menstruation and conception during lactation. *Journal of Obstetrics and Gynaecology of the British Empire* 61:824–829.
McNeilly, A. S., P. W. Howie, P. J. Houston, A. Cook, and H. Boyle
1982 Fertility after childbirth: Adequacy of post-partum luteal phases. *Clinical Endocrinology* 17:609–615.
McNeilly, A. S., A. F. Glasier, P. W. Howie, M. J. Houston, A. Cook, and H. Boyle
1983 Fertility after childbirth: Pregnancy associated with breast feeding. *Clinical Endocrinology* 18:167–173.
Palloni, A., and S. Millman
1986 Effects of inter-birth intervals and breastfeeding on infant and early childhood mortality. *Population Studies* 40:215–236.
Palloni, A., and M. Tienda
1986 The effects of breastfeeding and pace of childbearing on mortality at early ages. *Demography* 23:31–52.
Panter-Brick, C.
1989 Motherhood and subsistence work—the Tamang of rural Nepal. *Human Ecology* 17:205–228.
1991 Lactation, birth spacing and maternal work-loads among two castes in rural Nepal. *Journal of Biosocial Science* 23:137–154.
1992a Women's work and child nutrition: The food intake of 0–4 year old children in rural Nepal. *Ecology of Food and Nutrition* 29:11–24.
1992b Working mothers in rural Nepal. In *The Anthropology of Breast-Feeding*, edited by V. Maher, pp. 133–150. Oxford: Berg.
Pebley, A. R., S. L. Huffman, A. K. M. Chowdhury, and P. W. Stupp
1985 Intra-uterine mortality and maternal nutritional status in rural Bangladesh. *Population Studies* 39:425–440.
Peckham, C. H.
1934 An investigation of some effects of pregnancy noted six weeks and one year after delivery. *Bulletin of the Johns Hopkins Hospital* 54:186–207.
Potter, R. G., Jr., M. L. New, J. B. Wyon, and J. E. Gordon
1965 A fertility differential in eleven Punjab villages. *Milbank Memorial Fund Quarterly* 43:185–201.
Prema, K., A. N. Naidu, S. Neelakumari, and B. A. Ramalakshmi
1981 Nutrition-fertility interaction in lactating women of low income groups. *British Journal of Nutrition* 45:461–467.
Prentice, A., A. M. Prentice, and R. G. Whitehead

1981a Breast-milk fat concentrations of rural African women. 1. Short-term variations within individuals. *British Journal of Nutrition* 45:483–494.

1981b Breast-milk fat concentrations of rural African women. 2. Long-term variations within a community. *British Journal of Nutrition* 45:495–503.

Prentice, A. M., R. G. Whitehead, S. B. Roberts, A. A. Paul, M. Watkinson, A. Prentice, and A. A. Watkinson

1980 Dietary supplementation of Gambian nursing mothers and lactational performance. *Lancet* 2(8200):886–888.

Prentice, A. M., T. J. Cole, F. A. Foord, W. H. Lamb, and R. G. Whitehead

1987 Increased birthweight after prenatal dietary supplementation of rural African women. *American Journal of Clinical Nutrition* 46:912–925.

Retherford, R. D., M. K. Choe, S. Thapa, and B. B. Gubhaju

1989 To what extent does breastfeeding explain birth-interval effects on early childhood mortality? *Demography* 26:439–450.

Rivera, R., E. Ortiz, M. Barrera, K. Kennedy, and P. Bhiwandiwala

1985 Preliminary observations on the return of ovarian function among breast-feeding and post-partum non-breast-feeding women in a rural area of Mexico. *Journal of Biosocial Science Supplement* 9:127–136.

Roberts, S. B., A. A. Paul, T. J. Cole, and R. G. Whitehead

1982 Seasonal changes in activity, birth weight and lactational performance in rural Gambian women. *Transactions of the Royal Society of Tropical Medicine and Hygiene* 76:669–676.

Robyn, C., P. Delvoye, C. Van Exter, M. Vekemans, A. Caufriez, P. de Nayer, J. Delogne-Desnoeck, and M. L'Hermite

1976 Physiological and pharmacological factors influencing prolactin secretion and their relation to human reproduction. In *Prolactin and Human Reproduction*, edited by P. G. Crosignani and C. Robyn, pp. 71–96. New York: Academic Press.

Rutstein, S. O.

1983 Infant and child mortality: Levels, trends and demographic differentials. *WFS Comparative Studies*, No. 24. London: World Fertility Survey.

Santow, G.

1987 Reassessing the contraceptive effect of breastfeeding. *Population Studies* 41:147–160.

Sharman, A.

1951 Menstruation after childbirth. *Journal of Obstetrics and Gynaecology of the British Empire* 58:440–445.

Short, R.

1987 The biological basis for the contraceptive effects of breast feeding. *International Journal of Gynaecology and Obstetrics Supplement* 25:207–217.

Srinivasan, K., K. B. Pathak, and A. Pandey

1989 Determinants of breast-feeding and post-partum amenorrhea in Orissa. *Journal of Biosocial Science* 21:356–371.

Thapa, S., R. V. Short, and M. Potts

1988 Breast feeding, birth spacing and their effects on child survival. *Nature (London)* 335:679–682.

Topkins, P.

1943 The histologic appearance of the endometrium during lactation amenorrhea and its relationship to ovarian function. *American Journal of Obstetrics and Gynecology* 45:48–58.

Tracer, D. P.
1991 Fertility-related changes in maternal body composition among the Au of Papua New Guinea. *American Journal of Physical Anthropology* 85:393–405.

Trussell, J., and C. Hammerslough
1983 A hazards-model analysis of the covariates of infant and child mortality in Sri Lanka. *Demography* 20:1–26.

Tyson, J. E.
1977 Neuroendocrine control of lactational infertility. *Journal of Biosocial Science Supplement* 4:23–40.

Udesky, I. C.
1950 Ovulation in lactating women. *American Journal of Obstetrics and Gynecology* 59:843–851.

Van Ginneken, J. K.
1977 The chance of conception during lactation. *Journal of Biosocial Science Supplement* 4:41–54.

Vitzthum, V. J.
1989 Nursing behavior and its relation to duration of post-partum amenorrhoea in an Andean community. *Journal of Biosocial Science* 21:145–160.
1992 Infant nutrition and the consequences of differential market access in Nuñoa, Peru. *Ecology of Food and Nutrition* 28:45–63.

Weaver, L. T., and S. Beckerleg
1993 Is health a sustainable state? A village study in The Gambia. *Lancet* 341:1327–1330.

Wenlock, R. W.
1977 Birth spacing and prolonged lactation in rural Zambia. *Journal of Biosocial Science* 9:481–485.

Wood, J. W., D. Lai, P. L. Johnson, K. L. Campbell, and I. A. Maslar
1985 Lactation and birth spacing in highland New Guinea. *Journal of Biosocial Science Supplement* 9:159–173.

Worthman, C. M., C. L. Jenkins, J. F. Stallings, and D. Lai
1993 Attenuation of nursing-related ovarian suppression and high fertility in well-nourished, intensively breastfeeding Amele women of lowland Papua New Guinea. *Journal of Biosocial Science* 25:425–443.

12

Breast Cancer, Reproductive Biology, and Breastfeeding

Marc S. Micozzi

THE PROBLEM OF BREAST CANCER IN BIOCULTURAL PERSPECTIVE

The epidemiologic evidence is not yet clear or consistent as to all the major risk factors for breast cancer. To many women, and to those doing research in breast cancer, the reaction has been one of concern: "We still don't know what causes breast cancer," while incidence rates in the United States have continued to climb. During the last decade of studies on the epidemiology of breast cancer, incidence rates have increased from 1:11 to 1:9 U.S. women. Whether this represents a higher detection rate due to improvements in breast cancer screening, a genuine increase in cancer cases, or a combination of the two, remains a subject of debate. But to a considerable extent, we have had an idea about some of the correlates of breast cancer in modern populations for quite some time: the complex associations between early age at menarche, late age at first pregnancy, low parity, and lack of infant suckling.

Evolutionary biology (Potter, 1992) would suggest that for the preponderance of human evolutionary history, most women spent much of their adult lives pregnant or lactating. This is not the case in the twentieth-century United States, where medical students hear surgeons routinely refer to the breast as a "premalignant organ." However, *is* the nonpregnant, nonlactating breast to be considered "premalignant" in attempts to prevent breast cancer?

Demographic transition theory postulates that through time, populations shift from (1) high fertility/high mortality, to (2) high fertility/low mortality, to (3) low fertility/low mortality. The middle stage, where much of the world remains today, is held responsible for the tremendous world population growth of the last century, while western Europe and North America have made the final transition. If the increasing rates of breast cancer in this country during this century are inevitable correlates of fundamental demographic shifts to lower fertility rates, what is the role of specific risk factors such as breastfeeding?

If, for example, dietary modification to prevent breast cancer remains difficult and problematic, or proves to be inefficacious, are we justified in giving drugs (such as Tamoxifen) to prevent breast cancer (Love, 1992)? That is, will we be treating well women with "normal" breast tissue medically (if not surgically) with powerful and potentially dangerous chemopreventive agents in an effort to prevent breast cancer (a kind of medical "prophylactic mastectomy")? The current clinical trial to study prevention of breast cancer with Tamoxifen, which requires individual administration of an expensive, potentially toxic drug under ongoing medical supervision, is an example of what I have called the "medicalization of prevention" in contrast to traditional population-based efforts at prevention, e.g., diet and lifestyle.

If we come to view human behavior as an adaptation to the environment, and the epidemiology of breast cancer as evidence of human maladaptation (as in Potter, 1992), we may begin to consider human experience for the preponderance of human evolutionary history as a clue to the type of lifestyle to which human metabolism may be adapted (and which may help prevent cancer if followed, or contribute to cancer if not).

For example, archaeologists can reconstruct some human lifestyle and dietary patterns from prehistoric remains (just as modern urban archaeologists can validate contemporary dietary surveys by looking through refuse). Modern theories of human evolution and studies of nonhuman primates and hunter–gatherer societies also provide some models. Certainly, until the development of agriculture and animal domestication approximately 10,000 years ago, omnivorous humans had available to eat only those plants and animals that appeared in the wild. While we have tended toward a concept of "man the hunter" as somehow characteristic of early human experience, "woman the gatherer" may ultimately be a more accurate account. While big game hunting was a part of early human experience in some areas, its social significance may have been as great or greater than its nutritional significance much of the time. Furthermore, wild game, with 4–6% body fat, is nutritionally quite different from modern domesticated animals, with up to 40–60% body fat, the latter condition largely a phenomenon of the twentieth century in industrialized countries where cattle are grain-fed in feed lots.

Evolutionary biology might tell us that a healthy lifestyle and diet are simply the lifestyle and diet that well-nourished humans had "in the wild" (before the advent of agriculture and animal domestication). Agriculture, especially irrigation agriculture, has been regarded traditionally as a central force in human settlement and the origin of complex civilization, as well as a strongly positive development in human nutritional and health status. However, paleopathologists have recently uncovered evidence that sedentism and agriculture were associated with *increased* disease and malnutrition in human populations (Cohen, 1989). Some argue, however, that bioarchaeologic evidence is equally consistent with improvements *or* declines in health and nutritional status with the advent of agriculture (Wood, Milner, Harpending and Weiss, 1992). Some also argue that cancer is a relatively recent disease in human evolutionary history. Is cancer a result of leaving behind the heritage of our traditional gathering–hunting diet and lifestyle? The actual evidence for cancer in animals and humans in the Old World before Byzantium, and the New World before Columbus, is weak or nonexistent, even in many circumstances where cancer should be readily identifiable paleopathologically if present (Micozzi, 1991).

The national agenda for cancer research and health policy will not likely be set by greater understanding of human evolutionary biology or history, or by solely conducting experiments on animals to help answer questions about human health. Better insights into modern human biology and culture in the context of epidemiologic observations are needed to help understand the causes (and develop methods of prevention) of chronic diseases such as breast cancer.

In this broad context, the relations between breast cancer and breastfeeding must be considered in at least two regards: (1) the influence of breastfeeding and other reproductive practices in the subsequent development of breast cancer in women (who do or do not breastfeed), and (2) the effects of breastfeeding or lack of breastfeeding in infancy and the long-term risk of breast cancer in adulthood (in individuals who were or were not breastfed).

DIMENSIONS OF THE PROBLEM AND CROSS-CULTURAL ASPECTS

Historically, breast cancer has been the most frequent cancer in women and the leading cause of cancer death in women in the United States. The precise etiology of breast cancer is understood less than that of many other cancers, and specific major risk factors have been difficult to identify (Table 12.1). A few risk factors for breast cancer are associated

Table 12.1. Summary of Breast Cancer Risk Factors for the General Population

Risk factors	*Relative risk estimates*
Age (older)	>4
Premenopausal status	>4
Contralateral breast cancer	>4
First degree relative with bilateral, premenopausal breast cancer	>4
North American or European	>4
Sister with postmenopausal, unilateral breast cancer	1–2
Early age at menarche	1–2
Late age at first full-term pregnancy	2–4
Late age at menopause	1–2
Single marital staus	1–4
Upper Socioeconomic class	1–4
Urban residence	1–4
Obesity (older, postmenopausal)	1–4
Chest radiation	1–4
Ovarian cancer	1–4
Endometrial cancer	1–4
White (vs. black) ethnicity	1–4
Nonremoval of ovaries with hysterectomy	1–4

with significant relative risks, defined as a magnitude of risk differential greater than 4.0; that is, women who have the factor are more than four times more likely to develop breast cancer than those without the factor. These factors include increasing age, history of cancer in the opposite breast, history of bilateral premenopausal breast cancer in a first-degree relative, and residence from an early age in North America or Northern Europe (as compared to Africa or Asia). Other risk factors are associated with small but significant relative risks (magnitude of risk differentials between 1.0 and 3.9). These include early age at menarche, late age at first full-term pregnancy, late age at menopause, single marital status, upper socioeconomic status, urban residence, obesity, high dose radiation to the chest (e.g., for prior treatment of tuberculosis), previous ovarian or endometrial cancer, whether or not the ovaries have been surgically removed, and white (as compared to black) ethnicity. Although the identified risk factors distinguish women at increased risk of breast cancer, they do not entirely explain the rates of breast cancer among women around the world (Kelsey and Gammon, 1991).

International differences in breast cancer morbidity and mortality, and studies on migrant populations, point to the importance of environmental and lifestyle factors in the etiology of breast cancer. Data on breast cancer can be obtained from national (Kurihara, Aoki and

Tominaga, 1984) or regional (Waterhouse, Muir, Shanmugaratnam and Powell, 1982) cancer registries around the world, and two types of cancer data can be considered based upon either incidence or mortality rates. Incidence data are better linked to etiology, but are probably less accurate due to difficulties in ascertaining diagnosis in many countries or populations.

Mortality data are more accurate (being based upon death certification), but are less directly linked to etiology due to variations in screening, detection, diagnosis, treatment, and survival in different countries and among different populations. The use of age-specific data allows reasonable distinction between premenopausal and postmenopausal cancer rates in different populations.

Overall age-adjusted cancer rates allow comparison of breast cancer in populations of women with different age-distribution, longevity, and risk. Comparison of age-adjusted breast cancer incidence (Table 12.2) and mortality rates (Table 12.3) among different populations around the world shows marked variation. For example, breast cancer rates are five times higher among women in the United States than in Japan. These differences cannot be explained solely on the basis of genetic factors, since there is a higher incidence of breast cancer in Japanese-American women than in Japanese women living in Japan (Buell and Dunn, 1965; Buell, 1973; Dunn, 1977; Hirayama, 1978). In fact, some of the strongest evidence for the role of environmental and lifestyle factors in breast cancer comes from epidemiologic studies on Japanese migrants to the United States and Japanese living in Japan.

First (Isei), second (Nisei), and third (Sansei) generation Japanese-American women are present in California and in Hawaii in sufficient numbers to allow meaningful comparisons of breast cancer rates with those of women living in Japan, where breast cancer rates have historically been low. In migrant studies, genetic factors may be considered relatively constant, although the extent to which migrant populations are a selected group, and the effects of inbreeding reduction and interbreeding on successive generations must be considered. Migrants experience rapid changes in environmental risk factors and lifestyle, and changes in health outcomes through time and space (Albanes, Schatzkin and Micozzi, 1987). Migrant studies may be conducted synchronically (cross-sectionally), at one point in time, or diachronically (longitudinally), through time, in one or more places. Such descriptive studies have provided useful observations about environmental risk factors and breast cancer.

Breast cancer rates have increased in succeeding generations of Japanese migrants to the United States (Buell and Dunn, 1965). Age-standardized breast cancer incidence rates have been relatively low in

Table 12.2. Cross-National Comparison of Breast Cancer Incidence Rates[a]

Country	*Year of study*	*Breast cancer incidence per 100,000 population: age-standardized rates*
Senegal	1969	11.8
Singapore (Malays)	1973–1977	14.7
Japan	1973–1977	17.5
Poland (rural)	1973–1977	17.7
India	1973–1975	21.2
Singapore (Chinese)	1973–1977	21.9
Hungary (rural)	1973–1977	29.2
Puerto Rico	1963	29.5
Romania	1974–1978	30.1
Czechoslovakia	1973–1977	30.3
Hong Kong (Chinese)	1974–1977	31.1
Columbia	1972–1976	33.2
Yugoslavia	1973–1976	34.2
Spain	1973–1977	36.5
Poland (urban)	1973–1977	36.5
Jamaica	1973–1977	39.0
Finland	1971–1976	40.1
Norway	1973–1977	49.6
Australia	1973–1977	53.2
Denmark	1968–1972	54.4
France	1975–1977	54.5
Sweden	1973–1977	55.2
West Germany	1973–1977	55.7
Brazil	1973	56.2
U.S. (Asian)	1972–1977	57.3
Italy	1976–1977	57.6
Britain	1973–1977	58.4
Israel	1972–1976	59.9
New Zealand	1972–1976	62.6
Canada	1973–1977	63.2
U.S. (Black)	1973–1977	67.2
Switzerland	1964	76.1
U.S. (White)	1973–1977	83.7

[a] Adapted from Waterhouse et al. (1982).

Japan, intermediate in Japanese Hawaiians, compared to Caucasians in the United States (Table 12.4) (Waterhouse, Correa, Muir and Powell, 1976). There is an effect of time on the breast cancer incidence rates in Japanese Hawaiians. The rate increased from 23 per 100,000 during the period 1960–1964 (Doll, Muir and Waterhouse, 1970) to 44.2 per 100,000 during 1967–1971 (Waterhouse et al., 1976), and 57.3 per 100,000 during 1973–1977 (Waterhouse et al., 1982). During the period 1969–1973, the incidence of breast cancer among premenopausal Japanese women in

Table 12.3. Cross-National Comparison of Breast Cancer Mortality Rates[a]

Country	*Breast cancer deaths per 100,000 population: age-standardized rates*
Japan	6.5
Hong Kong	9.0
Singapore	10.2
Yugoslavia	15.2
Romania	15.6
Spain	17.8
Poland	18.0
Bulgaria	18.9
Greece	20.1
U.S. (Black)	21.2
Finland	22.6
Israel	24.0
Australia	24.0
Italy	28.1
Canada	28.1
New Zealand	29.1
France	30.3
Hungary	32.3
Norway	32.5
Austria	33.7
Sweden	34.5
Netherlands	37.2
West Germany	37.3
Switzerland	39.5
Denmark	41.3
Belgium	42.0
Great Britain	47.6
U.S. (White)	52.1

[a] Adapted from Kurihara et al. (1984).

California (41.0 per 100,000) was almost as high as that among premenopausal Caucasians (55.7 per 100,000) (Dunn, 1977).

In Japan itself, there have also been recent increases in breast cancer rates that correspond to "westernization" of lifestyle (Hirayama, 1978). The annual number of breast cancer deaths in Japan doubled during the period between 1955 and 1975. Normalized to the increased population, the rate of death from breast cancer has steadily increased from 3.5 per 100,000 in 1955 to 5.8 per 100,000 in 1975. The increase has been greatest among women 45 to 59 years of age, and among higher socioeconomic groups in urban areas (Hirayama, 1978).

In addition to ecological and geochemical features, the environment

Table 12.4. Breast Cancer: Age Standardized Incidence Rates[a]

Group	Locale	Incidence rates (per 100,000)
Japanese	Osaka	12.2
	Miyogi	13.0
	Okayama	16.6
Japanese	Hawaii	44.2
	California	47.0
Caucasian	Detroit	65.7
	Alameda	76.1
	San Francisco	79.4
Caucasian	Hawaii	80.3

[a] Adapted from Waterhouse et al. (1976).

includes cultural factors, such as health beliefs and behaviors, which also may be related to human health outcomes. With respect to cancer risk factors, breast cancer incidence rates in Japanese migrants appear to be related to the degree of acculturation to western lifestyle and diet.

In the Japan–Hawaii Cancer Study, Nomura, Henderson and Lee (1978) compared the diet of Japanese men whose wives had developed breast cancer with the diets of Japanese men whose wives did not. If it is assumed that the diets of husbands and wives were similar, the result indicated that the women who developed breast cancer followed a more western-style diet (more beef or other meat, butter/margarine/cheese, corn, and hot dogs, and less Japanese foods) than the control group. Moolgavkar, Day and Stevens (1980) suggested that the increasing incidence of breast cancer among Japanese-American women is associated with changes in lifestyle, including diet, in successive generations (cross-generational acculturation).

In a descriptive study of migrants, Buell (1973) also noted the increasing incidence of breast cancer in successive generations of Japanese women in America compared to those in Japan. The increasing rates were attributed to acculturation of diet and to increased height and weight. However, year of migration and age at migration can be independently related to the year of acculturation and age at acculturation, respectively. Although the distribution of ages among migrants in a given year of migration can be determined, different times of acculturation among different age groups may result in an irregular distribution of acculturated migrants (Albanes et al., 1987), making acculturation a difficult parameter to utilize.

The increasing cancer rates in Japanese-American women are reflected in age-specific cancer rates in Los Angeles. Younger Japanese-American women have higher breast cancer rates (like those of U.S. Caucasian women) than do older Japanese-American women (Waterhouse et al., 1982). Further, in San Francisco, the incidence of breast cancer among young Japanese-American women is almost as high as that among Caucasian women (Dunn 1977).

That young Japanese-American women have higher breast cancer rates than older Japanese-American women is consistent with a cohort effect. The cohort effect is also seen in the growth in stature of Japanese-American children born in 1940 compared to those born in 1955. The mean adult stature of Japanese-American women born in 1940 was 154 cm (Greulich, 1957), whereas that of Japanese-American women born in 1955 was 158 cm (Kondo and Eto, 1975). The generation of Japanese-American women with high breast cancer rates is the generation that had greater growth during childhood, and was probably exposed to a more western-style diet from infancy.

Thus, the time in life when environmental changes occur appears to be important to the long-term risk of breast cancer in women. It has been reported that persons who emigrate during childhood and adolescence experience the greatest changes in patterns of breast cancer (Buell, 1973). Buell's (1973) descriptive study also indicated a relation between height and weight and breast cancer risk within Japanese-American migrant groups. It appears that only the Nisei (second generation) and those Isei (first generation) who migrated before puberty attain greater stature, which, together with increased body weight, seems to be associated with an increased incidence of breast cancer (DeWaard, 1975). The migrant studies therefore suggest that acculturation early in life may be a critical factor in breast cancer risk (Miller, 1977).

RISK FACTORS FOR BREAST CANCER: EARLY NUTRITION AND BREASTFEEDING

Evidence for the Role of Nutrition

The dramatic environmental and temporal variations in cancer patterns, and the changing rates of cancer in migrants, suggest differential exposure of various populations to cancer risk factors. Although often it is not possible to pinpoint the environmental factors responsible for observed differences in cancer rates in the various ecologic and migrant studies, lifestyle and dietary and nutritional factors appear to play a prominent role.

Evidence for the role of nutrition in breast cancer relates primarily to relative dietary deficiencies of certain micronutrients (which may act as cancer protective factors), and relative dietary excesses of certain macronutrients (which may act as cancer-promoting factors). Two micronutrients of significance for human cancer are ß-carotene and selenium (Moon and Micozzi, 1989). The specific macronutrients of interest with respect to breast cancer risk are dietary fat, protein, and total calories, for which there are complex relationships with nutrition-mediated variables such as body size (Micozzi and Moon, 1992).

Timing of Nutritional Experiences

The timing of nutritional experiences appears important in the relation between dietary intake and breast cancer. Dietary patterns early in life may be related to the long-term risk of breast cancer (Miller, 1977), while effects of adult nutrition on body fat may mediate later hormonal influences on breast cancer. The effects of nutrition may also be partitioned anthropometrically by differentiation according to various measurements of body size (Micozzi, 1990).

Anthropometry provides information on past nutritional history and growth in human populations. Overnutrition during childhood is associated with increased stature and lean body mass, and accelerated rates of maturation. The former are reflected in increased height and body size in adults, and the latter by early age of menarche in women. Overnutrition in childhood is also related to increased deposition of adipose tissue. Obese and lean individuals differ in specific ways from infancy through old age. In general, fatter children are taller, heavier, and developmentally more advanced than their leaner counterparts. The obese are more advanced than the lean in skeletal and muscle mass, and in age at menarche by as much as 5 years. Obese children also tend to be tall at pubescence (Roche, 1984). It should be noted that these anthropometric observations are highly correlated with each other.

Breastfeeding and Influences in Early Life

Tendencies toward obesity begin early in postnatal life if nutritional intake is not properly balanced (Stini, 1978.) Excessive protein intake during the neonatal period may stimulate increased muscle growth, fat deposition, or most probably, both (Hahn and Koldovsky, 1966; Haymond, Karl and Pagliara, 1974). Thus, an environmental stimulus of overabundant nutrition during early growth and development may eventually lead to an adult whose body size is close to the maximum for that genotype (Stini, 1978).

Effects *in utero* may also be important. For example, women born to young mothers have a significantly lower risk of breast cancer than women born to older mothers (Rothman, MacMahon, Lin, Lowe, Mirra, Ravnihar, Salber, Trichopoulos and Yuasa, 1980). Whether a maternal age effect is transmitted through the fetal environment *in utero*, or through the neonatal environment through breastfeeding is not known; the older and younger mothers did not differ in breastfeeding practices. Alternatively, older mothers may be better established financially and can afford "better" nutrition, in this case, relative overnutrition.

A case-control study on over 200 children was undertaken to determine whether inadequate exposure to the immunological benefits of human milk may affect infant response to infection and increase susceptibility to childhood cancers. An increased risk for cancer was found among children breastfed less than 6 months or not breastfed at all, due largely to a six- to eightfold increased incidence of lymphoma (Davis, Savitz and Graubard, 1988).

Whether or not an infant is breastfed also has significant effects on neonatal nutrition and growth. Failure to breastfeed in early infancy may lead to overnutrition and overweight infants (Taitz, 1971). Human breast milk has among the lowest levels of protein of any mammalian milk, characteristic of species that suckle their young almost continuously. There is a positive relationship between the species-specific protein content of mammalian milk and the rate of early growth in neonates of the species. The percentage of protein in cows' milk, for example, is three times higher than in human milk. Early survival in most mammals demands rapid growth and maturation. However, humans are unlike most mammals in this respect (Stini, 1978). Cows' milk also differs from human milk in the type of protein present, as well as the concentration of total protein. Thus, the casein content of cows' milk is six times higher than that of human milk. Calcium and phosphorus are also much more abundant in cows' milk than in human milk.

Protein intake is a major environmental factor determining growth rate, size at a given age, and ultimate adult height. Some evidence also suggests that dietary protein intake at the time of maturity is a major environmental factor determining normal variation in growth and height. Conversely, among a wide range of anthropometric variables, height gains provide a good degree of discrimination among different levels of protein intake (Malcolm, 1979). Additionally, Kralj-Cercek (1956) and Wilson and Sutherland (1960) showed age at menarche to be closely related to higher animal protein intake, with early menarche in populations with high levels of protein intake.

Influence of Early Menarche

The common influence of increased nutrition early in life on both increased body size and early menarche is indicated by Malcolm's law (Newman, 1975), which states that "the later the average age at menarche, the smaller the average stature in the population" (e.g., Wilson and Sutherland, 1960). Increased body size and decreased age at menarche appear to share a common relation with nutritional patterns that may also place the individual at increased risk of breast cancer later in life. Since all these factors must be taken into account, it is important to examine the correlations among these risk factors, and to reconcile their common relation with breast cancer in a consistent fashion. Therefore, the effects of age at menarche on body size must be considered.

Eveleth and Tanner (1976) originally reviewed the relation of maturation to body size and shape. From infancy to adolescence, the trunk grows more slowly than the legs; however, at adolescence, the growth spurt is greater in sitting height than in leg length. Individuals who mature early have shorter legs in relation to the trunk since their preadolescent period (when the legs are growing relatively faster) is shorter. In terms of body shape, later maturers usually present a more linear body physique with relatively low weight-for-height, which may also be reflected in lean body mass.

In an early cancer study in women that used anthropometric dimensions beyond height and weight (or indices derived therefrom), Brinkley, Carpenter and Haybittle (1971) reported greater sitting height and frame size in breast cancer cases compared to controls. Therefore, while increased nutrition goes hand-in-hand with greater height, larger body size, and earlier age at menarche, the conjunction of these factors (which are, in turn, risk factors for breast cancer) produces an anthropometric pattern that may be distinctive. Increased sitting height, frame size, and lean body mass are the anthropometric variables correlated with the early nutritional pattern that places women at greater risk of breast cancer in later life. An increased intake of macronutrients early in life may be a critical factor for breast cancer. These anthropometric indicators are consistent with other known risk factors, and are consistent with available studies on breast cancer and body size.

Growth, Menarche, and Breast Cancer

Breast cancer has been proposed to be elevated in women who are obese and for those who had earlier menarche. The relations between these two risk factors can be explored, and both can be related to overfeeding during childhood. Epidemiologic evidence on nutrition, body size, and breast cancer presents a consistent pattern accounting for many breast cancer risk factors. DeWaard and colleagues (DeWaard, 1975; DeWaard and Banders-van Halewijn, 1974; DeWaard, Cornelius and Aichi, 1977) have shown that anthropometric variables, which may be correlated to excess nutrient intake in early life, are also correlated with increased risk for breast cancer in later life. For example, DeWaard first discovered that height accounts for much of the variability in breast cancer rates in adults and that weight is correlated primarily through its association with height. Large body mass and breast cancer may be independent consequences of the same nutritional pattern early in life, although as first shown by DeWaard, body weight alone is often not correlated with breast cancer risk in epidemiologic studies.

Overnutrition in the context of cancer is related to dietary excess of specific macronutrients. Miller (1977) argues that an increased intake of nutrients would be related to larger body size, rather than obesity per se. This hypothesis for humans is consistent with observations in laboratory animals by Ross, Bras and Lustbader (1983). The association between breast cancer and body size may, therefore, be indirect (Thomas, 1983).

Over the past several generations, many populations have increased in average body size, and have experienced a parallel trend toward earlier sexual maturation (Tanner, 1968; Tanner and Eveleth, 1975). The evidence that improved nutrition is an important factor in the decline in age at menarche is largely circumstantial. However, the close correlation of nutrition and physical growth, as well as results of animal experiments (Widdowson, 1974), lead to the conclusion that sexual development is advanced by increased nutrition (Malcolm, 1974). Increased body fat is also associated with an earlier age at menarche and later age at menopause. Menarcheal and menopausal ages may also have a common relationship to nutritional status and to constitutional factors that predate the onset of menarche and persist into later life (Sherman, Wallace, Bean and Schlabaugh, 1981).

Adult weight is related to nutritional factors, is negatively correlated with age at menarche, and is positively correlated with age at menopause (Sherman et al., 1981). Like body size, age at menarche and breast cancer risk may also be indirectly associated, with nutrition being the common risk factor (Staszewski, 1971). Therefore, the same nutritional pattern that is responsible for increased adolescent growth, increased attained (adult) height, and decreased age at menarche may be related to breast cancer risk in humans. Breastfeeding during infancy may play an important role in establishing nutritional and dietary patterns in early life that are related to the long-term risk of breast cancer in adulthood.

The importance of dietary excess should be considered with respect to the role of early nutrition in breast cancer, especially in developed countries. Overnutrition refers to an excessive intake of specific macronutrients, such as dietary fat, protein, and total calories, and their relationships to somatic conditions such as body size and obesity. The hypothesis that diet and overnutrition may play a role in breast cancer is supported by both animal experimental studies and human epidemiologic evidence.

Dietary Fat Intake

There is a popular scientific perception that excess dietary fat intake in "modern" as opposed to "traditional" human populations may be related to a number of negative health outcomes (Eaton and Konner, 1985), including cancer (Armstrong and Doll, 1975; Drasar and Irving, 1973; Hems, 1978).

Animal experimental evidence implicating dietary fat intake with breast cancer has been derived from studies of both spontaneous mammary tumors and chemically induced mammary tumors, as well as other site-specific tumors. Most of the data suggest that dietary fat promotes the growth of populations of cancer-initiated cells in the multistage process of carcinogenesis. The additional possibility that dietary fat plays an initiating role in carcinogenesis cannot be ruled out.

Human epidemiologic studies show high correlations between national levels of breast cancer and per capita consumption of total fat, animal fat, total protein, animal protein, and eggs (Drasar and Irving, 1973). For example, in Japan, per capita fat intake (especially animal fat and pork) is positively correlated with breast cancer mortality rates by geographic prefecture (Hirayama, 1978). In Britain, breast cancer mortality is positively related to per capita intake of animal fat and protein during the decade prior to death (Hems, 1978). In the United States, age-adjusted cancer mortality is positively correlated with per capita intake of fat, protein, beef, milk, and total calories (Gaskill, McGuire, Osborne and Stern, 1979). When nutrition-mediated factors such as height, weight, and age at menarche are statistically controlled, per capita intake of animal fat and protein maintains an independent correlation with breast cancer risk (Gray, Pike and Henderson, 1979). Increased consumption of fat, measured as total fat, animal fat, saturated fat, or unsaturated fat, is correlated with increased incidence of breast cancer among different ethnic groups in Hawaii (Kolonel, Hankin, Lee, Chi, Nomura and Hinds, 1981).

The first case-control study of diet and breast cancer was among Seventh-Day Adventists (Phillips, 1975). This study of 77 cases and 77 controls showed a positive association of life-style and dietary habits, including fat intake, with breast cancer, but the effect was somewhat weaker than suggested by correlation studies. The method of diet assessment did not permit quantification of dietary fat consumption; rather, it examined only the frequency of intake of various fat-containing foods. In a Canadian case-control study (Miller, Kelly, Choi, Matthews, Morgan, Munan, Burch, Feather, Howe and Jain, 1978), 400 breast cancer cases were characterized by an increased intake of all nutrients (total and saturated fat, and total calories). There was, however, little or no indication of a dose–response relationship with level of dietary fat intake in the breast cancer cases. Furthermore, the observation that more total calories were consumed by cases suggested the possibility of recall bias among cases. The percentage of fat in the diet of cases and controls could not be determined from the data. A third case-control study of 577 cases of breast cancer in Canada showed increased consumption of animal fat and protein (beef, pork, red meat) and sweet desserts in cases versus controls (Lubin, Burns, Blot, Ziegler, Lees and Fraumeni, 1981).

In a cohort study of 142,857 women in Japan, followed for 10 years beginning at age 40, increased breast cancer mortality was associated with high socioeconomic status and frequent meat consumption (Hirayama, 1978). Dietary fat intake among breast cancer cases came mainly from consumption of pork and animal fat. The risk of breast cancer among those with high fat intake was nearly 10 times higher than those with low fat intake.

Not all human studies of dietary fat intake and breast cancer have produced positive results. Some recent studies have reported no differences in estimated dietary fat intake between breast cancer cases and controls (Micozzi and Moon, 1992). The percentage of calories from fat cannot always be calculated in these studies, however, because total calories are not always estimated. In one study, no association was observed between fat intake and breast cancer incidence, although the study was not specifically designed to measure fat intake (Graham, Marshall, Mettlin, Rzepka, Nemoto and Byers, 1982).

Studies of the relation between fat and breast cancer, including other cohort studies, are still in progress. However, the most informative results may come from intervention studies. Dietary fat reduction trials have been undertaken but results are not yet available (Prentice, 1992).

Dietary Protein Intake

Excess dietary protein may also have a role in breast cancer. Animal experimental studies have shown an effect of increased dietary protein on tumor promotion in both spontaneous and chemically induced tumors, including mammary tumors. Lower dietary protein apparently inhibits the growth of spontaneous and chemically induced tumors (Ross, 1977), while evidence supports a tumor-promoting role for protein in dietary carcinogenesis (Clinton, Truex and Visek, 1979).

Ross and Bras (1965, 1971) observed an increasing incidence of spontaneous tumors, including mammary tumors, with increasing dietary protein intake in rats fed various isocaloric casein/sucrose ratios. Since sucrose was subsequently shown not to be a carcinogen (FASEB, 1976), this experiment was apparently testing the tumorigenic effect of protein. In animals with identical caloric intake, more tumors were found in groups with higher protein intake. Higher levels of protein intake early in life contributed to both a high tumor risk and a high mature weight in laboratory animals (Ross, 1977). This finding suggests that diet-mediated, early-life process involved in the regulation and duration of growth are also related to susceptibility to spontaneous tumor formation in rats (Ross et al., 1983).

In human epidemiologic studies, the possibility of a dietary effect of protein on cancer mortality or survival, as well as cancer incidence, has been suggested (Armstrong and Doll, 1975). With breast cancer specifically, there was a stronger association with animal protein than with total protein (possibly explained by the dietary association of animal protein consumption with fat consumption), but the correlation with total protein consumption was as strong as with total fat consumption. With other risk factors controlled, per capita intake of animal protein has also been related to breast cancer rates among different populations (Gray et al., 1979), including the United States (Gaskill et al., 1979). While breast cancer mortality was correlated with level of per capita food intake (protein, fat, and animal products) from the prior decade (Hems, 1978), the time-trend in Britain indicated that fat consumption was somewhat better correlated with breast cancer mortality than was protein consumption (Hems, 1980).

While early case-control studies (Phillips, 1975; Miller et al., 1978) did not find an association between protein consumption per se and breast cancer, a later, somewhat larger, case-control study (Lubin et al., 1981) clearly indicated that both animal fat consumption and protein consumption are risk factors. From both human and animal studies, an independent effect of protein consumption on breast cancer risk should thus be considered.

Energy Intake

While the precise composition of the diet appears to be important for breast cancer risk, the total amount of food consumed may also be an important variable. Total caloric intake is a less precise variable than dietary fat or protein intake because it is difficult to determine whether effects brought about by changing the quantity of the diet are due to resulting changes in caloric intake or to changed distribution of specific nutrients. Further, the concept of excess dietary intake of calories requires knowledge of calories expended, as well as calories consumed. Thus, level of energy expenditure (i.e., physical activity in various forms) is necessary to determine the level of excess caloric intake in an individual or population. Some measurements of physical activity do not directly address total caloric expenditure (Montoye and Taylor, 1984) and may be focused on determination of "fitness" relative to cardiovascular disease (LaPorte, Adams, Savage, Brenes, Dearwater and Cook, 1984).

Much of the animal experimental evidence and human epidemiologic studies, previously reviewed in the sections on dietary fat and protein intake, have also considered the effects of total caloric intake on cancer risk. Variable results have been reported, and appropriate controls have not always been used; thus, these results are difficult to evaluate. Ross and Bras (1971) found that caloric restriction early in the life of the rat is associated with a decreased prevalence of spontaneous tumors later in life. Berg (1975) has suggested that the international pattern of distribution of some cancers appears to be related to socioeconomic status, and affluent diets. Armstrong and Doll (1975) and Gaskill et al. (1979) also found that total caloric intake is related to cancer incidence and mortality, including breast cancer. The case-control study of breast cancer by Miller et al. (1978) found a higher mean intake of total calories in cases than in controls.

Excess intake of total calories, as well as fat and protein, may be reflected in measurements of body size. From this view, caloric intake may be related to anthropometric variables, such as weight and fatness, absolute or relative. The level of caloric intake (together with protein intake) may also have an effect on height, lean body mass, and other variables mediated during growth.

Lactose Intolerance

Lactose intolerance rates in various populations have also been related to the risk of breast cancer. In ecologic studies, populations that have no traditional or modern dairy industry and do not consume milk or milk products also have low rates of breast cancer, as in China. Breast cancer mortality has been directly correlated with the proportions of various populations that continue to secrete lactase in adulthood (Gaskill et al., 1979). The biocultural corollary, that breast cancer rates are related to per capita consumption of milk and dairy products among different human populations, is suggested by a number of studies (Micozzi and Moon, 1992). While Japanese populations have a high proportion of lactose intolerance (Johnson, Bowman and Schwitters, 1984), the recent increase in milk drinking in Japanese schools has been identified as a possible influence on the increased growth of Japanese children (Takahashi, 1984).

Societies with a high rate of lactose intolerance may exploit dairy food sources through consumption of yogurt, rather than raw milk. Large quantities of yogurt are consumed by some lactase-deficient populations (Simoons, 1969). Yogurt contains organisms that may digest lactose and facilitate intestinal absorption, thus making yogurt more digestible to lactase-deficient populations. The organisms in yogurt may also prevent formation of carcinogenic substances from the diet in the gastrointestinal tract (e.g., Goldin and Gorbach, 1984). Thus, lactase-deficient populations may be protected against some cancers by consumption of dairy products in the form of yogurt, rather than milk.

Overview of Overnutrition

The evidence linking excess dietary intake of macronutrients and breast cancer in case-control studies has not been as strong as results from ecologic, descriptive, and correlation studies. Since the dietary relation with breast cancer appears stronger in correlation studies than in case-control or cohort studies, the important dietary events relevant to breast cancer risk may occur early in life (Miller and Bulbrook, 1980). For example, dietary acculturation among Japanese migrants early in life appears central to the role of nutrition in the etiology of breast cancer (Miller, 1977). If nutrient intake in early life is a critical variable for long-term breast cancer risk, case-control studies on elderly women with breast cancer may not be the most appropriate manner of detecting a relation (Micozzi and Schatzkin, 1985).

The pattern of human epidemiologic evidence of breast cancer in women appears consistent with a role for excess dietary fat, protein, and total caloric intake early in life (Miller 1977; Miller and Bulbrook, 1980; Micozzi and Schatzkin, 1985). Events early in life such as breastfeeding that relate to diet, nutrition, and growth may have an impact on subsequent cancer incidence in human populations, in addition to dietary patterns later in life. Furthermore, given the limitations of accurate dietary assessment (Micozzi and Moon, 1992), nutrition-mediated factors that can be accurately measured (such as various indices of body size) may also be meaningful for comparisons of breast cancer rates in human populations. To the extent that breastfeeding and human breast milk provide a more appropriate species-specific diet in human infants (resulting in lower early dietary intake of calories, fats, and proteins, and slower growth rates), nursing may serve as a protective factor against breast cancer in later life for individuals who were breastfed.

REPRODUCTIVE BIOLOGY, BREASTFEEDING, AND BREAST CANCER

Reproductive variables and reproductive history have a marked effect on breast cancer risk (Kelsey and Gammon, 1991). These factors are related to hormonal status, and increased estrogen levels (and decreased progestogen levels) have been hypothesized as contributing to increased breast cancer risk.

Early age at menarche and late age at menopause have relative risks for breast cancer in the range of 1.2 to 1.9, while late age at birth of the first child has a relative risk between 2.0 and 4.0 in some studies (e.g., Staszewski, 1971). However, the effects of late maternal age at birth may be complex; among women who develop breast cancer, the earlier the first child, the earlier the age at the time of breast cancer diagnosis (Juret, Couette, Burne and Vernhes, 1974). The protective effects of high parity in breast cancer appear related to early age at birth of the first child (MacMahon, Cole, Lin, Lowe, Mirra, Ravnihar, Salber, Valaoras and Yuasa, 1970).

Although the important influence of a woman's reproductive history on her risk of breast cancer is widely recognized, it has not been clear whether these observations are entirely explained by age at first full-term pregnancy, or whether there are additional, independent influences of breastfeeding and parity. A logistic regression analysis of nearly 5000 women in the U.S. Cancer and Steroid Hormone Study confirmed the strong influence of age at first full-term pregnancy while revealing that parity and duration of breastfeeding also had strong influences on the risk of breast cancer (Layde, Webster, Boughman, Wingo, Rubin and Ory, 1989).

In a recent, population-based, case-control study also designed primarily to investigate the role of oral contraceptives in breast cancer, it was observed that the risk of breast cancer fell with increasing duration of breastfeeding and with increasing numbers of babies breastfed among young women (Chilvers, 1993). In Australia, a study of nearly 500 breast cancer cases indicated that lactation may play a modest direct or indirect role in reducing the risk of breast cancer (Siskind, Schofield, Rice and Bain, 1989). A case-control study in King County, Washington, showed that the risk of breast cancer decreases with increasing duration of lifetime lactational experience (McTiernan and Thomas, 1986). Among nearly 500 women with breast cancer and over 1300 controls in Buffalo, New York, there was evidence of a negative association between length of nursing and breast cancer risk. It was not clear, however, whether this observation means that breastfeeding is protective or that some women who are unsuccessful at lactation are at increased risk for subsequent breast cancer (Byers, Graham, Rzepka and Marshall, 1985).

The relation between lactation and the risk of breast cancer was specifically examined in a prospective cohort of nearly 90,000 women aged 30–55 years in the Nurses Health Study (London, Colditz, Stampfer, Willett, Rosner, Corsano and Speizer, 1990). However, there was no independent association found between lactation and breast cancer risk.

While several epidemiologic studies conducted in Scandinavian countries have not individually confirmed an association between age at first full-term pregnancy (independent of parity) and breast cancer risk, a meta-analysis of 8 studies involving over 5500 breast cancer cases confirmed that both low parity and late age at first full-term pregnancy are independent and significant risk factors (Ewertz, Duffy, Adami, Kvale, Lund, Meirik, Mellemgaard, Soini and Tulinius, 1990). These findings point out that risk factors with low relative risks (as are many of the reproductive factors including breastfeeding) may not always be detected in studies with relatively small numbers of cases and inadequate statistical power.

A recent review by Kvale (1992) confirms that abundant epidemiologic evidence exists showing early menarche, late menopause, low parity, and late age at first full-term pregnancy to be related to increased risk of breast cancer. Kvale and Heuch (1988), in a study of over 50,000 parous women in Norway, concluded that breastfeeding is not strongly related to the risk of breast cancer or any other common cancer. Results reported from two large prospective studies also suggest that breastfeeding is not strongly related to the risk of breast cancer among Western populations (Kvale, 1992). In a discussion of whether these epidemiologic findings provide a basis for primary prevention of breast cancer, Kvale and Jacobsen (1990) considered several known and suspected risk factors, including lactation, and concluded that it is difficult to suggest any feasible intervention strategy that would have a high probability of reducing the occurrence of breast cancer in the general population.

However, recent evidence exists for a relation between breastfeeding and breast cancer in non-Western populations. Various studies on small numbers of cases around the world have attempted to differentiate the effects of lactation on overall breast cancer risk. For example, in a study of 52 breast cancer cases in Japan, lack of breastfeeding had a relative risk of 2.3 compared with a relative risk of 2.6 for prior benign breast disease; early age at menopause and early age at first full-term pregnancy were associated with lower risk of breast cancer (Tashiro, Nomura and Hisamatu, 1990). In a self-reported study of 500 breast cancer cases in Beijing, high parity and long duration of lactation were protective factors against breast cancer (Tao, Yu, Ross and Xiu, 1988). In Shanghai, over 500 breast cancer cases also showed long duration of breastfeeding to be positively associated with lower breast cancer risk (Yuan, Yu, Ross, Gao and Henderson, 1988). This study demonstrated a clear and independent effect on breast cancer risk of breastfeeding in the majority of women in a population characterized by a long cumulative duration of nursing.

Ing, Petrakis and Ho (1977) studied women in fishing villages in Hong Kong, who by custom breastfeed only from the right breast. While in the general population the ratio of cancer in the left/right breast is essentially one, women who have consistently breastfed from only one breast show a significantly lower risk for development of cancer in the suckled breast. The actual physical process of breastfeeding may help to protect the suckled breast against cancer. This remarkable research provides the ultimate example of a controlled study in that both breasts of each of the women had been exposed to identical reproductive history and environmental (including systemic hormonal) influences, with the only difference being presence or absence of breastfeeding in one breast versus the other.

The relatively short periods of lactation seen in women in Western countries generally do not appear to be associated with a significantly lower risk of breast cancer. However, more intensive and longer durations of breastfeeding as observed in China, Hong Kong, and elsewhere appear to reduce the subsequent risk of breast cancer.

Finally, a recent study (Newcomb, Storer, Longnecker, Mittendorf, Greenberg, Clapp, Burke, Willett and MacMahon, 1994) in Maine, Massachusetts, New Hampshire, and Wisconsin showed a distinction between women with premenopausal versus postmenopausal breast cancer. Overall, lactation was not associated with the risk of postmenopausal breast cancer. However, among premenopausal women, a slight inverse association was observed, and lactation at early maternal ages and for long duration was associated with more substantial reductions in risk.

This study indicates that even in Western populations, those mothers that do breastfeed at young ages and for long duration show a significant reduction in the risk of premenopausal breast cancer. The authors suggest that a 25% reduction in breast cancer incidence could be achieved if all women with children lactated for 24 months or more

(Newcomb et al., 1994). Menopausal status may influence the effects of breastfeeding on breast cancer, as it appears to do for certain other risk factors (Paffenbarger, Kampert and Chang, 1980).

Breastfeeding may not hitherto have been clearly identified as a protective factor against breast cancer in women who breastfeed in Western societies because in these societies women do not breastfeed in the "ancient" or traditional pattern, i.e., on demand, throughout the night, and for a duration of at least one year. Sporadic breastfeeding, or breastfeeding on the same time schedule as bottle feeding, probably does not have the same physiologic effect. The application of more rigorous epidemiologic methods in larger, non-Western cohorts and better definition of breastfeeding patterns in epidemiologic studies should help resolve this question in the future.

Endogenous and Exogenous Hormones

Various hormonal mechanisms have been investigated in an attempt to explain the observation that early age at menarche, late age at birth of the first child, lack of breastfeeding, and late age at menopause are associated with increased breast cancer risk. All of these factors would result in prolonged, unopposed estrogen stimulation of breast tissue. Moolgavkar et al. (1980) and Thomas (1983) have argued, however, that hormones per se are unlikely to be of primary importance in determining overall risk in populations, although they may influence the epidemiology of breast cancer through their actions on the growth of nonneoplastic breast tissue.

No differences in total estrogen levels have been observed between groups of women with high rates of breast cancer in England compared to those with low rates in Japan (Bulbrook, Swain, Wang, Hayward, Kumaoka, Takatani, Abe and Utsunomiya, 1976) and in populations elsewhere (Hill, Wynder, Helman, Hickman, Rona and Kuno, 1976). Hayward, Greenwood and Glober (1978) also studied hormonal status in British, Japanese, and Japanese-Hawaiian women and found no differences in estrogen levels among populations with different rates of breast cancer. However, Trichopoulos, Cole, Brown, Goldman and MacMahon (1980) found an association between increased levels of estrogens and breast cancer in Greece. Although most studies on total endogenous estrogens and breast cancer have been negative, endogenous estrogen fractions have been studied in association with body fatness (see below).

Exogenous hormones have been studied in the form of oral contraceptives in premenopausal women. Studies have presented conflicting results on the risk for breast cancer of oral contraceptive use in young women (Royal College of General Practitioners, 1981). A large, population-based, case-control study showed no association between oral contraceptive use and the risk of breast cancer (Centers for Disease Control Cancer and Steroid Hormone Study, 1983), but subsequent studies showed an association between "high-progestogen" combination-type oral contraceptives and breast cancer in women before the age of 37 years (Pike, Henderson, Krailo, Duke and Roy, 1983), and an association between oral contraceptives use prior to the first full-term birth and increased risk of breast cancer prior to age 45 years (McPherson, Neil, Vessey and Doll, 1983). The hazards of subset analysis must be considered in the interpretation of these results. Reanalysis of the CDC (1983) data showed no effect on breast cancer risk of high-progestogen oral contraceptives or of oral contraceptive use before the first full-term pregnancy.

Studies of replacement doses of estrogens given to postmenopausal women have also yielded inconsistent results with respect to the risk of breast cancer (e.g., Kaufman, Miller, Rosenberg, Helmrich, Stolley, Schottenfeld and Shapiro, 1984). A large, case-control study in a hospital-based population (Kaufman et al., 1984) indicated that exogenous estrogens did not appear to influence the risk of breast cancer, even when taken for many years, and even in subgroups of women with other defined risk factors. More epidemiological studies on exogenous hormones and breast cancer are unlikely to produce more definitive results (Hulka, 1984).

Body Fat and Hormones

Regulation of endogenous hormones may be influenced by dietary fat and body fat. Dietary fat intake may influence overall levels of endogenous hormones, while body fat content may influence endogenous metabolism of estrogens, especially in postmenopausal women. Grodin, Siiteri and MacDonald (1973) determined that conversion of androstenedione to estrone in adipose tissue was an important determinant of endogenous estrogen levels in postmenopausal women, and postulated that dietary fat contributed to increased body fat stores through excess caloric intake.

Diet also influences the excretion of estrogens in both premenopausal and postmenopausal women. Omnivores have higher plasma estrone and estradiol levels than do vegetarians (Goldin, Adlercreutz and Dwyer, 1981; Goldin, Adlercreutz, Gorbach, Warram, Dwyer, Swenson and Woods, 1982), and premenopausal South African women fed a high fat (Western-style) diet have an apparent increase in estradiol levels (Hill, Garbaczewski, Helman, Huskisson, Sporangisa and Wynder, 1980). Postmenopausal vegetarian women have lower urinary excretion of estriol and total estrogens than matched nonvegetarian women (Armstrong, Brown and Clarke, 1981). In postmenopausal women especially, endogenous estrogen balance is influenced by interconversion of hormones in adipose tissue. Thus, total body fat may also be an important variable for breast cancer among women, based upon hormonal mechanisms.

BREAST BIOLOGY, APOCRINE GLAND FUNCTION, AND BREAST CANCER

Breast secretory activity has been related to the risk of breast cancer. Breast secretory activity may be influenced both by nutritional patterns and endogenous hormone activity. Although difficult to measure reliably, studies on the relation of estrogens to breast endothelial activity and breast fluid secretion may shed light on the role of diet and endogenous estrogens in breast cancer (Petrakis, Dupuy, Lee, Lyon, Maack, Gruenke and Craig, 1982). While estrogen levels in plasma (e.g., Goldin et al., 1982) and urine (e.g., Armstrong et al., 1981) have been studied in relation to the risk of breast cancer, levels of estrogen in breast fluid should be the critical observation relative to breast cancer, since it reflects most directly the microenvironment of breast tissue.

Early menarche is associated with early breast secretory activity, and increased nutrition may lead to increased breast secretory activity. In turn, breast biology is influenced by dietary protein levels (De Souza, Morgan, Lewis, Raggatt, Salih and Hobbs, 1974; Berg, 1975). Based upon an observed relation between higher socioeconomic status and increased breast secretory activity, Petrakis et al. (1982) hypothesized a relation between increased dietary intake ("improved" nutrition) and increased breast secretory activity, as assessed by measuring the quantity of breast fluid aspirated from the nipple in the nonlactating breast.

The amount of breast fluid has also been related to the type of cerumen secreted from related apocrine glands (Petrakis, Mason, Lee, Sugimoto, Parson and Catchall, 1975), which is, in turn, correlated with breast cancer mortality rates (Petrakis, 1977). The association between secretory activity of the nonlactating breast and related apocrine glands (cerumen-type) may have significance for breast cancer risk, since exogenously derived substances that may act as carcinogens are secreted into breast fluid. The turnover rate of substances secreted in the breast fluid may be a primary determinant of exposure of the breast epithelium to environmental and endogenous carcinogens and promoters (Petrakis, Maack, Lee and Lyon, 1980; Petrakis et al., 1982). Breastfeeding, in turn, has a strong influence over the turnover rate of substances secreted in the breast fluid, and prolonged lactation should minimize the exposure of breast epithelium to carcinogens.

Apocrine Gland Function

Observations on apocrine gland function at the population level have been related to susceptibility to breast cancer. Physiologically, female breast secretory glands, certain axillary sweat glands, and ceruminous (ear wax) glands compose the apocrine glandular system of the human body. Matsunaga (1962) illustrated that human cerumen occurs in two phenotypic forms, wet (sticky) and dry (hard). These phenotypic forms are governed by a single gene with two alleles, wet or dry. The allele for the wet type is dominant over that for the dry type (Matsunaga, 1962). The recessive dry type is predominant among Native American and Asian women, and the wet type is predominant among African and European women (Matsunaga, 1962). Petrakis (1977) observed that the frequency of the allele for the wet type of wax is high in populations at high risk for breast cancer and low in populations at low risk for breast cancer. Petrakis et al. (1975) further determined that the frequency of the wet-type gene is related to frequency of breast fluid secretor status in nonlactating women among different populations. Studying women from African-American, Caucasian, Chinese, Filipino, Japanese, and Mexican-American populations in San Francisco, these investigators found the highest rates of breast fluid secretor status among Caucasian women, and the lowest rates among Chinese women. Breast secretory fluids could be obtained by nipple aspiration in 81% of premenopausal Caucasian women, but only in 30% of premenopausal Chinese women.

Age and menopausal status also have an effect on secretor status among women: 60% of postmenopausal Caucasians were secretors, and only 4% of postmenopausal Chinese were secretors. This pattern appears to parallel the decline in estrogen production associated with menopause and the decrease in breast secretory activity associated with advancing age (Petrakis et al., 1975). Lynch, Albano, Danes, Layton, Kimberling, Lynch, Cheng, Costello, Mulcahy, Wagner et al. (1984) noted that it would be important to determine if the estrogen profiles of women who are genetically susceptible to breast cancer (Fishman, Fukushima, O'Connor, Rosenfeld, Lynch, Lynch, Guirgis and Maloney, 1978) might be correlated with breast secretory activity or cerumen characteristics. The hormonal basis of breast cancer risk, including the relevancy of maternal age at birth of first offspring for breast cancer risk in both mother and offspring, has been covered earlier in this chapter.

Wynder, Hill, Laakso, Littner and Kettunen (1981) found no statistically significant influence of menopausal status on breast secretor status among 244 healthy Finnish women who had an overall secretor status frequency of 38%. Petrakis, Wrensch and Ernster (1987) subsequently observed an age-related increase in the frequency of the dry wax phenotype among Caucasian (but not Asian or African) women. The use of exogenous estrogens in postmenopausal women was also associated with an increased frequency of the dry phenotype among women.

Wynder, Laht and Laakso (1985) studied over 1000 women in New York City and found no association between breast cancer and breast-fluid secretor status. In terms of the classic risk factors for breast cancer, there was an association between early age of menarche and adult breast fluid secretor status. However, there was no association between secretor status and parity, age at first pregnancy, or body weight. One group of women with preneoplastic breast abnormalities had a greater proportion of breast-fluid secretors. Wynder et al. (1985) also noted, however, that the composition of secretory fluid (which was not actually assessed in their study) is important to the pathogenesis of breast cancer.

Breast Fluid Composition

Petrakis and co-workers (1980, 1981) noted mutagenic activity in nipple aspirates of human breast fluid and identified specific mutagens (Petrakis et al., 1982), including cholesterol-epoxide (Craig, Gruenke and Petrakis, 1982). Petrakis and King (1981) studied human breast fluid from nearly 1500 women, aged 20–70 years, in San Francisco. Cytologic abnormalities in exfoliated breast epithelial cells were found in women with severe constipation. The authors postulated a mechanism by which mutagenic substances originating in the dietary tract may enter the circulation and reach the breast, where they may be selectively concentrated in breast fluid by the actions of breast apocrine secretory epithelia. The production of fecal mutagens in the colon has been described (Petrakis and King, 1981), and the association between breast cancer and bowel function has been confirmed among U.S. women, as reported in the U.S. National Health and Nutrition Examination Survey Epidemiologic Follow-up Study (Micozzi, Carter, Albanes, Taylor and Licitra, 1989).

The production of cytologic abnormalities in breast fluid cells is related to epithelial dysplasia in breast tissue and is regarded as a preneoplastic lesion by Petrakis and King (1981), who observed abnormal cells in nipple aspiration fluid from women with diagnosed atypical proliferative breast disease. Women with atypical proliferative breast disease, particularly in combination with a positive family history for breast cancer, are at a significantly increased risk for the development of breast cancer (Dupont and Page, 1985). Petrakis and King (1981), in a study of over 1000 Caucasian and Asian women in San Francisco, found that the wet-cerumen type was associated with the presence of pre-neoplastic cytologic atypia in nipple aspiration fluid. It is assumed that the presence of atypical cells in breast fluid is a marker for the presence of epithelial atypical proliferation in the actual breast tissue of women who have positive secretory status (Page, Vander Zwaag, Rogers, Williams, Walker and Hartmann, 1978). In turn, subsets of women with atypical proliferative breast disease (Page et al., 1978; Hutchinson, Thomas, Hamlin, Roth, Peterson and Williams, 1980; Roberts, Jones, Elton, Fortt, Williams and Gravelle, 1984) appear to be at significantly increased risk of breast cancer (Dupont and Page, 1985; Carter, Corle, Micozzi, Schatzkin and Taylor, 1988).

The Petrakis model of the wet/dry cerumen polymorphism found in different populations may be an indication of predisposition to breast cancer at the population level (O'Rourke and Petersen, 1983). However, the final association with breast cancer itself remains to be proven and is dependent upon establishing several associations among individual women in epidemiologic studies.

Breast Tissue Microenvironment

In the more recent Petrakis studies, women who were lactating, who were parous, or who had breastfed had lower levels of cholesterol and potentially carcinogenic cholesterol-epoxide in breast fluid. These low levels persist for 2 years postpartum or postlactation. Since breast fluid levels of potential carcinogens are reduced for relatively long periods after pregnancy or lactation, it has been hypothesized that this biochemical mechanism may help explain the reduction of breast cancer risk associated with parity (Gruenke, Wrensch, Petrakis, Miike, Ernster and Craig, 1987) and breastfeeding.

In addition, low levels of breast fluid estrogens were found following full-term birth and lactation, which may also provide a mechanism to explain why childbearing and breastfeeding may reduce risk. Furthermore, estrogen levels in breast fluid were not significantly related to estrogen levels in blood, which may explain why other studies do not observe relations between blood estrogen levels and breast cancer (Petrakis et al., 1987). Estrogen levels in the breast fluid itself should be far more significant for breast cancer risk, as these are the hormone levels to which breast epithelial tissue is most directly and consistently exposed.

While Petrakis (1977) originally attempted to account for the associations among cerumen type, breast secretory activity, and breast cancer epidemiology on a genetic basis at the population level, the association between breast cancer risk factors and breast secretory activity (Petrakis et al., 1987) may also be partially explained on an environmental basis, including the effects of childbearing and breastfeeding.

It should seem obvious that the microenvironment to which normal breast tissue is exposed plays a prominent role in the propensity to develop breast cancer. Factors that promote the growth of breast tissue at the cellular level, such as estrogens and certain nutrients, are associated with the development of breast cancer in women in epidemiologic studies. Those reproductive factors associated with prolonged, unopposed estrogen stimulation of breast tissue are clearly risk factors for breast cancer (Table 12.1), and indeed the breast tissue in nonlactating, nonpregnant women appears to be at significantly greater risk for the development of cancer compared to women who spend much of their adult lives pregnant and lactating. Clearly, breastfeeding is associated with reproductive factors that appear to protect women from developing breast cancer.

A purely independent effect of breastfeeding has been more difficult to define, although the studies of Petrakis and co-workers point to the importance of the hormonal and nutritional microenvironment of breast tissue. The effects of pregnancy and lactation appear to produce a microenvironment that is less carcinogenic for breast tissue, and avoid conditions of stasis in the breast.

CONCLUSIONS

Breast cancer risk, while as yet incompletely defined, appears to be associated with a very complex array of biological and cultural factors. The dramatic variations in breast cancer risk observed among Japanese and Japanese-American women, for example, indicate the important role of behavioral and environmental influences, including acculturation of diet and lifestyle. Reproductive factors also appear to play an important role, including pregnancy and lactation. However, breastfeeding behavior among women has been only incompletely characterized in epidemiologic studies of breast cancer.

Breastfeeding may help lower the risk of breast cancer by two general mechanisms: one associated with whether a woman was breastfed as a baby (early nutritional influences) and the other associated with whether a woman breastfed her child(ren). Dietary events relevant to breast cancer risk may have an influence early in the life of the individual. If an individual is not breastfed (e.g., formula-fed), there is the risk of overnutrition in early life.

Formula fed infants are exposed to higher caloric, fat, and protein intake than those who are breastfed. They are also not exposed to the immunologic benefits of breast milk, which may lead to an increased incidence of childhood cancer. Numerous human and animal studies are consistent with the hypothesis that overnutrition in infancy is a risk factor for the later development of certain cancers, including breast cancer. Increased childhood nutrition and growth also lead to earlier menarche. Early maturers have a life-long increase in the risk of developing breast cancer.

In mature women, breastfeeding may affect breast cancer risk by influencing systemic hormone levels and by influencing the microenvironment of the breast tissue. A woman who breastfeeds in the "ancient" or traditional pattern (on demand, through the night, and for a duration of at least 1 year) will experience lactational amenorrhea, usually from 1 to 2 years duration, and corresponding high levels of prolactin. Nonpregnant, nonlactating women have higher levels of estrogens, which appear to be associated with increased risk of breast cancer.

Prolonged lactation has an effect on the microenvironment of breast tissue and may help minimize exposure of the breast epithelium to carcinogens.

Recent studies indicate that the ancient or traditional pattern of breastfeeding appears to lower the risk of breast cancer. Earlier epidemiologic studies in Western and other populations may not have shown a clear, independent effect of breastfeeding on breast cancer because (1) breastfeeding behavior was incompletely characterized, and/or (2) the breastfeeding that does occur in Western populations generally does not follow the ancient or traditional pattern.

Biologically, pregnancy and lactation are linked in both adaptive and physiologic ways. Rapid sociocultural developments have recently resulted in many more years of fertile adult life in women who are not pregnant or lactating, compared to past generations. Breast cancer may be one of the biologic consequences.

REFERENCES

Albanes, D. A., A. G. Schatzkin, and M. S. Micozzi

1987 A survey of time related factors in diet and cancer. *Journal of Chronic Disease* 40:395–445.

Armstrong, B., and R. Doll
1975 Environmental factors and cancer incidence and mortality in different countries, with special reference to dietary practices. *International Journal of Cancer* 15:617–631.

Armstrong, B., J. B. Brown, and H. T. Clarke
1981 Diet and reproductive hormones: A study of vegetarian and non-vegetarian postmenopausal women. *Journal of the National Cancer Institute* 67(4):761–767.

Berg, J. W.
1975 Can nutrition explain the pattern of international epidemiology of hormone-dependent cancers? *Cancer Research* 35:3345–3350.

Brinkley, D., R. G. Carpenter, and J. L. Haybittle
1971 An anthropometric study of women with cancer. *British Journal of Preventive and Social Medicine* 25:65–75.

Buell, P.
1973 Changing incidence of breast cancer in Japanese-American women. *Journal of the National Cancer Institute* 51:1479–1483.

Buell, P., and J. Dunn
1965 Cancer mortality of Japanese Isei and Nisei of California. *Cancer* 18:656–664.

Bulbrook, R. D., M. C. Swain, D. Y. Wang, J. L. Hayward, S. Kumaoka, O. Takatani, O. Abe, and J. Utsunomiya
1976 Breast cancer in Britain and Japan. *European Journal of Cancer* 12:725–735.

Byers, T., S. Graham, T. Rzepka, and J. Marshall
1985 Lactation and breast cancer: Evidence for a negative association in premenopausal women. *American Journal of Epidemiology* 121: 664–674.

Carter, C. L., D. K. Corle, M. S. Micozzi, A. Schatzkin, and P. R. Taylor
1988 A prospective study of the development of breast cancer in 16,692 women with benign breast disease. *American Journal of Epidemiology* 128(3):467–477.

Centers for Disease Control Cancer and Steroid Hormone Study (CDC)
1983 Long-term oral contraceptive use and the risk of breast cancer. *Journal of the American Medical Association* 249(12):1591–1595.

Chilvers, C.
1993 Breast feeding and risk of breast cancer in young women. United Kingdom National Case-Control Study Group. *British Medical Journal* 307:17–20.

Clinton, S. K., C. R. Truex, and W. J. Visek
1979 Dietary protein, aryl hydrocarbon hydroxylase and chemical carcinogenesis in rats. *Journal of Nutrition* 109:55–62.

Cohen, M. N.
1989 *Health and the Rise of Civilization*. New Haven: Yale University Press.

Craig, J. C., L. D. Gruenke, and N. L. Petrakis
1982 Measurement of cholesterol epoxide formation and turnover in human breast fluid. In *Synthesis and Applications of Isotopically Labeled Compounds*, edited by W. P. Duncan and A. B. Susas, pp. 297–298. Amsterdam: Elsevier.

Davis, M. K., D. A. Savitz, and B. I. Graubard
1988 Infant feeding and childhood cancer. *Lancet* 2:365–368.

De Souza, I., L. Morgan, U. L. Lewis, P. R. Raggatt, H. Salih, and J. R. Hobbs
1974 Growth hormone dependence among human breast cancers. *Lancet* 2:182–184.
DeWaard, F.
1975 Breast cancer incidence and nutritional status with particular reference to body weight and height. *Cancer Research* 35:3351–3356.
DeWaard, F., and E. A. Banders-van Halewijn
1974 A prospective study in general practice on breast cancer risk in postmenopausal women. *International Journal of Cancer* 14:153–160.
DeWaard, F., J. P. Cornelius, and K. Aichi
1977 Breast cancer incidence according to weight and height in two cities of the Netherlands and Japan. *Cancer* 40:1269–1277.
Doll, R., C. Muir, and J. Waterhouse
1970 *Cancer Incidence in Five Continents*, Vol. II. New York: Springer-Verlag.
Drasar, B. S., and D. Irving
1973 Environmental factors and cancer of the colon and breast. *British Journal of Cancer* 27:167–172.
Dunn, J. E.
1977 Breast Cancer among American Japanese in the San Francisco Bay area. *National Cancer Institute Monograph* 47:157–160.
Dupont, W. D., and D. L. Page
1985 Risk factors for breast cancer in women with proliferative breast disease. *New England Journal of Medicine* 312:146–151.
Eaton, S. B., and M. Konner
1985 Paleolithic nutrition: A consideration of its nature and current implications. *New England Journal of Medicine* 312:283–289.
Eveleth, P. B., and J. M. Tanner
1976 *Worldwide Variation in Human Growth*. Cambridge: Cambridge University Press.
Ewertz, M., S. W. Duffy, H. O. Adami, G. Kvale, E. Lund, O. Meirik, A. Mellemgaard, I. Soini, and H. Tulinius
1990 Age at first birth, parity and risk of breast cancer: A meta-analysis of 8 studies from the Nordic countries. *International Journal of Cancer* 46:597–603.
Federation of American Societies for Experimental Biology (FASEB)
1976 Evaluation of the health aspects of sucrose as a food ingredient. Unpublished manuscript P I-III, I–30.
Fishman, J., D. Fukushima, J. O'Connor, R. S. Rosenfeld, H. T. Lynch, J. F. Lynch, H. Guirgis, and K. Maloney
1978 Plasma hormone profiles of young women at risk for familial breast cancer. *Cancer Research* 38:4006–4011.
Gaskill, S. P., W. L. McGuire, C. K. Osborne, and M. P. Stern
1979 Breast cancer mortality and diet in the United States. *Cancer Research* 39:3628–3637.
Goldin, B. R., and S. H. Gorbach
1984 Alterations of the intestinal macroflora by diet, oral antibiotics, and Lactobacillus: Decreased production of free amines from aromatic nitro com-

pounds, azo dyes, and glucuronides. *Journal of the National Cancer Institute* 73:689–695.

Goldin, B. R., H. Adlercreutz, and J. T. Dwyer
1981 Effect of diet on excretion of estrogens in pre- and postmenopausal women. *Cancer Research* 41:3771–3773.

Goldin, B. R., H. Adlercreutz, S. L. Gorbach, J. H. Warram, J. T. Dwyer, L. Swenson, and M. N. Woods
1982 Estrogen excretion patterns and plasma levels in vegetarian and omnivorous women. *New England Journal of Medicine* 307:1542–1547.

Graham, S., J. Marshall, C. Mettlin, T. Rzepka, T. Nemoto, and T. Byers
1982 Diet in the epidemiology of breast cancer. *American Journal of Epidemiology* 116:68–75.

Gray, G. E., M. C. Pike, and B. E. Henderson
1979 Breast cancer incidence and mortality rates in different countries in relation to known risk factors and dietary practices. *British Journal of Cancer* 39:1–7.

Greulich, W. W.
1957 A comparison of the physical growth and development of American-born and native Japanese children. *American Journal of Physical Anthropology* 15:489–515.

Grodin, J. M., P. K. Siiteri, and P. C. MacDonald
1973 Source of estrogen production in postmenopausal women. *Journal of Clinical Endocrinology and Metabolism* 36:207–214.

Gruenke, L. D., M. R. Wrensch, N. L. Petrakis, R. Miike, V. L. Ernster, and J. C. Craig
1987 Breast fluid cholesterol and cholesterol epoxides: Relationships to breast cancer risk factors and other characteristics. *Cancer Research* 47:5483–5487.

Hahn, O., and O. Koldovsky
1966 *Utilization of Nutrients during Postnatal Development*. London: Pergamon Press.

Haymond, M. W., I. E. Karl, and A. S. Pagliara
1974 Increased gluconeogenic substrates in the small-for-gestational-age infant. *New England Journal of Medicine* 291(7):322–328.

Hayward, J. L., F. C. Greenwood, and G. A. Glober
1978 Hormonal status in normal British, Japanese and Hawaii-Japanese women. *European Journal of Cancer* 14:1221–1228.

Hems, G.
1978 Contributions of diet and childbearing to breast cancer rates. *British Journal of Cancer* 37:974–982.
1980 Associations between breast cancer mortality rates, childbearing and diet in the United Kingdom. *British Journal of Cancer* 41:429–437.

Hill, P., E. L. Wynder, P. Helman, R. Hickman, G. Rona, and K. Kuno
1976 Plasma hormone levels in different ethnic populations. *Cancer Research* 36:2297–2301.

Hill, P., L. Garbaczewski, P. Helman, J. Huskisson, E. Sporangisa, and E. L. Wynder
1980 Diet, lifestyles and menstrual activity. *American Journal of Clinical Nutrition* 33:1192–1198.

Hirayama, T.
1978 Epidemiology of breast cancer with special reference to the role of diet. *Preventive Medicine* 7:173–195.
Hulka, B. S.
1984 When is the evidence for 'no association' sufficient? *Journal of the American Medical Association* 252(1):81–82.
Hutchinson, W. B., D. B. Thomas, W. B. Hamlin, G. J. Roth, A. V. Peterson, and B. Williams
1980 Risk of breast cancer in women with benign breast disease. *Journal of the National Cancer Institute* 65:13–20.
Ing, R., N. L. Petrakis, and J. H. C. Ho
1977 Unilateral breast feeding and breast cancer. *Lancet* 2:124–127.
Johnson, R. C., K. S. Bowman, and S. Y. Schwitters
1984 Ethnic familial and environmental influences in lactose tolerance. *Human Biology* 56:307–316.
Juret, P., J. -E. Couette, D. Burne, and J. -C. Vernhes
1974 Age at first birth: An equivocal factor in human mammary carcinogenesis. *European Journal of Cancer* 10:591–594.
Kaufman, D. E., D. R. Miller, L. Rosenberg, S. P. Helmrich, P. Stolley, D. Schottenfeld, and S. Shapiro
1984 Non-contraceptive estrogen use and risk of breast cancer. *Journal of the American Medical Association* 252:63–67.
Kelsey, J. L., and M. D. Gammon
1991 The epidemiology of breast cancer. *CA-Cancer Journal for Clinicians* 41:146–165.
Kolonel, L. N., J. H. Hankin, J. Lee, S. Y. Chi, A. Nomura, and M. W. Hinds
1981 Nutrient intakes in relation to cancer incidence in Hawaii. *British Journal of Cancer* 44:331–339.
Kondo, S., and M. Eto
1975 Physical growth studies on Japanese-American Children in comparison with native Japanese. In *Proceedings of Meeting for Review and Seminar of the U.S.–Japan Cooperative Research on Human Adaptabilities*, pp. 13–45. JIBP synthesis, Vol. 1. Tokyo: University of Tokyo Press.
Kralj-Cercek, L.
1956 The influence of food, body build, and social origin on the age at menarche. *Human Biology* 28:393–406.
Kurihara, M., K. Aoki, and S. Tominaga
1984 *Cancer Mortality Statistics in the World*. Nayoga, Japan: University of Nayoga Press.
Kvale, G.
1992 Reproductive factors in breast cancer epidemiology. *Acta Oncologica* 31:187–194.
Kvale, G., and I. Heuch
1988 Lactation and cancer risk: Is there a relation specific to breast cancer? *Journal of Epidemiology and Community Health* 42:30–37.
Kvale, G., and B. K. Jacobsen
1990 Risk factors for breast cancer. Do epidemiologic findings provide a basis

for primary prevention? (Norwegian) *Tidsskrift for den Norske Laegeforening* 110:232–235.

LaPorte, R. E., L. L. Adams, D. D. Savage, G. Brenes, S. Dearwater, and T. Cook
1984 The spectrum of physical activity, cardiovascular disease and health: An epidemiologic perspective. *American Journal of Epidemiology* 120:507–517.

Layde, P. M., L. A. Webster, A. L. Boughman, P. A. Wingo, G. L. Rubin, and H. W. Ory
1989 The independent associations of parity, age at first full term pregnancy, and duration of breast feeding with the risk of breast cancer. Cancer and Steroid Hormone Study Group. *Journal of Clinical Epidemiology* 42:963–973.

London, S. J., G. A. Colditz, M. J. Stampfer, W. C. Willett, B. A. Rosner, K. Corsano, and F. E. Speizer
1990 Lactation and risk of breast cancer in a cohort of US women. *American Journal of Epidemiology* 132:17–26.

Love, R.
1992 Clinical trials on breast cancer. In *Macronutrients: Investigating Their Role in Cancer*, edited by M. S. Micozzi and T. E. Moon, pp. 377–406. New York: Marcel Dekker.

Lubin, J. H., P. E. Burns, W. Blot, R. G. Ziegler, A. W. Lees, and J. F. Fraumeni, Jr.
1981 Dietary factors and breast cancer risk. *International Journal of Cancer* 28:685–689.

Lynch, H. T., W. A. Albano, B. S. Danes, M. A. Layton, W. J. Kimberling, J. F. Lynch, S. C. Cheng, K. A. Costello, G. M. Mulcahy, C. A. Wagner et al.
1984 Genetic predisposition to breast cancer. *Cancer* 53:612–622.

MacMahon, B., P. Cole, T. M. Lin, C. R. Lowe, A. P. Mirra, B. Ravnihar, E. J. Salber, V. G. Valaoras, and S. Yuasa
1970 Age at first birth and breast cancer risk. *Bulletin of the World Health Organization* 43:209–221.

Malcolm, L. A.
1974 Ecological factors relating to child growth and nutritional status. In *Nutrition and Malnutrition*, edited by A.F. Roche and F. Falkner, pp. 329–353. New York: Plenum.
1979 Protein-energy malnutrition and growth. In *Human Growth*, Vol. 3, edited by F. Falkner and J. M. Tanner, pp. 361–372. New York: Plenum.

Matsunaga, E.
1962 The dimorphism in human normal cerumen. *Annals of Human Genetics* 25:273–286.

McPherson, K., A. Neil, M. P. Vessey, and R. Doll
1983 Oral contraceptive and breast cancer. *Lancet* 2:1414–1415 (letter).

McTiernan, A., and D. B. Thomas
1986 Evidence for a protective effect of lactation on risk of breast cancer in young women. *American Journal of Epidemiology* 124:353–358.

Micozzi, M. S.
1990 Applications of anthropometry to epidemiologic studies of nutrition and cancer. *American Journal of Human Biology* 2:727–739.

1991 Disease in antiquity: The case of cancer. *Archives of Pathology and Laboratory Medicine* 115:838–844.

Micozzi, M. S., and T. E. Moon

1992 *Macronutrients: Investigating Their Role in Cancer*. New York: Marcel Dekker, Inc.

Micozzi, M. S., and A. G. Schatzkin

1985 International correlation of anthropometric variables and adolescent growth patterns with breast cancer incidence. *American Journal of Physical Anthropology* 66:206–207 (abstract).

Micozzi, M. S., C. L. Carter, D. Albanes, P. R. Taylor, and L. M. Licitra

1989 Bowel function and breast cancer in U. S. women. *American Journal of Public Health* 79:73–75.

Miller, A. B.

1977 Role of nutrition in the etiology of breast cancer. *Cancer* 39:2704–2708.

Miller, A. B., and R. D. Bulbrook

1980 The epidemiology and etiology of breast cancer. *New England Journal of Medicine* 303:1246–1248.

Miller, A. B., A. Kelly, N. W. Choi, V. Matthews, R. W. Morgan, L. Munan, J. D. Burch, J. Feather, G. R. Howe, and M. Jain

1978 A study of diet and breast cancer. *American Journal of Epidemiology* 107:499–509.

Montoye, H. J., and H. L. Taylor

1984 Measurement of physical activity in population studies: A review. *Human Biology* 56:195–216.

Moolgavkar, S. H., N. E. Day, and R. G. Stevens

1980 Two-stage model for carcinogenesis: Epidemiology of breast cancer in females. *Journal of the National Cancer Institute* 65:559–569.

Moon, T. E., and M. S. Micozzi

1989 *Nutrition and Cancer Prevention: Investigating the Role of Micronutrients*. New York: Marcel Dekker.

Newcomb, P. A., B. E. Storer, M. P. Longnecker, R. Mittendorf, E. G. Greenberg, R. W. Clapp, K. P. Burke, W. C. Willett, and M. MacMahon

1994 Lactation and reduced risk of premenopausal breast cancer. *New England Journal of Medicine* 330:81–87.

Newman, M. T.

1975 Nutrition and adaptation in man. In *Physiological Anthropology*, edited by A. Damon, pp. 210–259. London: Oxford University Press.

Nomura, A., B. E. Henderson, and J. Lee

1978 Breast cancer and diet among the Japanese in Hawaii. *American Journal of Clinical Nutrition* 31:2020–2025.

O'Rourke, D. H., and G. M. Petersen

1983 Biological anthropology and genetic disease research. Introduction. *American Journal of Physical Anthropology* 62:1–2.

Paffenbarger, R. S., J. B. Kampert, and H. Chang

1980 Characteristics that predict the risk of cancer before and after menopause. *American Journal of Epidemiology* 112:258–268.

Page, D. L., R. Vander Zwaag, L. W. Rogers, L. T. Williams, W. E. Walker, and W. H. Hartmann
1978 Relation between component parts of fibrocystic disease complex and breast cancer. *Journal of the National Cancer Institute* 61:1055–1063.
Petrakis, N. L.
1977 Genetic cerumen type breast secretory activity and breast cancer epidemiology. In *Genetics of Human Cancer,* edited by J. J. Mulvhill, R. W. Miller, and J. F. Fraumeni, pp. 297–299. New York: Raven Press.
Petrakis, N. L., and E. B. King
1981 Cytological abnormalities in nipple aspirates of breast fluid from women with severe constipation. *Lancet* 2:1203–1205.
Petrakis, N. L., L. Mason, R. Lee, B. Sugimoto, S. Pawson, and F. Catchpool
1975 Association of race, age, menopausal status and cerumen type with breast fluid secretion in nonlactating women as determined by nipple aspiration. *Journal of the National Cancer Institute* 54:829–833.
Petrakis, N. L., C. A. Maack, R. E. Lee, and M. Lyon
1980 Mutagenic activity in nipple aspirates of human breast fluid. *Cancer Research* 40:188–189.
Petrakis, N. L., M. E. Dupuy, R. E. Lee, M. Lyon, C. A. Maack, L. D. Gruenke, and J. C. Craig
1982 Mutagens in nipple aspirates of breast fluids. *Banbury Report 13: Indicators of Genotoxic Exposure,* edited by B. A. Bridges, B. E. Butterworth, and I. B. Weinstein, pp. 67–82. Cold Spring Harbor, NY: Cold Spring Harbor Laboratory.
Petrakis, N. L., M. R. Wrensch, and V. L. Ernster
1987 Influence of pregnancy and lactation on serum and breast fluid estrogen levels: Implications for breast cancer risk. *International Journal of Cancer* 40:587–591.
Phillips, R. L.
1975 Role of lifestyle and dietary habits in risk of cancer among Seventh-Day Adventists. *Cancer Research* 35:3513–3522.
Pike, M. C., B. E. Henderson, M. D. Krailo, A. Duke, and S. Roy
1983 Breast cancer in young women and use of oral contraceptives: Possible modifying effect of formulation and age at use. *Lancet* 2:926–930.
Potter, J.
1992 Epidemiology of diet and cancer: Evidence of human maladaptation. In *Macronutrients: Investigating Their Role in Cancer,* edited by M. S. Micozzi and T. E. Moon, pp. 55–86. New York: Marcel Dekker.
Prentice, R.
1992 Rationale, feasibility, and design of a low fat diet intervention trial among postmenopausal women. In *Macronutrients: Investigating Their Role in Cancer,* edited by M. S. Micozzi and T. E. Moon, pp. 355–376. New York: Marcel Dekker.
Roberts, M. M., V. Jones, R. A. Elton, R. W. Fortt, S. Williams, and I. H. Gravelle
1984 Risk of breast cancer in women with history of benign disease of the breast. *British Medical Journal* 228:275–278.

Roche, A. F.
1984 Anthropometric methods: New and old. What they tell us. *International Journal of Obesity* 8:509–523.
Ross, M. H.
1977 Dietary behavior and longevity. *Nutrition Reviews* 35:257–265.
Ross, M. H., and G. Bras
1965 Tumor incidence patterns and nutrition in the rat. *Journal of Nutrition* 87:245–250.
1971 Lasting influence of early caloric restriction on prevalence of neoplasms in the rat. *Journal of the National Cancer Institute* 47:1095–1099.
Ross, M. H., G. Bras, and E. D. Lustbader
1983 Diet, body weight and tumor susceptibility. *Twenty-eighth Scientific Report, Institute for Cancer Research*, pp. 18–20. Philadelphia, PA: Fox Chase Cancer Center.
Rothman, K. J., B. MacMahon, T. M. Lin, C. R. Lowe, A. P. Mirra, B. Ravnihar, E. J. Salber, D. Trichopoulos, and S. Yuasa
1980 Maternal age and birth rank of women with breast cancer. *Journal of the National Cancer Institute* 65:719–722.
Royal College of General Practitioners
1981 Breast cancer and oral contraceptives. *British Medical Journal* 282:2089–2093.
Sherman, B., R. Wallace, J. Bean, and L. Schlabaugh
1981 Relationships of body weight to menarche and menopausal age: Implications for breast cancer risk. *Journal of Clinical Endocrinology and Metabolism* 52:488–493.
Simoons, F. J.
1969 Primary adult lactose intolerance and the milking habit: A problem in biological and cultural interrelations. I. Review of the medical literature. *American Journal of Digestive Disease* 14:819–836.
Siskind, V., F. Schofield, D. Rice, and C. Bain
1989 Breast cancer and breastfeeding: Results from an Australian case-control study. *American Journal of Epidemiology* 130:229–236.
Staszewski, J.
1971 Age at menarche and breast cancer. *Journal of the National Cancer Institute* 47:935–940.
Stini, W. A.
1978 Early nutrition, growth, disease and human longevity. *Nutrition and Cancer* 1:31–39.
Taitz, L. S.
1971 Overnutrition among artificially fed infants in Sheffield regions. *British Journal of Medicine* 1:315–316.
Takahashi, E.
1984 Secular trend in milk consumption and growth in Japan. *Human Biology* 56:427–437.
Tanner, J. M.
1968 Earlier maturation in man. *Scientific American* 218:21–27.
Tanner, J. M., and P. B. Eveleth
1975 Variability between populations in growth and development at puberty.

In *Puberty: Biologic and Psychosocial Components*, edited by S. R. Berenberg, pp. 256–273. Leiden: H. E. Stenfert Kroese B. V.

Tao, S. C., M. C. Yu, R. K. Ross, and R. W. Xiu
1988 Risk factors for breast cancer in Chinese women of Beijing. *International Journal of Cancer* 42:495–498.

Tashiro, H., Y. Nomura, and K. Hisamatu
1990 A case-control study of risk factors of breast cancer detected by mass screening (Japanese). *Gan No Rinsho* 36: 2127–2130.

Thomas, D. B.
1983 Factors that promote the development of human breast cancer. *Environmental Health Perspective* 50:209–218.

Trichopoulos, D., P. Cole, J. B. Brown, M. B. Goldman, and B. MacMahon
1980 Estrogen profiles of primiparous and nulliparous women in Athens, Greece. *Journal of the National Cancer Institute* 55:43–46.

Waterhouse, J., P. Correa, C. Muir, and J. Powell
1976 *Cancer Incidence in Five Continents*, Vol. III. Lyons, France: International Agency for Research on Cancer.

Waterhouse, J., C. Muir, K. Shanmugaratnam, and J. Powell
1982 *Cancer incidence in Five Continents*, Vol. IV. Lyons, France: International Agency for Research on Cancer.

Widdowson, E. M.
1974 Changes in pigs due to undernutrition before birth and for one, two, and three years afterward, and the effects of rehabilitation. In *Nutrition and Malnutrition: Identification and Measurement*, edited by A. F. Roche and F. Falkner, pp. 165–181. *Advances in Experimental Medicine and Biology*, Vol. 49. New York: Plenum Press.

Wilson, D. C., and I. Sutherland
1960 Further observations on the age of menarche. *British Medical Journal* 2:864–867.

Wood, J. W., G. R. Milner, H. C. Harpending, and K. M. Weiss
1992 The osteological paradox: Problems of inferring prehistoric health from skeletal samples. *Current Anthropology* 33:343–370.

Wynder, E. L., P. Hill, K. Laakso, R. Littner, and K. Kettunen
1981 Breast secretion in Finnish women: A metabolic epidemiologic study. *Cancer* 47(6):1444–1450.

Wynder, E. L., H. Laht, and K. Laakso
1985 Nipple aspirates of breast fluid and the epidemiology of breast disease. *Cancer* 56:1473–1479.

Yuan, J. M., M. C. Yu, R. K. Ross, Y. T. Gao, and B. E. Henderson
1988 Risk factors for breast cancer in Chinese women in Shanghai. *Cancer Research* 48:1949–1953.

13

Commentary
Breastfeeding: Biocultural Perspectives

Sheila Kitzinger

FIRST THOUGHTS

This book focuses on the lives of women and their babies in the intimate reciprocity of breastfeeding. Rather than simply recording whether or not women breastfeed, whether and when supplementary foods are given, and when weaning occurs, the contributors to this volume explore relationships between the breastfeeding mother and her child through the 24 hours, and the seasonal variations—linked with agricultural work and the harvest, or with arid and rainy seasons, for example—that exist in some societies. The contributors reveal what Ellison describes as "the choreography of nursing." Analysis at this level means that we get a clearer picture than ever before of the contexts and styles of nursing in those traditional societies in which breastfeeding is more conspicuously successful than anywhere in urban, industrial, technocratic culture.

Understanding of the dynamics of breastfeeding is important not only because it enables babies to be nourished on the best possible and readily available food, but because human milk is one of the world's major economic resources. It is also "ecology, with love" (Kitzinger, 1980). It has been estimated, for example, that an American artificially fed baby uses 150 cans of formula each year. This adds up to approximately 70,000 tons of metal for the nation as a whole (Jelliffe and Jelliffe, 1978).

In spite of the lip-service to the importance of breastfeeding for infant well-being, the economic aspect of breastfeeding is largely unacknowledged by governments, as it is by medical systems and by doctors who have taken responsibility for women's and children's health. Even where the unique value of human milk is recognized, it is treated as an exploitable natural product, with mere glancing reference to the lives of the women who are the ones who make it. Breastfeeding, and failure to breastfeed, can be understood only within the context of wealth and poverty, female labor, the exploitation of women in the service of men, and the social systems that reinforce male power.

It should not be assumed that because lactation is a mammalian characteristic that breastfeeding is "natural." It is natural only in the sense that childbirth can also be claimed to be natural, and this is how Dettwyler refers to it in Chapter 2. Yet both these physiological processes are shaped by society and function within a complex system of social controls, in the same way that defecation and urination, sexual behavior, and food consumption are also socially constructed. There are wide cultural variations in practice, some of which make birth and breastfeeding more traumatic, others of which make each of these female activities easier and more satisfying (Kitzinger, 1994a). The context and pattern of breastfeeding are to a large extent controlled and dictated by men, and nowhere more so than where birth and breastfeeding are medicalized, and when technology has been developed, such as the manufacture of infant formula, which it is in the interest of large international corporations to promote and expand.

Following childbirth, there is for many women a window of opportunity in which lactation can be stimulated by suckling, and in which failure of stimulation eventually leads to suppression of lactation. Although adopting mothers are sometimes able to breastfeed, and grandmothers to induce lactation when grandchildren are left in their care, or when a breastfeeding daughter is sick or dies, this kind of commitment to nursing is rare in Western cultures. A more usual situation is that after a period in which the option to breastfeed is available—which lasts for some women not more than 5 to 6 weeks—a woman who has chosen not to breastfeed, or one who believes that she cannot make enough milk, or who has breast problems that she finds insurmountable, has to rely on alternative foods of one kind of another. If formula is introduced during this period, the chances of a woman succeeding in breastfeeding are much reduced. A randomized controlled trial has shown that babies given supplementary artificial milk[1] or other fluids are five times more likely to be formula-fed by the end of the first week of life than those who are exclusively breastfed (de Chateau, Holmberg, Jakobsson and Winberg, 1977; Winberg and de Chateau, 1979).

Companies that manufacture and promote infant formula engage in the wholesale destruction of the basic economic resource of human milk. Babies are exposed to bacterial infection, suffer gastrointestinal, respiratory and other diseases, and often die as a result. Cunningham (Chapter

9) also cites paralytic poliomyelitis, liver disease, reduced bone mass in young women, and increased exposure to radioactivity as other consequences of bottle-feeding.

Because women who would otherwise experience lactation anovulation for periods of up to 4 years in countries where they do not have access to effective means of contraception, there is increased risk of pregnancies occurring in rapid succession when mothers bottle-feed. Ellison draws on the work of the demographer Louis Henry to suggest that lactation may be the primary determinant of fertility variation in societies where there is no conscious birth control method. On the other hand, women in a wide range of societies are aware that breastfeeding has a contraceptive effect, if only because sexual intercourse is prohibited during lactation. As one lactating Jamaican mother said to me when asked if she used birth control: "Yes, me no have man this year." She was probably unaware that the frequent suckling she offered her baby because of her strong belief, shared with other Caribbean peasant women, that babies should never be left to cry, had the effect of preventing ovulation (Kitzinger, 1994b). In some cultures women are well aware of the contraceptive effect of breastfeeding; poor women in Istanbul state this as their main reason for choosing to breastfeed (Kocturk, 1988).

The side-effects of the promotion of artificial feeding are ill-health and poverty not only for the babies directly concerned, but for families and entire communities. Running a relief agency from our home to send food and other goods to the former Yugoslavia, we observed that in Croatia in June of 1993, the cost of feeding a baby infant formula came to 60% of the average income when one partner was employed. In fact, most people were unemployed. So babies were fed bread and water and artificial milk or ordinary cows' milk was diluted. Since then inflation has increased the cost of replacing mother's milk.

A standard practice of formula companies is to promote their products through funding of research projects, medical school departments, medical conferences, and freebies for doctors and nurses. In one year (1993) in the United States, for example, companies funded conferences, workshops, and fellowships for the Association of Women's Health, Obstetric and Neonatal Nurses, the National Association of Neonatal Nurses, and the American Academy of Pediatrics.

EXPERT ADVICE

The advice given to women by so-called *experts* has been, from the 1920s on, the main stumbling-block to successful breastfeeding. Truby-King, a New Zealand doctor who specialized in calf-rearing, was the primary proponent of a system of four-hourly, strictly regulated breastfeeding, which dictated the pattern of professional advice until very recently. He warned against overfeeding, "coddling," cuddling, and rocking babies, and states that it was unnatural for a baby to feed at any time between midnight and sunrise (Kitzinger, 1994a).

In most traditional societies, in contrast, the rhythms of breastfeeding are partly baby-led, partly a counterpoint to work tasks that can be performed with the baby nestled in a sling against the mother's body or lying close by her, tasks that are punctuated with breastfeeding whenever the baby signals readiness to feed. Frequent feeds maximize the fat content of milk, and—as Woolridge points out in Chapter 8—the baby is more likely to be satisfied and settled.

In Western cultures nighttime feeding is treated as undesirable by professional advisors, family members, and many mothers themselves. The goal is to "train a baby to go through the night." The first question people often ask of a new mother concerns nighttime waking, the implication being that a well-fed, "good" baby will not wake for feeds during the hours of darkness. In traditional cultures, where babies sleep beside or near their mothers, night feeds are taken for granted, and a baby may obtain a larger proportion of milk during the night than in the daytime. In Thailand, for example, night feeds persist through the first year of life, though daytime feeds are reduced. This does not lead to sleep problems. "Sleep dysfunction," Woolridge asserts, "is largely absent from such cultures."

Quandt refers to what she calls "the adoption of European practices of early feeding of paps and porridges" in slave societies in the Caribbean, where women's forced labor prevented them from breastfeeding during working hours (Chapter 5). Yet it is doubtful whether this was imitation of European practices. More likely it was an adaptation to the demands of conditions of slavery, which formed a pattern that persists to this day. Babies are often cared for by grandmothers in the daytime, but peasant woman sleep with their babies, who breastfeed on and off all night. When interviewing mothers in health clinics in rural Jamaica, where heavy emphasis was placed on teaching about the introduction of solid foods toward the end of the first year, I learned that they were reluctant to admit breastfeeding during the night. Yet these same women, interviewed in their own homes, revealed that though they offered the baby porridge and mashed banana in the day, their babies slept against their bodies in the night and suckled freely (Kitzinger, 1994a).

Mother–infant co-sleeping and breastfeeding through the first year of life may have a protective function against sudden infant death syndrome (SIDS). Co-sleeping and breastfeeding are elements in an adaptive complex that not only ensures that babies are fed, and close physical contact enables them to feel secure, but that may result in increased safety. Mckenna and Bernshaw (Chapter 10) reveal that sounds and movements made by the mother regularly arouse the baby from deep sleep, and thus stimulate breathing. Periods of apnea are most likely to occur during deep sleep, and what they term "arousal overlap" between mother and baby means that these periods of deep sleep are reduced when there is co-sleeping.

THE TRANSITION TO MOTHERHOOD

In traditional societies there is a transitional period following birth, which often lasts 40 days, during which mother and baby get to know each other and work out the steps of the "dance" of breastfeeding. In the earlier part of this period the woman is in partial or complete seclusion with her infant, and other women take over her responsibilities in the home and on the land. She is often fed specially nourishing foods, including those believed to increase and enrich breast milk, lies beside or over a "fire bath" or has steam baths, and is massaged by women family members and friends responsible for nurturing her.

The technocratic culture of North America lays great stress on the socialization of babies from birth so that they do not interfere with adult working lives and other commitments, and on inculcating in children habits of independence. Infant dependency is perceived as something to escape from as soon as possible. Although nursing may be acknowledged as appropriate in the first months of life, provided that mothers do it in private, and do not appear to make an exhibitionist sexual display of their breasts, many people express distaste at witnessing a toddler or older child at the breast. It may be suggested that the mother is unwilling to cut the emotional umbilical cord with her child because of her own dependency needs, or that she is deriving illicit sexual pleasure from the breastfeeding relationship. In short, her behavior is treated as pathological. Dettwyler (Chapter 2) refers to a court case in the United States in which custody of a young child was awarded to a father on divorce because it is claimed that the mother had failed to wean at an appropriate time, and must therefore be psychologically unstable.

FUTURE RESEARCH DIRECTIONS

There are many aspects of breastfeeding that need to be explored further. Most important of these is the *meaning* that breastfeeding has for mothers in each society and each culture within a society. Breast milk has symbolic significance as well as practical use.

Imagery of Healing and Poisoning

Human milk may be used to heal—it is a preferred remedy for eye injuries and sores in the Caribbean, for example—and to sustain the old and sick. It is often ascribed a purity similar to that of tears. At the same time, like menstrual blood, breast milk is potent with female energy, and represents women's power to generate and nurture. Because male and female essences, semen and breast milk, must be kept separate, in many societies there are taboos on sexual intercourse during lactation. This is not primarily because it is thought that the baby may sicken, but that man may we weakened, and his penis wither and drop off. Within the context of medicalized childbirth, breast milk frequently has been considered unsuitable for babies, because it is too weak or too rich, because there is not enough of it, or it is too plentiful, or because it is believed to be poisonous. Joseph De Lee, the Chicago obstetrician who established the twentieth-century medical model of childbirth, warned against "abnormal milk," and wrote that it acted as "an irritant intestinal poison, and fatalities have been reported" (De Lee, 1904). Mothers are usually blamed for whatever goes wrong with their children, and when a baby does not thrive, doctors have often seen the mother as responsible because of her ignorance or selfishness. De Lee went on to say that in his own experience, "these cases have all been neurotic mothers." However, the alternative he proposed was not a substitute milk but a wet-nurse. If the baby still failed to thrive, another wet-nurse should be selected (De Lee, 1904).

In many cultures colostrum is seen as too "strong," or as dangerous for the newborn. So it is expressed and thrown away, while the baby is breastfed by other women or fed coconut water or other substitute fluids until there is evidence of mature milk. Perhaps we should understand such a custom in terms of the reinforcement of relationships between women. For the social effect of this practice is to engage other women in the group in the active care of mother and baby. It thus has a cohesive function. The infant is not simply the child of its biological mother, but of a group of women linked in commitment to each other.

Fildes (Chapter 4) lists a range of foods given to newborn babies. These are often ritual substances, for example, clarified butter, honey, leaf juice and gold dust, fed to babies in ancient India. The avowed purpose is also to clear meconium from the baby's bowels. The purging of newborn babies was standard practice in eighteenth- and nineteenth-century Europe. It was introduced to Jamaica by slave managers, and peasant babies there are still purged with castor oil.

If a mother is under stress it may also be believed that her milk can become poisoned. When a peasant mother in north Africa is overworked and exhausted, her baby gets "bad milk" which makes the child sick (Creyghton, 1992). If she is too hot, too cold, angry, depressed, or sick she should not breastfeed because her milk will be bad. Historically in Europe husbands were enjoined to check that the wet-nurse was healthy and emotionally calm and to see that she was treated well, lest her milk poison the baby. A seventeenth-century Bishop of Exeter counseled that "manie a disease and ill qualitie is drawne with the milk from a bad nurse" (cited in McLaren, 1984:68). There were special warnings about redheads, who were likely to be of such a passionate nature that their milk would be poisonous.

The Monster Baby

To understand feeding practices we also need to understand how adults think about babies, and how they interpret their behavior and respond to their signals. A baby crying for the breast may be perceived as dangerously out of parental control, as a tyrant trying to dominate the mother, and as fundamentally evil. In those cultures of childrearing where it is believed that babies are born in a state of original sin, the process of acculturation entails conflict between the will of the parents and that of the child. Saint Augustin wrote: "Is it not a sin to lust after the breast and wail, for if I now lust with similar ardor after a food appropriate to my age, people would ridicule me. . . . It is therefore an evil desire, since in growing up we tear it out and cast it aside" (cited in Badinter, 1980:31). Medical men writing in books of advice about mothercraft have often counseled a mother to show a baby "who is master."

From medieval sages to behaviorist psychologists—and beyond—mothers have never been short of advice on how to discipline their babies and limit the time spent at the breast. In breastfeeding, as in the conduct of childbirth, the tyranny of clock-watching has intruded on the spontaneous physiological rhythms (Millard, 1990). The clock is a simple, familiar, apparently innocuous, but potentially dangerous technology that, though it has been around for a long time, has only within the past 80 years been used to direct and dominate the female processes of birthing and breastfeeding (Kitzinger, 1994a).

Woman-to-Woman

Another theme that needs to be explored cross-culturally is the nature of support for the nursing couple, and the lack of it in many Western societies (Raphael, 1981). When women talk about their breastfeeding experiences, this is a major topic—the need for acceptance, encouragement, and practical help. They often seek help from another woman, and for many this is missing (Locklin and Nabor, 1993).

In traditional cultures, worldwide, a new mother is given woman-to-woman support. This is not suddenly introduced once the baby has arrived. Other women share with her the experience of pregnancy, give skilled companionship during childbirth, and nurture her for some weeks after the birth. In medieval Europe a woman called her *god sibs*—literally "sisters in God"—when she started labor, and they hurried to her side to give her both emotional and physical support in childbirth and to care for her afterward (Kitzinger, 1994a). We need to explore further how such support groups function in different societies, how they are modified by urban living, and how new forms can evolve in industrial societies—as they frequently do, for example, in cultural minorities in North American cities.

Social Values and Women's Lives

Anthropologists need to examine further the values in different cultures and the social pressures on women that result in women choosing to bottle-feed or being unable to breastfeed. In some societies those with the most wealth and status have their babies suckled by wet-nurses, introduce other foods very early, or use substitute milks, with the result that infant mortality rates are often higher in such families than among the poor. This was common practice in England from the seventeenth century on. Breastfeeding avoidance is frequently part of a system of values that stresses the conjugal relationship at the expense of the mother–baby relationship, and that puts priority on the sexual privileges of men, and the use of a woman to display men's status and wealth.

Where reproduction has been medicalized, pregnancy and childbirth constitute a rite of passage that reflects and reinforces the core values of a society in which women are expected to rely on technology and powerful patriarchal institutions in the most intimate moments of their lives. Their bodies are treated as machines always at risk of break-down (Davis-Floyd, 1992). Birth and breastfeeding are medically "managed." Women go into labor and attempt to breastfeed under the constant threat of failure. When they lose confidence, cannot trust their bodies to attain a standard performance, and are given the implicit message that they are damaging their babies, they have an actively managed labor or a Cesarean section, or both, or switch from breastfeeding to formula. Both birth and infant feeding have been incorporated into a technocratic system under the control of men.

The contributors to the volume, coming from multidisciplinary backgrounds, point a way toward recording the behavior and understanding the values implicit in breastfeeding in diverse cultures, and reveal the role of breastfeeding in infant and maternal well-being, the developing mother–child relationship, and women's control over and confidence in their bodies.

NOTE

1. I use the term "artificial milk" to mean milk that has been modified by a manufacturing process. By the term "substitute milk" I mean either artificial milk or the milk of an animal such as a cow or goat.

REFERENCES

Badinter, E.
1980 *The Myth of Motherhood*. London: Souvenir Press.
Creyghton, M-L.
1992 Breast-feeding and *baraka* in Northern Tunisia. In The *Anthropology of Breast-Feeding*, edited by V. Maher, pp. 37–58. Oxford: Berg.
Davis-Floyd, R.
1992 *Birth as an American Rite of Passage*. Berkeley: University of California Press.
de Chateau, P., H. Holmberg, K. Jakobsson, and J. Winberg
1977 A study of factors promoting and inhibiting lactation. *Developmental Medicine and Child Neurology* 19:575–587.
De Lee, J.
1904 *Obstetrics for Nurses*. Philadelphia, PA: Saunders.
Jelliffe, D. B., and E. F. P. Jelliffe
1978 *Human Milk in the Modern World*. London: Oxford University Press.
Kitzinger, S.
1980 *The Experience of Breastfeeding*. New York: Penguin.
1994a *Ourselves as Mothers*. New York: Addison Wesley.
1994b The social context of birth: Some comparisons between childbirth in Jamaica and Britain. In *Ethnography of Fertility and Birth*, 2nd ed., edited by C. P. MacCormack. Prospect Heights, IL: Waveland Press.

Kocturk, T.
1988 Advantages of breastfeeding according to Turkish mothers living in Istanbul and Stockholm. *Social Science and Medicine* 27(4):405–410.
Locklin, M. P., and S. J. Nabor
1993 Does breastfeeding empower women? *Birth* 20(1):30–35.
McLaren, A.
1984 *Reproductive Rituals*. London: Metheun.
Millard, A. V.
1990 The place of the clock in pediatric advice: Rationales, cultural themes, and impediments to breastfeeding. *Social Science and Medicine* 31(2):211–221.
Raphael, D.
1981 The midwife as doula: A guide to mothering the mother. *Journal of Nurse-Midwifery* 26(6):13.
Winberg, J., and P. de Chateau
1979 Attempts to increase breastfeeding. *Psychosomatic Medicine in Obstetrics and Gynaecology*, 5th International Congress, Rome, pp. 851–854.

14

Commentary
Breastfeeding Is More Than Just Good Nutrition

Ruth A. Lawrence

INTRODUCTION

Breastfeeding is not new nor are the issues and controversies new to history or medicine. The rediscovery of breastfeeding in western countries was begun in the late 1940s and early 1950s by a few physicians who were exploring the role of women, of parents, and of child rearing away from the laboratory and the science of nutrition. A vocal and innovative group at Yale New Haven Hospital, Drs. Edith Jackson and Grover Powers, established the rooming-in unit and childbirth without fear with the Department of Obstetrics (Jackson, 1950; Jackson, Wilkin and Auerbach, 1956). Later the work of Niles Newton and her obstetrician husband, Michael, addressed the psychology and physiology of human lactation and its interrelationship with other stages in the physiology of reproduction (Newton and Modahl, 1989; Newton and Newton, 1948, 1950). The interest in breastfeeding was also flamed by women themselves who challenged the scientific wisdom that suggested that infant feeding was a problem for the chemist and involved finding the right chemical formula. Women began to educate themselves about their bodies, childbirth, and infant care. They challenged the use of medication in labor and interventions during childbirth, and they challenged the routine suppression of lactation and the substitution of a bovine-based formula to nourish their young. Women, well-educated and well-read, took back the birthing process of which breastfeeding is part. Many of these efforts were formalized by the development of groups and organizations, the best known of which became La Leche League International (La Leche League International, 1990) and the International Childbirth Education Association. Both of these groups are women support groups that have become international. Similar groups sprang up independently across the country and around the world. They have demanded that childbirth be changed back to a natural process, and that women make an informed choice about infant feeding.

Breastfeeding is the natural completion of the reproductive cycle that has resulted in the birth of a normal infant who requires further nourishment and nurturing (Lawrence, 1994). The breast prepares for lactation throughout the reproductive years beginning with the development of the breast early in puberty. The hormones that develop the uterus and stimulate the ovaries and uterine lining to produce the menstrual cycle also stimulate the breast to develop a ductal system and elaborate the areola and nipple and their ability to become erect. The response of the breast to the menstrual cycle continues throughout the reproductive years. When pregnancy occurs, the breast promptly responds to the new hormonal milieu and begins preparation for full lactation. A marked increase in ductular sprouting and branching occurs with lobular formation and the production of lacteal cells that line the acini. From the third month of gestation, secretory material resembling colostrum appears in the acini, and by 16 weeks gestation, the breast is capable of full lactation (milk production) whenever the conceptus is delivered. With the delivery of the placenta, which has produced a hormone that keeps the breast from responding to the high levels of prolactin present during pregnancy, the breast is able to respond to prolactin by making milk and to oxytocin by secreting or ejecting the milk. A key to establishing a good milk supply is the "ejection reflex" that is triggered by the infant suckling at the breast (see Figure 14.1). This sends a message via the nervous system and the spinal column to the pituitary and hypothalamus where the oxytocin is released. It stimulates the myoepithelial cells that surround the acini and ducts to contract sequentially, moving the milk along the ducts and ejecting it through the nipple. The oxytocin also causes the myoepithelial cells in the uterus to contract and thus advances the physiological postpartum involution of the uterus during the first few weeks postpartum. Suckling also results in the release of prolactin from the hypothalamus. Prolactin stimulates the lacteal cells to make milk. Each time the infant is put to breast, the reflex is initiated and milk is produced and released.

The physiologic process of lactation impacts many phases of life itself. Beginning with infancy, the process of being breastfed provides a special relationship of the infant with his mother that can be imitated by bottle feeding but not duplicated. The work of Swedish investigators has documented that newly born infants can locate and latch on to the breast unassisted if placed on the mother's abdomen once the umbilical cord is

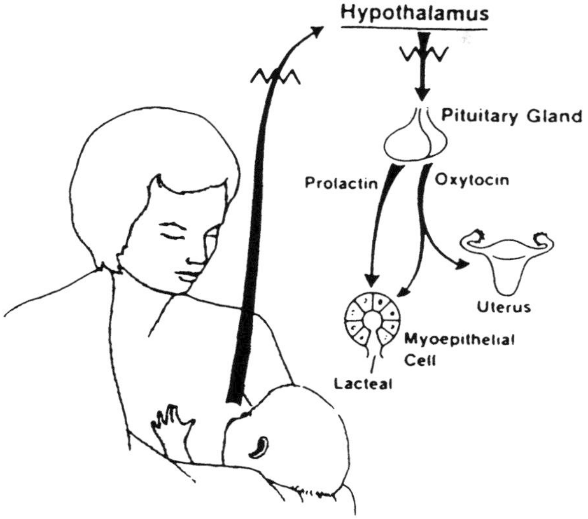

Figure 14.1. Diagrammatic outline of ejection reflex arc. When the infant suckles the breast, he stimulates mechanoreceptors in the nipple and areola that send a stimulus along nerve pathways to the hypothalamus, which stimulates the posterior pituitary to release oxytocin. Oxytocin is carried via the bloodstream to the breast and uterus. Oxytocin stimulates myoepithelial cells in the breast to contract and eject milk from the alveolus. Prolactin is responsible for milk production in the alveolus and is secreted by the anterior pituitary gland in response to suckling. Stress such as pain and anxiety can inhibit the let-down reflex; the sight or cry of the infant can stimulate it. Reproduced by permission of C.V. Mosby Publishing Co., from Lawrence, R.A. *Breastfeeding: A Guide for the Medical Profession*, 4th ed., 1994.

cut and clamped (Righard, 1990). The infant is born with the necessary instincts and reflexes to locate and latch onto the breast, suckle, swallow, and digest breast milk. The ejection reflex is automatic. Women on the other hand have to learn how to facilitate proper suckling. Positioning one's self and presenting the breast is not a reflex, it is a learned skill. Prior to the formula feeding revolution, all women learned about breastfeeding from other women and by growing up with breastfeeding. Everyone breastfed and families lived in close knit groups, one generation with the next, so that witnessing and learning about breastfeeding were inherent in growing up.

The process of being breastfed is the source of the first human bond formed outside the womb. The distance from the infant to the mother is perfect for the newborns to visualize the maternal face. The closeness against the chest wall allows the infant to experience the maternal heartbeat, a familiar intrauterine sound. The warmth of the lactating breast replaces the familiar warmth of the uterus. Hunger is satiated by suckling. Does all this matter? Little study has been directed at the impact of this experience repeated many times day and night for weeks and months. Little study has been directed at the impact of not having this experience but being nourished through an inanimate object by a myriad of caregivers in various degrees of intimacy. Newton, however, did study a group of 3 year olds whose mothers were matched for age, parity, ethnicity, education, and socioeconomic status. Those infants who were breastfed for 6 months or longer compared with those who were bottle-fed, were more advanced developmentally, more outgoing and assertive, and socialized better. Other studies have suggested that exclusively breastfed infants move along the developmental scale more quickly.

Paleonutrition, the anthropologic study of diet and nutrition of ancient peoples, is described in Chapter 3 by Stuart-Macadam. The question of whether breast milk has a unique isotopic signature that could be used to trace lactation patterns in prehistoric times is being tested. The measurement of strontium–calcium (Sr/Ca) ratios is a possible key to weaning patterns since the Sr/Ca ratio is low in human milk and high in solid foods according to Stuart-Macadam. Such studies were consistent with ethnographic information on traditional Palestinian Arab communities, in which she indicates that children were weaned between 2 and 3 years of age. The effect of breastfeeding on the mother has had little attention as well, partly because it is difficult to "study" breastfeeding. It is very difficult to do a randomized control where a group of women are assigned to breastfeed or not to breastfeed. Anthropologists McLorg and Bryant (1989) did, however, report on a group of young mothers enrolled in the WIC Program (Women, Infants, and Children Nutrition Program of the United States Department of Agriculture) in Kentucky. Prenatally, they were randomly assigned to one of two groups. One group was taught about breastfeeding, encouraged to breastfeed, and supported during the breastfeeding. The other group had the same number of contacts and as much support postpartum, but breastfeeding was not mentioned. Prenatally, the women were evaluated psychologically and measurements of self-esteem were performed. All women scored prenatally in the same range. At 1 year postpartum when the tests were repeated, those who had breastfed had higher self-esteem and had developed confidence. Their interactions with their infants were more mature and reflective of a secure bond between mother and child. From a practical standpoint, the breastfeeders had gotten their lives together, finished school, gotten a job, or accomplished some other achievement.

Biologically, breastfeeding suppresses ovulation and extends the period of interpregnancy infertility making some degree of child spacing a natural phenomenon, further demonstrating the balance between breastfeeding and the reproductive cycle. The longer the night feedings continue, the longer infertility continues.

The cultural context of the human breast is a complex summation of a variety of beliefs. Dettwyler (in Chapter 7) refers to the "Culture of Misinformation" as a cause of women's indecision about breastfeeding. This misinformation includes the notion that breasts are primarily sexual objects, and that breastfeeding has limited nutritional value and is to be carried out only in private. Furthermore, much of the misinformation is perpetuated by the trusted physician. While the argument that in the United States the mammary gland is viewed as a sexual object is well accepted, the association of breastfeeding with sexual pleasure for the mother has only recently surfaced in public discussion. For most women, most of the time, Dettwyler points out that the physical act of breastfeeding is neither particularly pleasurable nor particularly uncomfortable. It is neutral. Furthermore, she continues, breastfeeding is not "one thing" for all women for all children at all times. Breasts should be restored to their rightful place as the most important point of contact between mother and child after birth.

EXTERNAL INFLUENCES ON BREASTFEEDING

Historically, breastfeeding has been influenced by the fashion of the day as socially elite women often wished to be free of the burden and responsibility of nourishing their infant. Substitute milks from other species were associated with a very high infant death rate because of contamination, so that wet nursing, an ancient custom, was utilized until the beginning of the twentieth century. Wet nursing is the term used for nursing an infant who is not the mother's, probably properly termed surrogate nursing now. The careful selection of such a substitute was written about in the early treatises on infant care. Fildes discusses wet nursing in Chapter 4. The important point is, however, that other arrangements for feeding the infant have always been needed whether the mother dies in childbirth, is too ill to feed, or does not wish to do so. The poor woman has always had to nurse her infant as alternatives (wet nursing or animal milks) were costly. The death rates among infants not nursed by their own mother has always been extremely high. Among infants in foundling homes, the rate is above 90% in the first year of life. In third world countries today, the death rate is 50% among infants not breastfed in the first year of life. At last in the recent five decades, an inexpensive (but not cheap) and relatively safe alternative, infant formula, has been available to all women. Pressures beyond an individual woman's wish to be free of the responsibility have been at work. Science has pursued an alternative feeding to replace the nutritional benefits of human milk. Working from a bovine milk base, formulas have been designed to fulfill the perceived nutritional needs in terms of basic protein, fat, carbohydrate, and micronutrients such as iron, copper, and zinc, and vitamins. The formulas are carefully manufactured and quality controlled. Every drop is the same as every other drop quite in contrast to human milk where constituents change feeding to feeding, day by day, and over time. The fat content of human milk is a classic example of these changes increasing through a given feeding, being higher early in the morning and decreasing after 6 months postpartum. All of the nutrients in human milk are readily bioavailable and easily digested and absorbed. Human milk, as with the fresh untreated milk of all species, contains active enzymes that facilitate the digestion and absorption of nutrients, stimulate the infant gut to mature, protect the gut from infection and other stresses, and provide an immunologic barrier to disease (Lucas, Morley, Cole, Lister and Leeson-Payne, 1992). Formulas do not have these properties.

Scientists are diligently working to reproduce the protective elements identified in human milk such as nucleotides to be placed in infant formulas to mimic some of the infection-protection qualities of human milk. Efforts to produce a formula that does not produce an allergic response have also been extensive. Human milk has been the model, the gold standard. Although there is a large gap between the most ideal formula and human milk, all manufacturers claim their product is closest to human milk.

The commercial aspects of formula marketing have changed the picture for the woman making a decision about infant feeding. The "Madison Avenue" approach to formula marketing has made women the target of slick high-pressure misleading information about the risk/benefit ratio of formula versus mother's milk. The health care professional has been replaced by television and magazine advertising. Well-educated women who wish to breastfeed usually manage to overcome this pressure, but many do not. A woman who gets all her information from television gets barraged with advertisements about infant formula. She also receives unsolicited samples in the mail.

The infants who would most benefit by being breastfed, the infants of young low income, undereducated women, are not being breastfed (Bryant, Coreil, D'Angelo, Bailey and Lazarov, 1992). They are the infants with the most malnutrition, infection, illness, and psychologic deprivation. A woman who has breastfed her infant has not been known to abuse her infant.

Many of these low income, poorly educated women are clients of WIC. WIC provides formula feeding women with vouchers for formula valued at least at $60 a month, an offering hard to resist. Nationally, WIC spends over 500 million dollars a year of tax money on formula whereas only 8 million dollars is available to promote and support breastfeeding women, nearly a one hundred-fold difference in spite of the commitment to breastfeeding of most WIC staff.

STRIKING A BALANCE

As pointed out by Fildes, there are complex interactions between the biology and the culture of breastfeeding and the method of infant feeding can have a profound effect on health and disease. Choosing a method of infant feeding is a mother's decision. She should have enough straightforward information to make an informed decision. All studies have shown today that women who are well-educated, higher socioeconomic status, in a stable relationship (married) of all ethnic groups, choose to breastfeed when provided adequate information to make an informed decision. Furthermore, breastfeeding goes well and continues for months or years when there is adequate information and support, especially from the significant other. The success is dependent upon the mother's personal resources balanced against the external pressures of advertising of formula, free samples especially from hospitals and doctors' offices, and negative reinforcement from one's family.

The role of the physician is supportive, perhaps providing the information base, and facilitating a successful introduction following the birth in the hospital or home and responding to problems with knowledge and experience to preserve breastfeeding. The nurses who work with the mother during labor, delivery, and postpartum provide the practical knowledge and experience to assist the mother in putting the infant to the breast and latching on. Outside of the network of obstetrician, pediatrician, midwife, and perinatal and office nurses, the mother may need a doula. A doula as first described by Dana Raphael is "a friend from across the street" (Raphael, 1973:23 and 147). She is someone who is there, is supportive, not to prescribe and not to diagnose, but to support. Mother-to-mother programs such as that provided by La Leche League are a rich source of this support. A peer support program can be just that. The first peer support program among WIC clients was started in Georgia by Wanda Grogan, R.D., Ph.D. in the early 1980s. Peer support programs have gradually spread. The key is *peer*. Programs that are initiated in the community and involve community members from the beginning succeed. They succeed especially if the program is designed so that the peer support person is there through pregnancy, delivery, and beyond to encourage and support the woman to get good prenatal care, keep appointments, and follow the advice given, until the child goes to school. Breastfeeding then fits into the total perinatal picture as a natural bridge between carrying the fetus *in utero* and totally weaning the infant to food and drink.

WHAT IS NORMAL BREASTFEEDING?

The most appropriate patterns of breastfeeding and feeding management are not known according to Woolridge but are probably a function of culturally acceptable norms. In his discussion of night feedings, he points out that prolactin levels are higher at night and sustaining night feeds is the best way to maintain lactational amenorrhea. In western cultures, however, an effort is made to eliminate night feedings as quickly as possible. Pediatric textbooks reflect a change in medical view since the early 1900s when feeding every 2 hours but only once at night was recommended. Then the rigid 4-hour schedule with no night feeds was recommended. It was finally acknowledged that a rigid schedule was contrary to the natural needs of the infant. Mothers were the major forces urging that infants be fed "on demand" or as needed.

Volume and fat content have been matters of great concern. Woolridge reports in his chapter regarding "Baby-Controlled Breastfeeding: Biocultural Implications," that the greater the interval between feeds, the lower the average fat content and thus the more frequent the feeds, the higher the fat content. The fat content varies across a 24-hour period and the pattern is different depending on the geographic location. The author further asserts that "the most explicit factor with which the magnitude of change in fat concentration from the start to the end of the feed is related is the volume of milk removed." It has been well-documented that residual milk remains in the breast even after a feeding, suggesting that infants actually exercise appetite control even in the face of poor growth. There is discordance between the pattern of feeding that is biologically optimal and that which culture imposes. This is true for the bottle fed as well. Thus, the frequency of feeds and the duration and patterns of breast usage should be controlled by the infant not mandated by society.

In a discussion of the sociocultural aspects of breastfeeding, Quandt states that the most important dimensions of breastfeeding are whether or not breastfeeding is initiated, the duration of exclusive breastfeeding, and the frequency, duration, and temporal distribution of breastfeeding episodes. The biobehavioral interactions in breastfeeding are critical because breastfeeding is distinct from other domains of food behaviors according to Quandt because the availability of adequate quantity and quality of milk is dependent upon the interactions. The more suckling, the more milk. "Breastfeeding Style" has been used to describe the key behaviors that affect milk volume, composition, and maternal reproductive status.

Other chapters document the remarkable benefits of breast milk and breastfeeding. Beginning with the detailed work of Cunningham, the reader quickly finds evidence to support the conviction that breast milk is protective against gastrointestinal disease, respiratory illness, otitis media, sepsis, and a host of other infections. The immunoprotective effects noted include inflammatory bowel disease, Henoch-Schonlein purpura, juvenile diabetes, childhood malignancies, allergies, and coronary artery disease. For the mother, the prolongation of postpartum infertility, reduced incidence of long-term calcium deficiency, and the reduced risk of breast cancer serve as major secondary benefits as described by Ellison and Micozzi.

Why then are not all infants breastfed everywhere? Why are not all health professionals working tirelessly to encourage and support women to breastfeed successfully? Understanding history provides insights; looking to other cultures and searching for the forces of industry and the powers that work against breastfeeding provide explanations and excuses.

Breastfeeding has nutritional, medical, sociologic, anthropologic, political, and cultural significance. Breastfeeding is more than just good nutrition. Governments, communities, professionals, families, and women should guard this precious resource and promote breastfeeding. Affordable health care begins with breastfeeding.

REFERENCES

Bryant, C. A., J. Coreil, S. L. D'Angelo, D. F. Bailey, and M. Lazarov
1992 A strategy for promoting breastfeeding among economically disadvantaged women and adolescents. *NAACOGS Clinical Issues in Perinatal and Women's Health Nursing* 3(4):723–730.

Jackson, E. B.
1950 Pediatric and psychiatric aspects of the Yale rooming-in project. *Connecticut Medical Journal* 14:616–621.

Jackson, E. B., L. C. Wilkin, and H. Auerbach
1956 Statistical report on the incidence and duration of breastfeeding in relation to personal-social and hospital maternity factors. *Pediatrics* 17:700–715.
La Leche League International
1990 *The Womanly Art of Breastfeeding,* 5th ed. Franklin Park, IL: La Leche League International.
Lawrence, R. A.
1993 The pediatrician's role in infant feeding decision-making. *Pediatrics in Review* 14:265–272.
1994. *Breastfeeding: A Guide for the Medical Profession,* 4th ed. St. Louis: C. V. Mosby.
Lucas, A., R. Morley, T. J. Cole, G. Lister, and C. Leeson-Payne
1992 Breast milk and subsequent intelligence quotient in children born preterm. *Lancet* 339:261–264.
McLorg, P. A., and C. A. Bryant
1989 Influence of social network members and health care professionals on infant feeding practices of economically disadvantaged mothers. *Medical Anthropology* 10(4):265–278.
Newton, N., and C. Modahl
1989 New frontiers of oxytocin research. In *The Free Woman: Women's Health in the 1990s,* edited by E. V. van Hall and W. Everaerd, pp. 308–318. Carnforth, England: Parthenon Publishing Group.
Newton, M., and N. Newton
1948 The let-down reflex in human lactation. *Journal of Pediatrics* 33:693–704.
Newton, N., and M. Newton
1950 Relation of the let-down reflex to the ability to breastfeed. *Pediatrics* 5:726–733.
Raphael, D.
1973 *The Tender Gift: Breastfeeding*. New York: Schocken Books.
Righard, L.
1990 Newborn attachment to the breast. *Lancet* 336:1105–1107.

15

Commentary
Breastfeeding Study Design Problems—Health Policy, Epidemiologic and Pediatric Perspectives

Doren Fredrickson

INTRODUCTION

As a practitioner of twentieth-century pediatrics and epidemiology, I am intrigued by the controversies surrounding breastfeeding, and note the sometimes discrepant research findings that this book's authors have endeavored to piece together to make sense out of the whole thing. Recent findings of important health benefits related to breastfeeding reviewed by the previous authors include reductions in maternal breast cancer and postpartum fertility, as well as reductions in child morbidity and mortality, and enhancements in child cognitive function.

It is both fascinating and a terrible condemnation of Western medical practice that breastfeeding—closely linked to age-old concepts of goodness such as motherhood and family formation—should be surrounded by as much variation in medical practice and scientific pronouncement as it is. This is fascinating because it clearly portrays the limitations of breastfeeding epidemiologic method as currently developed, and terrible because of necessary suspicions that arise regarding companies and health professionals who profit from the current confusion.

Breastfeeding as a personal activity with health consequences is involved in a triangle of culture, health science, and fiscal economy. These three factors are mutually interactive, and anyone with a keen eye for human biology or anthropology must keep such relationships in mind when considering the scientific controversies of breastfeeding. The efforts by this book's authors to make plain the current understandings and misunderstandings related to breastfeeding are pertinent and refreshing. They are pertinent because of the potential health cost savings that breastfeeding may offer to developed and developing nations alike. They are refreshing because the findings imply an empowerment of the family and individual to achieve, at low cost, diverse benefits that high-cost medical practice cannot currently offer. The amazing thing is that such an empowerment comes by living according to the manner for which we appear to be biologically constructed. Reviewing these chapters should make us identify breastfeeding as "doing the right thing," and as a social and biological good. Indeed, one is struck that there should be a moral imperative to breastfeed for mother's benefit, for baby's benefit, and for society's benefit.

Because lactation originated with and defines mammalian species, there can be little doubt that it must provide complex survival advantages to both mother and infant that have been millions of years in the making. It is inconceivable that evolutionary economy would allow as much hormonal, developmental, cognitive, immunological, and nutritional biological activity as breastfeeding requires to be conserved over thousands of generations without clear survival advantages to be derived. How, then, did the current array of controversies arise?

Specifically, I want to address two controversies that appear here in previous chapters: weaning and sudden infant death syndrome (SIDS). I will discuss important issues from the vantage point of pediatrics and epidemiology. This will require perusal of the histories of breastfeeding study design, breastfeeding epidemiology, infant-feeding profit motives, biological models of disease, the refinement of disease theory during the last century, and the influence of each upon the others. An examination of the epidemiology and study design features of breastfeeding health benefit studies will be used to reflect on weaning studies. Although the following comments pertain exclusively to infant health benefits, examples could easily be found to illustrate similar issues in regard to maternal health benefits as well.

WEANING, EPIDEMIOLOGY, AND STUDY DESIGN

At least 15 early studies conducted in Europe and the United States between 1895 and 1947, (Knodel, 1977, cited by Lawrence, 1994), showed a large infant survival advantage caused by breastfeeding. These analyses relied on comparison of proportions surviving between those babies classified dichotomously as breastfed or nonbreastfed. The tradition of dichotomous transformation of breastfeeding, inherently a continuous variable, into a simple binary yes–no variable has continued to this day with great loss of statistical power. Breastfeeding is not a dichotomous variable, but rather a continuous variable whose effects can be assumed to vary directly in proportion to the length of time to weaning and the daily dose of breastfeeding. Steps for measurement of daily dose have been described (Labbok and Krasovec, 1990). These two factors, duration (of weeks or months to weaning age) and daily dose, must be evaluated concurrently to produce a cumulative dose-type variable, rather than a grossly oversimplified dichotomous variable (Fredrickson, n.d.).

The reasons for the extensive use of the dichotomous definition of breastfeeding in so many epidemiological studies are understandable if we review the history of epidemiology itself. Epidemiology is a new science, scarcely a hundred years old, which arose out of studies of infectious disease epidemics and toxic-exposure cancer epidemics, and only recently has been used to investigate health behaviors and chronic diseases. Subjects of epidemic disease studies such as John Snow's exemplary treatise on cholera were labeled as dead or alive, exposed or nonexposed, in dichotomous fashion for obvious reasons (Snow, 1855). Likewise, early studies of lung cancer and tobacco smoking labeled subjects in dichotomous fashion as smokers or nonsmokers (Fielding, 1992). Naturally, when bacteria or viruses are virulent enough, and when carcinogen exposure is uniformly high enough, such labeling does not hide the health effects in question. Thus, although a dose–response would be an interesting thing to know, one may choose to collapse all dose data into a single dichotomous variable without excessive loss of significance.

Similarly, when breastfeeding was uniformly of reasonably long duration, as it was at the turn of the nineteenth to twentieth centuries, then any breastfeeding was long-duration breastfeeding and the health benefits were easily detectable. We know that breastfeeding duration as well as incidence were formerly high but rapidly decreased among North American mothers following the 1940s (American Academy of Pediatrics, 1982). This partly explains why breastfeeding studies early in the century could show such clear survival advantages even when breastfeeding was classified as a dichotomous variable. It was because breastfed infants at the time uniformly received a large cumulative dose of breastfeeding. In such a situation, any comparison between bottle and breastfed infants involved a comparison between babies who did or did not receive a large dose of breast milk, providing easily detectable differences. However, as breastfeeding duration (weaning age) declined, the health benefits associated with progressively smaller doses declined as well. And as breastfeeding duration progressively shortened during the post-World War II period, health benefit effects became harder, if not downright impossible, to sort out, when treating breastfeeding as a traditional dichotomous variable.

Also, the infant mortality rate among bottle-fed infants fell from six to eight times higher than breastfed infants, down to twice as high as breastfed infants, during the years when antibiotics and immunizations were introduced, water supplies became cleaner, and human milk substitutes better formulated and policed (Knodel, 1977). Smaller margins of difference such as these are more likely to be statistically insignificant unless sample size is significantly increased. These necessary increases in sample size drastically increase research costs because of the additional resources required to recruit subjects, assess outcomes, and enter data for a larger subject pool. Use of a continuous variable to describe breastfeeding could potentially then greatly reduce the cost, since fewer data are wasted.

The final reason for historical reliance upon dichotomous variables in breastfeeding epidemiology is the ease by which simple statistics can be employed for calculation of significance. When dichotomous exposures are compared to dichotomous outcomes, simple Chi-square analysis suffices. This can be calculated using a published table and pencil and paper. Calculating dose effects using continuous variables requires more complex statistics such as multiple regression, logistic regression, and survival analyses that are most feasible only with computers. Of course, computers did not exist in meaningful numbers until the 1980s.

Other methodological issues in 20 studies published between 1970 and 1984 that attempted to measure the impact of breastfeeding upon infection were reviewed by Bauchner, Leventhal and Shapiro (1986). These authors noted concerns that most studies did not fully comply with criteria of interest to health outcomes researchers. The concerns dealt primarily with sample size and confounders that can independently affect infant health: maternal and family smoking, family size, and socioeconomic status (e.g., maternal education). The authors also recommended a clear definition of breastfeeding as a variable but did not advocate changing the measurement of the variable itself from dichotomous to continuous.

At least one recently published study in which Leventhal participated (Rubin, Leventhal, Krasilnikoff, Kuo, Jekel, Weile, Levee, Kurzon and Berget, 1990), and that reported no benefit of breastfeeding in a Copenhagen suburb, has been criticized for not addressing breastfeeding in a sound manner (Hopkinson, 1991). Critics noted that the authors classified partially breastfeeding mothers as bottle feeding to increase the number of bottle-feeding mothers to produce an adequate sample size. This produced a major misclassification bias and hid the protective effects of breastfeeding.

Table 15.1. Breastfeeding Health Benefit Studies Showing Dose–Response in Developed Nations[a]

Study	*Focus of study*	*Breastfeeding duration categories*
Rogan and Gladen (1993)	Intelligence	0, 0–9, 10–19, 20–49, 50+ weeks
Labbok and Hendershot (1987)	Malocclusion	0–3, 4–6, 7–9, 10–12, >12 months
Howie, Forsyth, Ogston, Clark and Florey (1990)	Hospitalization, gastrointestinal disease	0, 1–13, 14–26, 27–39, 40–52, >52 weeks
Fredrickson et al. (1993)	SIDS	0, 1, 2, 3, 4, 5, 6 months
Mitchell et al. (1991)	SIDS	0, 1, 2–5 days
Duncan, Ey, Golberg, Wright, Martinez and Taussig (1993)	Otitis media	0–1, 2–4, 5–6, >6 months
Davis, Savitz and Graubard (1988)	Childhood cancer	0, 1–6, >6 months
Virtanen, Rasanen, Aro, Lindstrom, Sippola, Lounamaa, Toivanen, Tuomilehto and Akerblom (1991)	Type I diabetes	0–2, 3, 4, 5, 6, 7, 8, >9 months

[a] In each of these studies, the greater the duration of breastfeeding, the greater the health benefit.

Eight studies incorporating recommended criteria and even utilizing a continuous variable definition for breastfeeding have been performed in the United States and Europe and reported in the literature (Table 15.1). These will probably remain few in number pending adequate interest by federal funding sources to promote further investigation. Only three of the eight studies included a subsample with breastfeeding duration greater than 12 months. In these three studies all infants who had received breastfeeding durations greater than 12 months were lumped together. These groups could thus conceivably comprise infants breastfed 13 months to 5 years or longer, although we cannot know that. Each study demonstrated increasing dose–response in health benefits during the weaning times under analysis. That is, health benefits increased as duration of breastfeeding increased. Unfortunately these studies can shed no light on the optimum weaning time for infants, or even whether there *is* a time when health benefits cease. None reported the range of breastfeeding duration for study mothers, so we have no idea about the relative numbers breastfeeding past 13 months, up to 2 to 5 years. However, the studies cited do indicate that weaning should not be considered until at least 12 months, and there is no reason to assume that these benefits would cease after 12 months if breastfeeding were to continue. Relatively few women in the regions (United States, Scotland, and Finland), and during the years when these studies were conducted, breastfed long enough to make long duration subject pools large enough to have statistical power. In fact, the United States experiences the lowest breastfeeding rate of all industrialized countries with the exception of Ireland (Helsing, 1990; Ryan, Rush, Krieger and Lewandowski, 1991). Clearly, to obtain sufficient data to adequately describe optimum weaning time for health benefits, we need studies that recruit women who breastfeed longer than the current United States norm.

Many breastfeeding studies conducted in developing countries during the 1960s–1980s reported highly protective breastfeeding effects while continuing to use breastfeeding as a binary variable (Cunningham, Jelliffe and Jelliffe, 1991). However, findings of these studies like those of Europe and the United States during the 1895–1947 era (Lawrence, 1994) may not be persuasive to families, health product regulators, and health providers in modern developed nations who may assume that water chlorination, sewage treatment, and improved human milk substitutes may eventually make human milk substitutes equally beneficial compared to human milk.

Two researchers have reviewed the history of controlled marketing negotiated between formula manufacturers, the American Medical Association, and the American Academy of Pediatrics. They imply that there was a long history of joint financial benefit deriving from negotiated hospital distribution and marketing of human milk substitutes by health professionals. This negotiated activity was not officially halted until the 1980s (Greer and Apple, 1991).

Nor is the baby formula industry a small one: a recent report indicates that annual United States sales result in $2.4 billion in earnings, of which 81% are profit (Pear, 1993). Human milk substitute purchase has been estimated to potentially cost the average United States family $500–$1000 in the first year of an infant's life. These estimates do not include costs related to higher infant illness (Batten, Hirschman and Thomas, 1990).

Still, health providers and families would hardly have embraced human milk substitutes with such fervor if the disease transmission and control theories of the time had not supported such departures from the long established ways of motherhood and nature. We need to recall that disease transmission and causation were seen in the light of the then-recent discoveries of bacteriologists such as Henle, Pasteur, and Koch, and the work of military surgeons who had discovered decontamination as an effective approach to war wound infection control. It may have seemed a logical step to conclude that absolute sterility was a laudable goal, especially until the early 1940s when the first antibiotics became available in the United States. Pasteurized or boiled human milk substitutes may have seemed to be safe foods for babies because of their lack of culturable bacteria, while human milk with its culturable (endogenous normal flora) bacterial strains could be considered suspect.

Ideas of those early years now appear naive. Experience with immune suppression among patients undergoing transplant or chemotherapy or Acquired Immune Deficiency Syndrome has brought new awareness to clinicians during the 1970s–1990s. These experiences have shown us that when immune-compromised patients become infected, it is of little use to sterilize or administer antibiotics in the absence of immune competence. This was not widely recognized until the last 30 years of the twentieth century.

We have long known about the high concentrations of maternal white cells and antibodies in human milk (Lawrence, 1994). However, the function of lymphocytes beyond passive immune protection was not well understood. We know that children do not achieve adult immune status until the age of 5 to 6 years. That is, children—especially infants—are susceptible to numerous viral and bacterial infections, and blood immunoglobulin levels do not approximate adult levels until that age (Behrman, Kliegman, Vaughan and Nelson, 1992). Recent reports indicate that breastfeeding serves a powerful immune-enhancing and modulating role during this period of relative immune incompetence (Hahn-Zoric, Fulconis, Minoli, Moro, Carlsson, Bottiger, Raiha and Hanson, 1990; Pabst and Spady, 1990). These studies indicate that the immune systems of the mother and child are linked by breastfeeding, with the naivete and incompetence of the child's own immune system bolstered and enhanced by direct stimulation induced by maternal breastmilk lymphocytes. In short, the infant's immune system seems to be strengthened and *taught* what to attack. At the same time, the large number of studies reporting reduced allergic and autoimmune disease among breastfed children (Hanson, Carlsson, Ekre, Hahn-Zoric, Osterhaus and Roberton, 1989; Lawrence, 1994) indicate that the infant's immune system is *taught* what *not* to attack as well.

These advances in studying human milk constituents show that breast milk can quite readily be described as broad-spectrum medicine as well as nutrition. It has high concentrations of important antiinfective properties, active immune modulators such as various fractions of white blood cells and lymphokines, growth factors, and unique nerve growth enhancers (Lawrence, 1994). As such, it deserves treatment like any other medicine in epidemiologic studies. Based on this, I will repeat here that it deserves to be measured as a continuous variable for analysis of dose–response effects.

There is another reason beyond data conservation for describing breastfeeding as a continuous variable. This second reason arises from the biological models of the health outcome in question. Many health outcomes occur as a result of many causes. These causes may act separately or together. The biological models that describe these causative pathways must be kept in mind when confounders are chosen for research. When such a web of multicausation is present, it is crucial to utilize the enhanced precision of measurement offered by continuous variables rather than dichotomous variables so that interactions and confounder collinearity can be calculated (Hennekens and Buring, 1987).

SUDDEN INFANT DEATH SYNDROME

Sudden infant death syndrome (SIDS) offers a case in point for discussion. We know that SIDS is most certainly multifactorial. Biological models with verification studies exist showing that SIDS can be caused by gastroesophageal reflux (Jolley, Halpern, Tunell, Johnson and Sterling, 1991), undetected congenital heart defects, sudden cardiac arrhythmia, early presymptomatic respiratory syncytial virus (RSV) infections, afebrile undetected meningitis and sepsis, infant botulism, carbon dioxide intoxication and hypoxemia, and aggravated periodic breathing secondary to immature brain stem respiratory drive (Carroll and Loughlin, 1993; Kraus and Bulterys, 1991). Carbon dioxide intoxication/hypoxemia is also known as the "laying prone" risk factor, and derives from the immature brain stem respiratory drive center's inability to detect significant variations in inspired oxygen. It is similar to prolonged periodic breathing. The effects of many of these causes are in turn aggravated by cigarette smoke exposure in interactive fashion.

It is logical to assume that breastfeeding would assist in preventing some of these causes, perhaps most of them, but not all. Especially the risk of infectious causes (RSV and other viral pneumonias, undetected meningitis and sepsis) would certainly be reduced as a result of breast milk's active and passive immune protection. Likewise the risk of gastroesophageal reflux would be practically eliminated because breastfed infants experience faster gut maturation, controlled satiety, and virtually no clinically significant gastroesophageal reflux. If we are to believe the mounting data suggesting that breastfeeding augments neuroproliferation and central nervous system development (Lawrence, 1994; Rogan and Gladen, 1993), then risk of SIDS due to immature brain stem, and even carbon dioxide intoxication/hypoxemia would be reduced by exposure to breastfeeding. However, the effects of undetected congenital heart defects and arrhythmias would probably not be reduced. The exact proportion of all SIDS cases attributable to each of these causes is not known with absolute certainty. Preliminary estimates suggest that infectious diseases and immature brain stem (in the form of periodic breathing or carbon dioxide intoxication/hypoxemia) may cause the major proportion of SIDS cases (Kraus and Bulterys, 1991). Thus breastfeeding can be postulated to provide quite significant protection from SIDS. Research conducted using the National Maternal and Infant Health Survey data set has supported such an hypothesis (Fredrickson, Sorenson, Biddle and Kotelchuck, 1993). The multicausal nature of SIDS must be kept in mind, however. The discussion of the biological models and supporting research suggests that breastfeeding may protect against most SIDS, but not all SIDS.

It is important to become acquainted with the scientific milieu within which epidemiologists study disease. It may surprise many nonepidemiologists to consider breastfeeding as an exposure. Whereas common usage of "exposure" refers to something bad or toxic, epidemiologists use "exposure" to discuss contact with beneficial forces as well. This arises because any independent variable under epidemiologic study can be seen two ways, each of which is inversely equivalent. While exposure to a toxic substance causes disease, nonexposure to the same toxic substance would be shown to prevent disease. Likewise exposure to a beneficial substance would be shown to prevent disease, while lack of exposure to this substance would conversely be seen to cause disease. By these means, beneficial factors such as breastfeeding, moderate exercise, and dietary fiber are considered "good" exposures that prevent disease among humans, compared to the lack of such exposures that are linked to elevated disease risk. Breastfeeding researchers thus may refer to breastfeeding as a beneficial exposure, or equivalently to lack of breastfeeding as a harmful exposure.

Other epidemiologic issues related to future studies include the need to evaluate confounding and collinearity carefully using established epidemiological techniques (Hennekens and Buring, 1987). In relation to SIDS and co-sleeping (as a protective exposure) studies must carefully control confounding variables linked in separate causative pathways to SIDS. Cigarette smoking by either parent, but especially the mother, must be carefully controlled to evaluate interaction with co-sleeping. Any protective effect provided by co-sleeping might be wiped out or even reversed by the intense tobacco smoke exposure provided by parental, and especially maternal, smoking in the sleeping room (Mitchell, Scragg, Stewart, Becroft, Taylor, Ford, Hassall, Barry, Allen and Roberts, 1991).

SIDS is an especially terrifying and unexplainable loss of infant life accounting for over one-third of postneonatal infant deaths in the United States (Kraus and Bulterys, 1991). If simple low-cost interventions such as supine sleeping, co-sleeping, and breastfeeding can be shown to prevent SIDS, then this would be an important discovery. With strong biological models for co-sleeping and breastfeeding to prevent these major causes of SIDS, it is hoped that further studies will be conducted that appropriately measure breastfeeding to determine the exact effects. No data sets exist in 1995 that contain all variables in adequate fashion for the necessary analysis.

FISCAL CONSIDERATIONS

Reports from the United States Department of Commerce indicate that, despite cost-containment efforts using Diagnosis-Related Groups (DRGs) during the last 6 years, the cost of medical care has continued upward. It increased 20% during 1992 alone, when total U.S. health care expenditure exceeded $838 billion. This figure represents 14% of the gross domestic product, a percentage approximately double that of any other developed nation (Pear, 1993). This high cost reduces the competitiveness of products produced by U.S. businesses, and drains the national economy of financial resources urgently needed to refinance national debt and invest in infrastructure, research, and development. Such conditions create an opportune time for business, health insurance, and government leaders to incorporate breastfeeding as an affordable health intervention that can assist in meeting these needs.

The potential health and cost savings produced by breastfeeding's health advantages should be of immediate interest to the entire health and business sectors. Unlike some preventive health measures, breastfeeding costs little beyond providing proper nutrition, encouragement, and some medical support to all breastfeeding mothers, and modern workplace accommodations for breastfeeding mothers who work outside the home. And unlike many preventive measures such as smoking cessation that take decades to appreciate health cost savings, breastfeeding produces cost savings within the first year due to decreased illness.

Health and business groups most able to generate immediate financial advantage from breastfeeding include capitated health insurance systems, such as Health Maintenance Organizations (HMOs), and self-insured corporations. For these groups, any reduction in illness and/or worker–parent absenteeism provided by breastfeeding will produce an immediate increase in profits. This is especially obvious in the case of HMOs. And although employers generally have been reported to provide little support to working women who breastfeed (Barber-Madden, Petschek and Pakter, 1987), a preliminary breastfeeding support trial by Dow Chemical and American Telephone and Telegraph has shown impressive savings in infant illness and parent absenteeism (*Wall Street Journal*, 1993).

The early 1990s saw some preliminary attempts to offer preventive services in the form of quit-smoking counseling within HMOs. Amidst skyrocketing health costs these attempts have been abandoned, however, after employers began annual insurance switching in order to force insurers into rival bidding price cuts (M.R. Greenlick, personal communication). When insured groups of patients began to be switched from one plan to another on an annual basis, the incentive for HMOs to invest in smoking cessation disappeared, since the cost benefits accruing on account of reduced illness would then be enjoyed by a competitor during the next year. After getting their fingers burned in this manner, most HMOs are reluctant to perform any nonmandated preventive services at all. However, breastfeeding is likely to be very different from smoking cessation in view of the rapid same-year profit return potentially caused by breastfeeding health benefits during an infant's first year of life. We should expect to see increased breastfeeding support services offered by well-managed capitated systems as HMOs catch on to this concept and work to increase breastfeeding among their insured families during the next decade.

The same is not as true for traditional fee-for-service medical provider systems, which profit primarily when individuals are sick. It is perhaps not surprising that physicians (Michelman, Faden, Gielen and Buxton, 1990) and nurses (Anderson and Geden, 1990) have been reported to be poorly trained and motivated to support breastfeeding, or that this century's rise in formula marketing and cultural acceptance of bottle-feeding derived "not from any motive of altruism, philanthropy or paternalism, but rather from a spirit of enlightened self-interest and cooperation (between formula companies and physicians)" (Greer and Apple, 1991).

Because of this, it appears to be imperative to include breastfeeding in national health policy consideration within industrialized nations. This is especially true for deliberations on health care reform within the United States. Even as late as 1994, breastfeeding was ignored during health reform debate. It seems patently unwise to omit from consideration such a simple, low-cost intervention with immediate cost savings and diverse health benefits. The Department of Health and Human Services' Health Objectives for the Year 2000 advocate approximately doubling the number of mothers breastfeeding (United States Public Health Service, 1991), but these objectives are nonbinding. It is especially sad that breastfeeding would be ignored by health policy planners, while large corporations and a fee-for-service health care system derive considerable financial advantage resulting from formula feeding and the nation desperately struggles to pay for diseases apparently partly derived from formula feeding.

REFERENCES

Anderson, E., and E. Geden
1990 Nurses' knowledge of breastfeeding. *Journal of Obstetric, Gynecologic and Neonatal Nursing* 20(1):58–64.

American Academy of Pediatrics
1982 Policy statement based on task force report: The promotion of breastfeeding. *Pediatrics* 69(5):654–661.

Barber-Madden, R., M. A. Petschek, and J. Pakter
1987 Breastfeeding and the working mother: Barriers and intervention strategies. *Journal of Public Health Policy* Winter:531–541.

Batten, S., J. Hirschman, and D. Thomas
1990 Impact of the special supplemental food program on infants. *Journal of Pediatrics* 117(2Pt2):S101–109.

Bauchner, H., J. M. Leventhal, and E. D. Shapiro
1986 Studies of breast-feeding and infections: How good is the evidence? *Journal of the American Medical Association* 256:887–892.

Behrman, R. E., R. M. Kliegman, V. C. Vaughan, and W. E. Nelson, eds.
1992 *Nelson Textbook of Pediatrics,* 14th ed. Philadelphia: W. B. Saunders.

Carroll, J. L., and G. M. Loughlin
1993 Sudden infant death syndrome. *Pediatrics in Review* 14(3):83–93.

Cunningham, A. S., D. B. Jelliffe, and E. F. P. Jelliffe
1991 Breastfeeding and health in the 1980s: A global epidemiologic review. *Journal of Pediatrics* 118(5):659–666.

Davis, M. K., D. A. Savitz, and B. I. Graubard
1988 Infant feeding and childhood cancer. *Lancet* 2(8607):365–368.

Duncan, B., J. Ey, C. J. Golberg, A. L. Wright, F. D. Martinez, and L. M. Taussig
1993 Exclusive breast-feeding for at least 4 months protects against otitis media. *Pediatrics* 91(5):867–872.

Fielding, J. E.
1992 Smoking: Health effects and control. In *Maxcy-Rosenau-Last Public Health and Preventive Medicine,* 13th ed., edited by J. M. Maxcy, and R. B. Wallace, pp. 715–740. Norwalk: Appleton and Lange.

Fredrickson, D. D.
n.d. Breastmilk as medicine: A new 2-dimensional cumulative dose variable for breastfeeding. Manuscript in preparation. University of Kansas School of Medicine.

Fredrickson, D. D., J. R. Sorenson, A. K. Biddle, and M. Kotelchuck
1993 Relationship between sudden infant death syndrome and breastfeeding intensity and duration. *American Journal of Diseases of Children* 147(May):460.
Greenlick, M. R.
1993 Director, Center for Health Research, Kaiser Permanent, Portland, Oregon. Personal communication to Doren Fredrickson.
Greer, F. R., and R. D. Apple
1991 Physicians, formula companies, and advertising: A historical perspective. *American Journal of Diseases of Children* 145:282–286.
Hahn-Zoric, M., F. Fulconis, I. Minoli, G. Moro, B. Carlsson, M. Bottiger, N. Raiha, and L. A. Hanson
1990 Antibody responses to parenteral and oral vaccines are impaired by conventional and low protein formulas as compared to breast-feeding. *Acta Paediatrica Scandinavica* 79:1137–1142.
Hanson, L. A., B. Carlsson, H. P. Ekre, M. Hahn-Zoric, A. D. Osterhaus, and D. Roberton
1989 Immunoregulation mother-fetus/newborn, a role for anti-idiotype antibodies. *Acta Paediatrica Scandinavica Supplement* 351:38–41.
Helsing, E.
1990 Supporting breastfeeding: What governments and health workers can do—European experiences. *International Journal of Gynecology and Obstetrics* 31(Suppl. 1):69–76.
Hennekens, C. H., and J. E. Buring
1987 *Epidemiology in Medicine*. Boston: Little, Brown.
Hopkinson, J.
1991 Breast-feeding and infectious illness, power and confidence intervals (letter). *Pediatrics* 88:1079–1080.
Howie, P. W., J. S. Forsyth, S. A. Ogston, A. Clark, and C. D. Florey
1990 Protective effect of breast feeding against infection. *British Medical Journal* 300:11–16.
Jolley, S. G., L. M. Halpern, W. P. Tunell, D. G. Johnson, and C. E. Sterling
1991 Risk of sudden infant death from gastroesophageal reflux. *Journal of Pediatric Surgery* 26(6):691–696.
Knodel, J.
1977 Breast feeding and population growth. *Science* 198:1111 (Cited in R. A. Lawrence, 1994).
Kraus, J. F., and M. Bulterys
1991 Epidemiology of sudden infant death syndrome. In *Reproductive and Perinatal Epidemiology*, edited by M. Kiely, pp. 219–249. Boca Raton, FL: CRC Press.
Labbok, M. H., and G. E. Hendershot
1987 Does breast-feeding protect against malocclusion? An analysis of the 1981 Child Health Supplement to the National Health Interview Survey. *American Journal of Preventive Medicine* 3(4):227–232.

Labbok, M., and K. Krasovec
1990 Toward consistency in breastfeeding definitions. *Studies in Family Planning* 21(4):226–230.
Lawrence, R. A.
1994 *Breastfeeding: A Guide for the Medical Profession*, 4th ed. St. Louis: C. V. Mosby.
Michelman, D. F., R. R. Faden, A. C. Gielen, and K. S. Buxton
1990 Pediatricians and breastfeeding promotion: Attitudes, beliefs, and practices. *American Journal of Health Promotion* 4(3):181–186.
Mitchell E., R. Scragg, A. W. Stewart, D. M. Becroft, B. J. Taylor, R. P. Ford, I. B. Hassall, D. M. Barry, E. M. Allen, and A. P. Roberts
1991 Results from the first year of the New Zealand Cot Death Study. *New Zealand Medical Journal* 104:71–76.
Pabst, H. F., and D. W. Spady
1990 Effect of breast-feeding on antibody response to conjugate vaccine. *Lancet* 336:269–270.
Pear, R.
1993 Health-care costs up sharply again, posing new threat: Shadow on U.S. economy: Commerce Dept. puts '92 total at $838.5 billion, calling it new weight on business. *New York Times* Jan 5, Vol CXLII (49,202):1, col. 6.
Rogan, W. J., and B. C. Gladen
1993 Breast-feeding and cognitive development. *Early Human Development* 31:181–193.
Rubin, D. H., J. M. Leventhal, P. A. Krasilnikoff, H. S. Kuo, J. F. Jekel, B. Weile, A. Levee, M. Kurzon, and A. Berget
1990 Relationship between infant feeding and infectious illness: A prospective study of infants during the first year of life. *Pediatrics* 85:464–471.
Ryan, A. S., D. Rush, F. W. Krieger, and G. E. Lewandowski
1991 Recent declines in breast-feeding in the United States, 1984 through 1989. *Pediatrics* 88(4):719–727.
Snow, J.
1855 *On the Mode of Transmission of Cholera*, 2nd ed. London: Churchill.
United States Public Health Service—Department of Health and Human Services
1991 *Healthy People-2000*. DHHS Publication No.(PHS) 91-50212. Washington, DC: Superintendent of Documents, U. S. Government Printing Office.
Virtanen, S. M., L. Rasanen, A. Aro, J. Lindstrom, H. Sippola, R. Lounamaa, L. Toivanen, J. Tuomilehto, and H.K. Akerblom
1991 Infant feeding in Finnish children <7 yr of age with newly diagnosed IDDM. *Diabetes Care* 14(5):415–417.
Wall Street Journal
1993 Service aids employers with nursing mothers. *Wall Street Journal*, Tuesday, January 19, 1993, B1.

Biographical Sketches of the Contributors

Nicole J. Bernshaw, M.S.,IBCLC, is a Senior Research Specialist in the Department of Bioengineering at the University of Utah. She is the Area Professional Liaison Leader for La Leche League of Utah, the editor of the newsletter for the Utah Coalition to Promote Breastfeeding, an abstractor for *Breastfeeding Abstracts*, and the Book Review Editor for the *Journal of Human Lactation*. Her special interest is in the development of an interactive educational software program on human lactation for health professionals, which she started with funding from the National Institutes of Health.

Allan S. Cunningham, M.D., is Associate Professor of Pediatrics at the State University of New York Health Science Center, Syracuse. He is a member of the American Board of Pediatrics and the Professional Advisory Board of La Leche League International. He has practiced general pediatrics since 1971 and is the father of five breastfed children.

Katherine A. Dettwyler is Associate Professor of Anthropology at Texas A&M University. Most of her research focuses on the biocultural interactions between infant feeding beliefs and practices and the growth and health of children in Mali, West Africa. She is the author of *Dancing Skeletons: Life and Death in West Africa*, published by Waveland Press in 1994.

Peter T. Ellison is Professor of Anthropology and Chair of the Department of Anthropology at Harvard University. His research interests are centered on the ecology of human reproduction, particularly on the sensitivity of female ovarian physiology to age and energetics. He and his collaborators have conducted field research on five continents using methods of salivary steroid analysis that have been developed in his laboratory.

Valerie Fildes has been engaged in research into infant care and wet nursing prior to 1800 at the Wellcome Institute for the History of Medicine in London and later with the Cambridge Group for the History of Population and Social Structure. She has authored and edited a number of books including *Breasts, Bottles and Babies: A History of Infant Feeding* (1986) and *Wet Nursing: A History from Antiquity to the Present* (1988).

Doren Fredrickson, M.D., is board certified in Pediatrics and Preventive Medicine, and has earned a Ph.D. in Public Health-Epidemiology from the University of North Carolina-Chapel Hill. He is Assistant Professor at the Department of Preventive Medicine at the University of Kansas School of Medicine-Wichita, where he is Director of Research in Prevention and Primary Care. His research interests concern epidemiology, primary care, and health behaviors, with underlying concern for patient empowerment and cost-effective disease prevention.

Sheila Kitzinger has an international reputation as a social anthropologist, researcher, and advocate for women concerning their experiences of pregnancy, birth, and motherhood. Her research on childhood and midwifery spans cultures as varied as the Caribbean, North America, Europe, South Africa, New Zealand, and Japan. She is a Member of the Royal Society of Medicine, and sits on the advisory boards of a number of organizations. She is also an Honorary Professor at Thames Valley University. Her books include *Woman's Experience of Sex*, *Birth Over Thirty-five*, *Breastfeeding Your Baby*, *Homebirth and Other Alternatives to Hospital*, *Ourselves as Mothers*, and *Pregnancy and Childbirth*.

Ruth Lawrence, M.D., is a pediatrician, neonatologist, and clinical toxicologist, and Professor of Pediatrics and Gynecology at the University of Rochester, Chief of Newborn Nurseries, and Director of the Breastfeeding and Human Lactation Study Center. Her major published work on breastfeeding and human lactation is her textbook, *Breastfeeding: A Guide for the Medical Profession*, now in its fourth edition. She has also published many articles, abstracts, and chapters on various topics related to breastfeeding and human lactation, especially infant feeding choices and maternal lean body mass. Dr. Lawrence was a member of the Subcommittee on Nutrition During Lactation for the Institute of Medicine and serves as a consultant to several special committees for the Bureau of Maternal and Child Health. She is a member of the International Society for Research on Human Milk and Lactation. With Dr. Audrey Naylor, she helped to establish the Milk Club in association with the American Pediatric Society. She is a founding member of the newly established (1994) Academy of Breastfeeding Medicine, an international organization for physicians.

James J. McKenna is the E. Marshall and Elizabeth Hahn Chair of Social Science and Professor of Anthropology at Pomona College. He is internationally known for studies of child-care practices and SIDS. His research focus redefines what constitutes "normal" infant sleep and the importance of infant/parent co-sleeping. This research has challenged pediatric models of infant sleep. Professor McKenna's recent publications include "Mutual behavioral and physiological influences among solitary and co-sleeping mother-infant pairs: Implications for SIDS" (*Early Human Development*, 1994); "Co-sleeping mothers and infants influence each other's sleep physiology: Overview and implications for SIDS" (*Journal of Development Physiology*, 1994); "Sleep and arousal, synchrony and independence among mothers and infants sleeping apart and together: An experiment in evolutionary medicine" [*Acta Paediatrica*, 1994 (with Sarah Mosko)].

Marc S. Micozzi, M.D., has been Director of the National Museum of Health and Medicine since 1986 and a Distinguished Scientist in the American Registry of Pathology since 1992. Dr. Micozzi has a Ph.D. in Anthropology and has presented more than 100 scholarly papers at professional conferences and is the author of over 130 scientific publications. Among the places his work has been published are the *New England Journal of Medicine*, the *Journal of the American Medical Association*, the *American Journal of Public Health*, and the *Journal of the National Cancer Institute*. He has published several books and edited volumes on diet and nutrition, cancer prevention research, and medical anthropology.

Sara A. Quandt is Associate Professor of Public Health Sciences at Bowman Gray School of Medicine of Wake Forest University, with an adjunct appointment in the Department of Anthropology. She has served as President of the Council on Nutritional Anthropology, and was a member of the Subcommittee on Nutrition During Lactation for the Institute of Medicine. Her research interests have focused on nutrition through the life cycle in evolutionary and ecological perspectives. This has included issues of infant feeding and, most recently, nutritional strategies of the elderly.

Patricia Stuart-Macadam is Associate Professor of Anthropology at the University of Toronto. Her research focuses on an evolutionary and biocultural perspective of health, disease, and nutrition in prehistoric and contemporary human populations. Her current interests include human lactation, cancer, female "biological superiority," and gender differences in disease. She is the editor (with Susan Kent) of *Diet, Demography, and Disease: Changing Perspectives on Anemia* published by Aldine de Gruyter in 1992.

Penny Van Esterik is Associate Professor of Anthropology and co-director of the Thai Studies Project at York University, Toronto. Her teaching and research interests include gender and development in Southeast Asia, refugee studies, nutritional anthropology, and breastfeeding research. Most of her fieldwork has been in Thailand, where she has published on the Thai food system, infant feeding practices, and women and Buddhism. Recent publications include *Beyond the Breast-Bottle Controversy* (1989), *Women, Work and Breastfeeding* (1992), and *Taking Refuge: Lao Buddhists in North America* (York Lanes Press, 1993). She is currently the coordinator of the task force on breastfeeding and women's work for WABA (World Alliance for Breastfeeding Action).

Michael W. Woolridge, M.D., qualified in Zoology at the University of South Wales and Monmouthshire, Cardiff, then studied for his doctorate in animal behavior under Dr. Richard Dawkins at Oxford University. For the past 15 years, he has conducted research into the physiology of lactation, specializing recently in clinical problems of breastfeeding. He has published widely on the practical management of breastfeeding, and has contributed to efforts by the Royal College of Midwives to improve professional understanding and management of breastfeeding, mainly through publication of the handbook "*Successful Breastfeeding*" (Churchill Livingstone). He is currently National Director of UNICEF's "Baby Friendly Hospital Initiative" in the UK.

Index

Made in the USA
Las Vegas, NV
22 January 2022

42064768R10245